CANCER-CAUSING AGENTS
A PREVENTIVE GUIDE

CANCER - CAUSING AGENTS

A PREVENTIVE GUIDE

by
Ruth Winter

A HERBERT MICHELMAN BOOK
CROWN PUBLISHERS, INC., NEW YORK

To the memory of
Paul Nadan,
editor and friend

Printed in the United States of America
Published simultaneously in Canada by General Publishing Company Limited

Library of Congress Cataloging in Publication Data

Winter, Ruth, 1930–
    Cancer-causing agents.

    1. Carcinogens.   2. Cancer—Prevention.   I. Title.
RC268.6.W56   1979   616.9'94'05   79-12458
ISBN 0-517-53600-5
ISBN 0-517-53601-3 pbk.

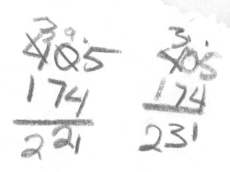

ACKNOWLEDGMENTS

The author wishes to thank Jane Brody of West Orange, New Jersey, for her assistance in the research for this book, and Robin Winter of Miami, Florida, for her help in typing and proofreading the manuscript.

The author gratefully acknowledges the following sources used in compiling this book:

- Brody, Jane E. *You Can Fight Cancer and Win*. New York: McGraw Hill, 1977.
- *Cancer Rates and Risks*, 2d ed. Washington, D.C.: U.S. Department of Health, Education and Welfare, 1974.
- *Cancer and the Worker*. Bill Boland, Executive Editor. New York: The New York Academy of Sciences, 1977.
- *Environmental Pollution and Carcinogenic Risks*. Geneva, Switzerland: International Agency for Research on Cancer, 1976.
- Hawley, Gessner G. *The Condensed Chemical Dictionary*. 9th ed. rev., New York: Van Nostrand Reinhold Company, 1977.
- *Health Hazards of the Human Environment*. Geneva, Switzerland: World Health Organization, 1972.
- *The Merck Index*. 8th ed. Edited by Paul G. Stecher. Rahway, N.J.: Merck, Sharp and Dohme Research Laboratories, 1968.
- *The Merck Manual*. 11th ed. Edited by Charles E. Lyght. Rahway, N.J.: Merck, Sharp and Dohme Research Laboratories, 1966.
- *Physicians' Desk Reference*. Oradell, N.J.: Medical Economics Company, 1978.

- Shimkin, Michael B., M.D., *Contrary to Nature*. Washington, D.C.: U.S. Department of Health, Education and Welfare, 1977.
- *Stedman's Medical Dictionary.* 21st ed. Baltimore, Md.: The Williams & Wilkins Company, 1966.
- Stellman, Jeanne, Ph.D., Daum, Susan, M.D. *Work Is Dangerous to Your Health.* New York: Pantheon Books, 1973.
- *Suspected Carcinogens: A Subfile of the NIOSH Toxic Substance List Tracor Jitco, Inc.* Rockville, Md.: U.S. Department of Health, Education and Welfare, June 1975.
- *Suspected Carcinogens: A Subfile of the Registry of Toxic Effects of Chemical Substances.* Cincinnati, Ohio: U.S. Department of Health, Education and Welfare, Public Health Service, Center for Disease Control, December, 1976.
- Symposium. Piscataway, N.J.: Waksman Institute of Microbiology, Detection and Action of Environmental Carcinogens, November 8, 1978. J. Oliver Lampen, director, Waksman Institute; Robert W. Simpson of the Institute; Irving Selikoff, director, Environmental Science Laboratory, Mt. Sinai School of Medicine, New York; Charles Heidelberger, Cancer Research Laboratory, University of Southern California; Otto Plescia of the Institute; I. Bernard Weinstein, Institute for Cancer Research, Columbia University Medical Center, New York; and John H. Weisburger, Naylor Dana Institute for Disease Prevention, Valhalla, New York.
- *Toxicants Occurring Naturally in Foods.* 2d ed. Washington, D.C.: National Academy of Sciences, 1973.

INTRODUCTION

This book contains information about known and suspected cancer-causing agents. Before you slam the cover shut and say, "Why bother? Everything causes cancer," consider this: Everything *does not* cause cancer! Only a small percentage of the physical and chemical substances to which we are exposed do. Unfortunately, many of these carcinogens are present in our daily lives—in almost every case unnecessarily, because there are safer alternatives.

You may be surprised at some of the known cancer causing-agents to which you may be exposed daily. Among them are certain fats, hormone pills, brake linings, beef, varnishes, solvents, pesticides, chlorine, mushrooms, weed killers, plastic food wraps, solder, mothproofers, wood dusts, and water softeners, not to mention your own emotions. Perhaps the most surprising causes of cancer are the anesthesia given during surgery and the very drugs used to treat cancer.

Scientists estimate that 70 to 90 percent of the new cases of cancer affecting 700,000 Americans each year are caused by carcinogens in our environment. Such agents are increasing primarily because of our penchant for producing synthetic chemicals. In the past 10 years alone, our production of man-made compounds has expanded 255 percent. There are now more than 80,000 chemicals being manufactured, and about 700 new ones are added to the list each year. Almost all of these "unnatural" products have never been tested for their cancer-causing tendencies. We have found out the hard way that some of them do cause the disease. Two of the more infamous examples are vinyl chloride, used to make plastics and now causing liver cancer in previously exposed workers, and DES, a synthetic estrogen, now causing cancer in some of the daughters of women given the drug years ago during pregnancy.

One in four Americans today is exposed to some hazardous substance while at work, according to a 1972–1974 survey taken by the Occupational Safety and Health Administration (OSHA) of the U.S. Department of Labor. OSHA found that one percent of the entire work force—880,000 people—has been exposed to one or more of the 17 carcinogens regulated by the agency. Thousands and thousands of other workers are currently exposed to the more than 2,000 substances known or suspected of causing cancer.

If you do not work in industry, don't breathe a sigh of relief, because there is disturbing evidence that industrial carcinogens can reach well beyond the factory gates and endanger workers' families and other residents of the community. Factory wastes can carry carcinogens into anyone's food, air, and water. A National Cancer Institute (NCI) study has found abnormally high rates of cancer in 39 counties across the country where there are major petroleum-refining centers. This leads to the suspicion that the petroleum industry that produces hydrocarbons and other potential carcinogens may be a chief contributor to environmental cancers. Other specific studies have shown that asbestos, vinyl chloride, beryllium, and arsenic are already associated with disease and deaths among people who have never worked with these substances.

Unfortunately, our nation's ability to produce carcinogens far outweighs our ability to detect and control them.

What is a carcinogen? A carcinogen is any agent that causes tumors in man or animals. It can be a chemical, physical, or viral substance that somehow sets off the genetic information within a cell and begins a process that if uncontrolled, ends in disaster.

The major advances in recognition of cancer-causing agents have come from epidemiological (relating to epidemics) studies. The data is collected from:

- *Descriptive Studies:* A cluster or change or difference in neoplasm (tumor) rates in a group—usually workers—is identified. Lung cancer among asbestos workers is an example.
- *Retrospective Studies:* Histories of cancer victims have revealed such occupational carcinogens as shale oil, chromates, 2-NA, benzidine, or drug carcinogens such as Thorotrast, and DES. Once a relationship between a substance and a human cancer is suspected or confirmed,

cohort studies are done to define more precisely the time relationship and the magnitude of the risk.

- *Prospective Studies:* These are follow-up investigations. The population studied is divided into groups, according to the degree and duration of exposure to a suspected or known carcinogen. In case-control studies, the groups, as far as possible, differ only in exposure to the carcinogen. Follow-up studies are then carried out to determine the incidence of cancer in the various exposure categories, and the risk is assessed by comparing results. The analysis also reveals the relationship between cancer occurrence and age at first exposure, as well as how long it takes for the cancer to develop. Care must be taken to screen out the influence of factors other than the suspected cancer-inducing agent. Finally, if a specific substance is determined a carcinogen, its removal from the environment should be followed by epidemiological evidence of a decline in the frequency of the cancer it causes.

Epidemiologists turn up a great deal of useful information by comparing the cancer rates in various countries and in various regions of the same country. In the 1940s, for example, it was found that cancer of the liver was very common in African blacks but not in American blacks. Japanese living in Japan had a high rate of stomach cancer and a low rate of colon cancer, but when they emigrated to the United States, they developed a low rate of stomach cancer and a high rate of colon cancer just like other Americans.

Investigators have found that death rates from all forms of cancer combined are higher in industrialized areas than in rural areas. They are not sure why. Is it life-style? Urban dwellers are known to use more tobacco and alcohol. Is it occupation? Working with industrial pollutants combined with the more polluted air and water of the cities may work in concert to increase the risk. Perhaps it is due to factors not yet identified. It is known only that in the northeastern and Great Lakes areas of the United States there is a higher death rate from all types of cancer combined than in other areas. But the death rates for specific types vary from one region to another. For instance, the southeast has a greater mortality rate from cancer of the uterine cervix than other parts of the country, and the south has an above-average occurrence rate for skin cancer, probably because of the greater exposure to sun in the "sun-belt" states.

Income and social class also show up on the epidemiologists' charts. Low socioeconomic groups have above-average incidence and death rates from all cancers combined. But again, variations appear in the statistics on specific types. For instance, although there are marked links between low socioeconomic status and cancer of the uterine cervix, esophagus, and stomach, there is a below-average incidence of breast cancer in low-income groups. Why? Is it life-style? Quality of medical care? Exposure to cancer-causing materials in the environment?

3

Cancer researchers are sure that for most major cancers, racial or hereditary factors are of much less importance than environmental factors. However, one of the outstanding characteristics of carcinogenesis (the production of cancer) is that there is a great variability in individual susceptibility to carcinogens. In a few cases, the answers are obvious. Redheads and blondes are more susceptible to skin cancer than brunettes because they have less melanin in their skins to protect them from ultraviolet radiation. But why does only one person out of 11 who smokes two packs of cigarettes a day get lung cancer while the other 10 do not?

Carcinogenesis is not a simple process. It results from the interaction of the cancer-causing agent with the biological target. The effect is influenced by the susceptibility of various cell types, various tissues or organs, and individual immunity. Factors such as age, sex, hormonal status, diet, inheritance, and individual variations in the metabolic handling of chemicals all contribute to determine the response of a human being to a carcinogen; differences in test animals as high as 100-fold or 1,000-fold can be obtained by changing only one factor at a time. Thus valid epidemiological studies are difficult to conduct because reactions to a single carcinogen may not appear in the study groups due to the varying degrees of susceptibility.

These difficulties are further complicated by the long period between exposure to a cancer-causing agent and the development of the cancer. It may take 2 to 40 years.

Vinyl chloride is a prime example. Large-scale production of it began in the 1950s, and production grew 15 percent per year until 4 billion pounds were manufactured in the United States. But more than half the vinyl-chloride workers who were diagnosed as having liver cancer in June 1974 had first been exposed prior to the 1950s. How many more cases of vinyl-chloride-induced liver cancer will appear in workers in the coming years? How many are living with a cancer time bomb?

In testimony before Labor Department hearings, OSHA representatives pointed out that generally the greater the exposure, the shorter the latency period. In one study of bladder tumors among 78 dye workers, the length of exposure appears to correlate inversely with the length of the latency period—the greater the exposure, the shorter the latency. But because so many factors influence latency, it is impossible to define the extent to which the length and degree of exposure may be important.

OSHA representatives said that latency poses difficult medical, social, and economic problems in identifying hazardous contaminants in the environment. Chemicals may appear safe for human exposure after they have been used for 10 to 15 years without obvious harm. With carcinogens, however, the lack of demonstrated damage to health even after this comparatively long period gives a false sense of security. Thirty or 40 years may be required before enough people have been exposed to a carcinogen to produce detectable cancer. The long delay between exposure and symptoms of the disease often makes it medically and scientifically impossible to identify carcinogens in the environment.

Detection difficulties posed by the latency period, for instance, are compounded by the mobility of our society: people in our country change jobs, residences, doctors, and hospitals frequently, so that even large-scale adverse health effects from latent disease may go undetected. Moreover, people are exposed to carcinogens in great variety and concentration, not only on the job but in their diets and surrounding environment. This multiplicity of exposure further complicates isolating the cause for any given cancer.

Another problem, according to OSHA investigators, is that epidemiological studies are difficult to conduct because it is seldom possible to separate out a single variable from the complex mix of chemical agents to which we are exposed in our work and other environments.

The Ad Hoc Committee of the NCI stated in 1970: "It has become increasingly obvious that the hazard from a single chemical carcinogen cannot be evaluated out of a context of total environmental exposure. Estimation of the 'cumulative carcinogenic dose' resulting from all possible chemical carcinogens is presently impossible."

How then do you go about proving something is a carcinogen? Russell Train, former administrator of the Environmental Protection Agency, (EPA) said when ordering the removal of the pesticides heptachlor and chlordane from the market in 1976: "I have noted some tendency not entirely absent from the record, to assert that any chemical, if fed in sufficiently large amounts will cause cancer in test animals. This is not true. A study sponsored by the National Cancer Institute tested 140 pesticides and industrial chemicals in two strains of mice and less than 10 percent of these were found to be carcinogenic."

It is, of course, unethical as well as illegal to deliberately test carcinogens on humans. Therefore, animal experiments must be used and the data extrapolated from results to evaluate human risks. This does involve uncertainties. Federal agencies consider any agent that produces tumors in animals a cancer hazard to humans if the results were achieved according to the established parameters of a valid carcinogenesis test.

In many animal experiments the type of cancer produced is exactly the same as that recorded in human studies. For example, bladder cancer is produced in man, hamster, dog, and monkey by 2-NA. In other instances species variations result in the induction of different types of cancer at different locations by the same cancer agent. Benzidine causes liver-cell carcinoma in the rat and bladder cancer in man and dog.

The fact that all human carcinogens—with the possible exception of arsenic—also cause tumors in animals encourages the belief that these tests are valid. However, there are significant differences in the numbers of exposed populations of humans and test animals and the age during which each is exposed. There are also metabolic differences in activation of the carcinogen. And while the majority of human carcinogens have been shown to cause cancer in animals, the reverse is not as clear. There are a number of recognized animal carcinogens such as penicillin that have not been found to cause cancer in man—at least not yet.

Government agencies maintain that for regulatory purposes, they must assume the results of tests in rodents will closely parallel tumor induction in humans, although they cannot be absolutely certain of this. Therefore, when an agent is carcinogenic in animals, mathematical formulas are used to extrapolate the dosages from animals to humans. Confirmation, if possible, is then based on epidemiological investigations in humans.

Dr. Samuel Epstein of Case Western Reserve, one of the world's leading experts on carcinogens, emphatically states that animal carcinogens are not less dangerous than human and that "there is no evidence of species specific carcinogens." He maintains that it is a myth that tumorigens (causes of tumors) are less dangerous than carcinogens; the existence of a tumor-inducing agent as opposed to a cancer-inducing agent has been vigorously proposed, particularly for the chlorinated hydrocarbon pesticides such as DDT and dieldrin, which have long been known to induce liver tumors in mice. He said tumorigens and carcinogens are synonymous and recognition of lung metastases from "benign" tumors in mice from designated tumorigens such as dieldrin proves it.

Animal studies do have their limitations. Cancer researchers are particularly concerned about chemicals that may cause 1,000 cases of cancer in the human population of 200 million, or about one case of cancer in about 200,000. Because of cost, most animal studies are limited to 250 to 1,000 animals. In such relatively small samples, a cancer-causing agent that would produce a malignancy in one person out of 200,000 would not even show up. Thus researchers increase dosages until results appear. Once animals in the group develop tumors, statisticians calculate what percentage would contract cancer from a smaller dose.

Imperfect as they are, animal tests do serve as a warning to humans. Had such warnings been heeded, many victims now dead of cancer would be alive today. As early as 1930, for example, scientists reported that exposure to vinyl chloride caused ill effects in laboratory animals. In 1970, Italian scientists noted that rats exposed to high levels of vinyl chloride for one year had developed tumors. But it wasn't until 1974, when an alert plant physician at B. F. Goodrich reported three cases of very rare liver cancers among workers at a single vinyl-chloride production plant, that the substance was first recognized as a serious cancer threat.

The same tale is told for DES, the synthetic estrogen. French researchers reported in 1938 that it caused mammary cancer in mice. Similar reports were made during the 1940s and 1950s; yet DES was added to feed, implanted in animals bred for human consumption, and given to pregnant women to prevent miscarriages. Had observant Massachusetts researchers not noticed rare cancers in young girls and made the correlation between those cancers and the synthetic estrogens taken by their mothers, the tragedy might have continued to escalate. It is still with us, of course, because no one knows how long the latency period is, how many offspring —both male and female—will eventually develop cancer, and if the mothers themselves are at risk because of the drug.

DES is still being added to animal feed, and traces of the drug are still found in meat brought to market. Because of legal red tape, as of this writing the Federal Drug Administration (FDA) has not been able to ban the use of this estrogen in animal feed.

Scientists were able to designate vinyl chloride and DES as human carcinogens because these two substances caused rare tumors. But what about the carcinogens that cause common tumors?

In these cases animal tests are vital. Whether or not we heed the results, they can predict a cancer hazard for humans. This is why so many scientists, consumer advocates, and labor leaders are urging more testing be done and why they strongly supported the Toxic Substances Control Act. That legislation was passed in 1976 after five years of debate, and opposition from the $113 billion-a-year chemical industry. The act gives the government authority to require certain chemicals be tested for health hazards before they are put on the market. Unfortunately, there is a shortage of money and personnel to conduct long-term testing. Animal studies take a minimum of two years and cost $100,000 and more. Because toxicologists are in short supply, they can demand salaries of $75,000 annually. The government estimates the testing needed just to catch up with untested organic chemicals known to be in the environment would cost $2 billion; another $300 million would be needed each year to test new chemicals.

There is one controversial partial solution. In the early 1970s, Dr. Bruce Ames, a biochemist at the University of California at Berkeley, developed a simple test using common bacteria that reveals whether a chemical is a mutagen. The test can be done quickly and is relatively inexpensive. Mutagens act by changing the genetic material that is transferred to daughter cells when cell division occurs. Carcinogens also act by fouling up the genetic material within a cell. There are scientists who vehemently deny that malignant transformation of cells has anything to do with mutations. A University of California molecular biologist described the Ames Screening Test as a "bit like looking under the lamppost for a coin lost a block away because of the availability of light."

The fact is, however, that almost all of the chemicals known to be carcinogenic have also been shown to be mutagenic in the Ames Test. These include beta-naphthylamine, benzidine, cigarette-smoke condensates, and vinyl chloride. On the other hand, some 46 noncarcinogenic common biochemicals were tested by the Ames method and were found not to be mutagenic. Therefore, it is likely that a chemical determined to be mutagenic will also be carcinogenic. This was true of mutagens such as 2-acetylaminofluorene, now banned, and the widely used industrial chemical and grain fumigant ethylene dibromide, which was subsequently tested and found to be carcinogenic.

There is further frightening evidence that carcinogens and mutagens may be two sides of the same coin. Mutagenic chemicals given to pregnant mice have been found to cause cancer not only in their "children" but in their "grandchildren" as well.

Are we dooming our children to cancer? Dr. William Wardell, director of the Center for the Study of Drug Development, speaking in Philadelphia, December 6, 1978, at a symposium on Public Issues and Private Medicine, told his colleagues that genes must be protected and that drugs and other environmental chemicals are potential ways in which the genes of mankind may be damaged. He also warned about the particular vulnerability of the young to carcinogens: "It has been shown quite conclusively that the younger a person the more susceptible he or she is to carcinogenesis. The child has a lifetime of latency in which the tumor can appear."

Indeed, two generation studies with saccharin showed that in animals. The artificial sweetener is a bladder carcinogen for male rats. According to the February 1979 report of the National Academy of Sciences, a significant increase in bladder cancer was found consistently in male offspring exposed continuously in utero and through life.

How much exposure to a carcinogen does it take to damage a gene or to cause cancer in a child or an adult? Can small amounts of a carcinogen be harmless? No one knows for certain. Some scientists, including a number who work for industry, argue that the amount or dose of a carcinogen is significant. They point to studies of certain high-risk groups of workers exposed to the same chemical, where only a certain percentage of them developed cancer. That percentage usually included those who had the greatest exposure. They believe this indicates that there may be a "threshold limit of exposure below which a carcinogen will not cause cancer."

There are others who believe that even the smallest amount of a carcinogen is not safe. The truth may lie somewhere in between. One of the most prevalent theories among cancer researchers today is that viruses and agents such as the X-ray are direct carcinogens, while chemical carcinogens require many steps to do their dirty work. Chemical carcinogens have to bypass our defenses of enzymes, membranes, and antibodies and overcome "modifiers" such as diet, age, intestinal flora, and heredity. If our defenses are weak, the tiniest amount of a carcinogen may destroy us. If they are strong, large amounts would be needed to breach the fortress. Furthermore, it is also believed that many human cancers are not due to one carcinogen but to a complex of carcinogens and "promoters" that work together to destroy our defenses.

Many researchers now believe that we may have cancer-causing agents in our systems for years, but unless a "promoter" comes along to "turn on" the cancer-causing agent, we do not develop cancer. For example, because tobacco smoke is a suspected promoter, asbestos workers with carcinogenic asbestos fibers in their lungs who smoke have a much higher incidence of cancer than asbestos workers who do not smoke. Then too, researchers have shown that they can give test animals the powerful carcinogen DMBA and nothing will happen. However, if they first give them DMBA and then croton oil, one week or even a year later the animals will quickly develop cancer. One of the great hopes is that science will be able to interfere with the cancer-producing process by stopping carcinogens from being turned on by promoters, thus rendering them harmless.

However, most occupational and government cancer experts believe there is no safe level as far as carcinogens are concerned. They have solid arguments to back them up. As mentioned earlier, even brief exposure to a cancer-causing agent can cause cancer many years later. This delay from time of exposure to time of disease may range from 2 to 40 years, but averages about 20.

OSHA experts point out that two biological characteristics distinguish carcinogens from other agents that cause chronic toxicity: the general irreversibility of effects *and* the long latent period between exposure to the carcinogen and manifestation of the effect—cancer.

Once a cell has been switched on (transformed) from its normal status to a neoplastic (potentially malignant) one, OSHA experts maintain this cell can replicate and produce neoplastic daughter cells. Only a few initially transformed neoplastic cells are needed to give rise to a growing tumor— there is experimental evidence that even a single cell can be transformed by chemicals to produce a malignant tumor. It is consistent with our knowledge of carcinogenesis, they say, that a relatively small number of molecules of the carcinogen may be sufficient to initiate the neoplastic change in a target cell. Following such an initial event, alterations lead ultimately to a cancer cell, which is then capable of autonomous growth. Thus a single biological event produced by a very small number of molecules may be sufficient to initiate the irreversible development of a tumor.

There is dramatic evidence to support this contention. For example, short exposure to benzidine has caused tumors in workers 30 years later. Brief exposure to asbestos has caused cancer in humans decades later. Vinyl chloride has been found in the bodies of highly exposed workers as long as 5 years after their last exposure. A number of other carcinogens such as dieldrin, DDT, PCBs, ethylene dichloride, ethylene dibromide, and beryllium also persist in the body tissues for long periods. Apparently, once a person is exposed, the potential for developing cancer continues indefinitely.

Industry spokesmen say there is no such thing as a risk-free environment and that cancer-causing properties of some substances are more potent than others. Thus limited exposure to low-potency substances might not be so dangerous as to warrent eliminating all exposure. OSHA and the FDA do not recognize such differences and maintain there is no safe level of exposure to a cancer-causing agent.

The famous or infamous Delaney Amendment, depending on your point of view, was part of the 1958 Food Additives Amendment Law. Written by Congressman James Delaney, the law specifically states that no additive may be permitted in any amount if tests show that it produces cancer when fed to man or animals. Despite repeated attacks by industry, politicans, and some scientists, the FDA has held fast.

Are we protected from carcinogens? Cancer and the Worker, published in 1977 by the New York Academy of Sciences, points out the following:

More than 200 years ago, a British surgeon, Sir Percivall Pott, recognized the association between chimney sweeps' exposure to soot, and their scrotal cancer. Today, coke-oven workers in the steel industry are exposed to similar coal-combustion products and are dying from cancer at the rate of 10 times that of other steel workers.

More than 130 years after cancer was first discovered among copper smelters exposed to arsenic, some 1.5 million American workers are inhaling the same substance. They are also dying at twice the rate of lung cancer and 8 times the rate of lymphatic cancer as others in the nation.

More than 80 years ago, scientists discovered that aromatic amines caused bladder cancer among German dye workers. Such amines as benzidine and beta-naphthylamine were banned or taken off the market decades ago in the United Kingdom, Japan, Switzerland, Italy, and the Soviet Union. Yet in 1973 thousands of Americans were still literally sloshing around in these chemicals. The workers are now developing, and will continue to develop, bladder tumors at an epidemic rate. In 1974 half of the former employees at one benzidine plant had developed bladder cancer.

More than 75 years ago asbestos was known to cause a fatal lung disease. It was identified more than 25 years ago as a potent cause of lung cancer. But until recently, workers in dozens of asbestos factories and in hundreds of asbestos-related trades were laboring in asbestos dust so thick it blocked out the light. An expected 300,000 to 400,000 current and former asbestos workers in this country will die of cancer at more than double the national rate.

The U.S. Department of Labor estimates that in a single year, one in 10 workers have a work-related illness, disease, accident, or death. Whenever additional regulations are suggested, commercial enterprises always threaten that they will cost money and jobs.

Once again, vinyl chloride serves as an example. During the long hearings in the mid-1970s, the industry argued against the government's proposed restrictions on these chemicals, contending that they would mean the loss of 2 million jobs and an end to production worth $65 billion a year. Despite the gradual adoption of tighter rules for workers exposed to vinyl chloride, however, a spokesman for the plastics industry told the *Wall Street Journal*, March 4, 1978, that production in 1977 was 8 percent greater than in 1974.

When government agencies took up an offensive against carcinogens in the workplace, 90 companies and 60 trade associations formed the American Industrial Health Council to lobby against the government's efforts to tighten regulations. When New Jersey was designated "cancer alley" in 1977, because of the high rate of the disease among workers, the state government made efforts to tighten exposure to carcinogens in the workplace. The companies again threatened a choice between jobs or cancer. A New Jersey senator, in a slip of the lip, answered: "There's no reason why we can't have both." He explained later to reporters that he meant that a cleanup of the state's environment, particularly of chemicals known to cause cancer, did not necessarily mean that the state would lose jobs. Industry spokesmen of course disagreed. They said too zealous a crackdown on pollution could force plants to close.

We now have to determine whether exposure to carcinogens must be eliminated or reduced, when possible, regardless of the cost in dollars. The alternative—cancer—is too high a price to pay.

Monitoring work health hazards and providing medical tests and counseling could cost as much as $2 billion a year, according to government experts. By comparison, $3 to $5 billion is being spent annually for all types of cancer treatment. Add that to lost earnings and productivity and the bill adds up to a whopping $12 billion annually.

Who protects us from cancer-causing agents at work? at home? in the marketplace? The ABCs of government regulation of carcinogens fall into —and sometimes between—several federal agencies:

OCCUPATIONAL SAFETY AND HEALTH ADMINISTRATION (OSHA). Created in 1971 as a branch of the Department of Labor, it is supposed to recognize and regulate the 20,000 to 84,000 compounds in the workplace. OSHA has 1,561 inspectors of whom 980 are safety specialists, 520 are health specialists, and 61 discrimination officers (protecting the rights of workers who complain of work conditions). With this number of inspectors, OSHA is charged with protecting more than 62 million workers in 5 million workplaces. Chances of a business being inspected are about one in 1,300. OSHA tries, therefore, to concentrate on identified high-risk businesses. OSHA's director of Health Standards Program, Grover Wrenn, testifying in hearings at the Labor Department, said that any attempt to improve control over occupational carcinogenesis "does not mean, as some parties to this proceeding have erroneously characterized as 'OSHA's view,' that OSHA is attempting by this proposal to establish a risk-free workplace. It means merely that workers should not be subject to risk of irreversible illness when it is feasible for that risk to be reduced." OSHA's 1978 proposals would categorize chemicals. Those which have been found to cause cancer in humans or in two species of mammalian test animals, such as rats and mice, or in one species in which the results have been reconfirmed, would trigger emergency temporary standards to control exposure at the lowest level feasible. A permanent standard would be mandated within six months. OSHA now regulates 17 chemicals. About 200 chemicals would fall into this new category.

ENVIRONMENTAL PROTECTION AGENCY (EPA). It regulates 35,000 pesticides composed of about 1,500 chemical entities. This agency, created in 1970, also oversees control of pollutants such as auto emissions, or chemical wastes that make their way into air and water.

FOOD AND DRUG ADMINISTRATION (FDA). With a staff of 1,265 inspectors and 350 scientists, the agency regulates about 2,500 food additives and thousands of unintentional contaminants in food, drugs, and cosmetics. They oversee more than 20,000 prescription drugs, 300,000 over-the-counter drugs, and 4,000 ingredients used in cosmetics. In 1977, FDA inspectors made 18,236 food inspections, 6,510 drug inspections, 2,123 medical-device inspections, 600 cosmetic inspections, 4,001 biological (vaccines) inspections, and 245 radiological-health inspections.

U.S. DEPARTMENT OF AGRICULTURE (USDA). A division that shares the FDA authority over meat products that contain such known and suspected carcinogens as nitrites and DES.

CONSUMER PRODUCT SAFETY COMMISSION (CPSC). Formed in the 1970s, it has jurisdiction over unreasonable risk of injury in more than 2.5 million manufacturing, distributing, retailing, and importing companies. About half of all businesses in this country fall into this category. The fabric chemical Tris, a flame retardant found to be carcinogenic, fell under this commission's jurisdiction.

NATIONAL INSTITUTE FOR OCCUPATIONAL SAFETY AND HEALTH (NI-OSH). Congress set up this institute in 1970 to play a key role in helping to protect workers and their health on the job. The agency was to conduct occupational-health research; to inspect manufacturers' plants at employers' and workers' requests, and for its own studies, and to recommend standards for safe exposure to hazardous substances. NIOSH is supposed to work closely with OSHA, the organization responsible for setting the legally permitted exposures to hazards in the workplace. NIOSH, through its investigations into plant conditions and studies of already available data, provides OSHA with the scientific background needed to determine these rules. When a workplace crisis arises, the two agencies often work in tandem to find out how the workers were harmed and to help the industry correct the problem. Under the law, NIOSH documents summarizing its findings about a hazard should be used by OSHA to help in setting health and safety regulations for industry. But although NIOSH has sent its sister agency almost 90 of these criteria documents, only a few of the former's recommendations have been used in the OSHA standards issued so far.

NUCLEAR REGULATORY COMMISSION (NRC). It became a separate federal agency when the Atomic Energy Commission was disbanded and was subsequently incorporated into the new Department of Energy. It oversees the safety of atomic-power plants and their emissions, nuclear reactors, and nuclear gadgetry in industry.

Unfortunately, even with all these agencies and the best efforts of government and industry officials, many workers are still exposed to carcinogens every day. As Dr. J. William Lloyd, formerly with NIOSH and now an epidemiologist with the United Steel Workers, said: "Almost everything we know now about occupational cancer comes from counting dead bodies."

The truth is that many persons with cancer never learn that their tumors are work related. This is especially true if the workers are employed at small plants.

Tumor outbreaks among workers, if publicly reported, are published in technical journals with a two-year lag after discovery. The companies are usually not identified by name.

The following recommendations have been made by OSHA and National Academy of Sciences experts and should be enforced:

- All chemicals suspected as potential cancer-causing agents should be tested before marketing.
- All producers and users of carcinogens should be licensed and inspected periodically to determine proper safety precautions.
- Strict protective measures should be enforced in industrial plants, schools, and elsewhere when chemicals are worked with.
- Information should be available to permit workers to decide whether they want to continue working in a high-risk area in a particular workplace and if so, how they can reduce the hazard to themselves.
- Carcinogens should be identified by generic as well as trade names, and easily understood data should be provided including risks, description of the disease in humans, routes of exposure in the workplace, and measures to reduce exposure.
- There should be a central national source of information about the hazards of specific substances in the workplace.
- In addition to protective measures taken in industry, there are safety

precautions that should be enforced to protect the public at large.

- Hospitals and private physicians should be required to report every new tumor case to a central registry. Patients' names need not be used, but pertinent information should be fed into a computer such as employment, family and medical histories, diet, personal habits, hobbies, etc. This data could provide epidemiologists with clues to carcinogens in the environment and ultimately the causes of various cancers.
- Before new chemicals are added to foods, they should be tested for carcinogenicity and efficacy. If they provide no real benefit to the consumer, they should not be added to our chemical burden.
- All water supplies should be tested repeatedly for chemical carcinogens.
- Industries must be responsible for disposing of their toxic wastes by means other than public sewage systems, waterways, and dumps where the carcinogens may pollute air and water.
- All chemicals being used in manufacturing, including "trade secrets," should be reported to the appropriate government agencies and inserted in a computerized system so that when a carcinogen is identified, the public can be alerted immediately and will know exactly what products may contain the substance.
- The government should withdraw support from tobacco growers and provide them with financing and encouragement to switch to other crops.
- The media should voluntarily refuse to promote cigarette smoking.

All the substances listed in this book have been identified at least once as a carcinogen. Some of the older studies would not stand up to scientific scrutiny today, and the designated substances may not be carcinogens. Others listed in the book are extremely dangerous and have been proven to cause lethal cancers in humans.

Every listing, when possible, provides you with a source to refer to should you wish to further investigate a particular carcinogen.

Definitions of types of cancers and chemical terms are supplied.

In addition to using this book to inform yourself about what is known and suspected concerning agents that cause cancer, you must ask yourself some difficult questions:

- Are you working at a job in which you have little protection against exposure to known cancer-causing agents? Are you willing to pay the price required to change the situation?—even if it means changing jobs? If you live near an industry that is polluting the air and water and government regulations are ineffective, will you move? help organize a group to take action against the polluter?

- Are you willing to change your habits? reduce the fat and increase the fiber in your diet? give up cigarettes? forgo sunbathing? stop buying sodium-nitrite-laced processed meats?
- Are the conveniences of plastics or the attractions of certain shades of dye worth the price in terms of workers' health and your own safety?

Life is not without risk. We want convenience and quality. We must always, however, weigh risks against benefits. The anticancer drugs, for example, are worth the risk. If you needed them and did not take them, you would be dead and the risk of developing cancer 20 years hence would be unimportant. On the other hand, is a certain shade of hair dye worth the risk of developing cancer?

If you are a woman, can you arrange to have your first child, if you plan to have children, before the age of 30. Are you willing to have annual physical checkups, including a Pap test and breast and proctoscopic examinations? If you are a man, will you undergo regular physical exams, including prostate and proctoscopic examinations. If after consulting this book you think you may have one of the precancerous conditions, will you make an appointment right away with your physician?

No claim is made that every chemical mentioned poses an imminent danger of producing cancer. No claim is made that everything known to cause cancer is listed. This text serves only to provide information about many of the known and suspected cancer-causing agents you may encounter in your daily life. The search for and the recognition of carcinogens is just beginning. Unfortunately, for many, it is already too late. But as the search progresses and more and more information is compiled, the odds that we and our children will develop this dread disease are greatly reduced. Prevention is the best weapon against cancer. You must demand and support the ongoing search and heed the warnings produced. Chances are one out of four that your life depends upon it.

REFERENCES FOR THE INTRODUCTION

David Burnham, "Plan on Labeling for Carcinogens Arouses Dispute," *New York Times,* March 5, 1978, p. 1.

Cancer Rates and Risks, 2d ed., U. S. Department of Health, Education and Welfare, Washington, D.C., 1974.

Cancer and the Worker, New York Academy of Sciences, New York, 1977.

Guidelines for Carcinogen Bioassay in Small Rodents, National Cancer Institute Carcinogenesis Technical Report Series No. 1, May 19, 1976.

Health Hazards of the Human Environment, World Health Organization, Washington, D.C., 1972.

John Higginson, "The Importance of Environmental Factors in Cancer," Inserm Symposia Series, vol. 52, 1976, p. 261.

"Identification, Classification and Regulation of Toxic Substances Posing a Potential Occupational Carcinogenic Risk," *Federal Register,* October 4, 1977.

Douglas Martin, "Search for Toxic Chemicals in Environment Gets a Slow Start: Is Proving Difficult and Expensive," *Wall Street Journal,* May 9, 1978.

Thomas Maugh II, "Carcinogens in the Workplace: Where to Start Cleaning Up," *Science,* September 23, 1977.

Mary Jo Patterson and Joan Whitlow, "Workers Often Kept in Dark on Chemical Risk," *Newark Star Ledger,* January 13, 1978.

P. Shubik and D. Clayson, "Application of the Results of Carcinogen Bioassays to Man," Inserm Symposia Series, vol. 52, 1976, p. 241.

L. Tomatis, "Extrapolation of Test Results to Man," Inserm Symposia Series, Vol. 52, 1976, p. 261.

AAF. *See* 2-Acetylaminofluorene.

ACETAMIDE. *Acetic acid amide.* Colorless deliquescent crystals with a mousy odor derived from ethyl acetate and ammonium hydroxide. Used as a reactant, peroxide stabilizer, and general solvent in lacquers, explosives, soldering flux; as a hygroscopic, wetting, or penetrating agent; and to denature alcohol. It is a mild irritant with low toxicity. Has caused liver cancer when given orally to rats in doses of 5,000 milligrams per kilogram of body weight.[1,2,3]

2-ACETAMIDOFLUORENE. *See* 2-Acetylaminofluorene.

ACETANILIDE. *Trimethylactanilide.* White shiny leaflets or powder, odorless and derived from aniline *(see)*. Used as a rubber accelerator, inhibitor in hydrogen peroxide, a stabilizer for cellulose ester coatings, as a synthetic camphor, in pharmaceutical chemicals, and in dyestuffs. It is also a precursor of penicillin, and it is used as an antiseptic. It caused tumors when given orally to rats in doses of 3,500 milligrams per kilogram of body weight.[4]

ACETIC ACID. *Bromo, chromium salt, diazo-, and dehydro-.* A clear colorless liquid with a pungent odor. It occurs naturally in apples, cheese, cocoa, grapes, skimmed milk, oranges, peaches, pineapples, strawberries, and a variety of other fruits and plants. It is an organic acid solvent for gums, resins, volatile oil; It is used in freckle lotions, hand creams, and hair

17

dyes, as a scalp stimulator in hair products, and to stop bleeding. In solution it is mildly irritating to the skin. It is highly irritating to the skin in its glacial form (without much water), and its vapors are capable of producing lung obstruction. Used as a synthetic flavoring agent, it is one of the earliest known food additives. Generally recognized as safe for packaging only. It caused cancer in rats and mice when given orally or by injection.[5]

2-ACETYLAMINOFLUORENE. *AAF, FAA; 2-FAA, 2-fluorenylacetamide, 2-acetamidofluorene, and N-acetylaminophenanthrene.* A light tan crystal or solid, it has been demonstrated to cause cancer in humans. The one major chemical company making the substance ceased production when OSHA issued an occupational standard, setting forth the legally allowable exposure to it. However, the chemical had been patented as a pesticide in 1940. Although reportedly never used, it reappeared in other industrial or laboratory processes as a contaminant. According to OSHA, it is used today only in cancer research laboratories. This substance induces a high rate of cancer in laboratory animals,[6] and OSHA has a strict standard for the protection of laboratory workers and manufacturing workers who may handle substances containing more than one percent of 2-acetylaminofluorene.

N-ACETYLAMINOPHENANTHRENE. *See* 2-Acetylaminofluorene.

ACID BLUE. *Sodium salt, CI acid blue 3, blue URS.* An acid dye widely used as an inexpensive coloring for plastics, wools, silk, varnishes, and some pigments. The ability of this dye to color and remain fast during washing and exposure to light is good. It caused tumors in rats when injected under the skin in doses of 960 milligrams per kilogram of body weight.[7]

ACID LEATHER ORANGE. *See* Benzenesulfonic Acid.

ACRIDINE. *1'-Ethyl-1,2,5,6-dibenzacridine.* Small colorless needles derived from coal tar and used in the manufacture of dyes; derivatives, especially acriflavine and proflavine *(see),* are used as analytical reagents. They caused tumors and cancers in mice when injected under the skin in doses of 60 milligrams per kilogram of body weight.[8]

ACRIDINE RED. *3H-Xanthen-6-amine, N-methyl-3-(methylamino)-, hydrochloride.* Derived from anthracene (coal tar), it has red crystals. It is highly irritating to the skin and mucous membranes and causes sneezing on inhalation. Used in the manufacture of dyes, its derivatives are employed to analyze certain chemicals. Some dyes from it are used for antiseptics. It caused cancer when injected under the skin in rats in doses of 1,350 milligrams per kilogram of body weight, and there is an OSHA standard for it as a carcinogenic agent.[9]

ACRILAN. *See* Acrylonitrile.

ACRYLONITRILE. About 1.5 billion pounds of this substance are produced in the United States each year and used in acrylic and other synthetic fibers with such trade names as Orlon, Acrilan, Creslan, Acrylan, Elura, and Verel. It is also used in resin, plastics, latexes, and fumigants. In January 1978 the U.S. Department of Labor announced an "emergency action" to reduce worker exposure, saying that 10,000 workers were directly exposed and that another 125,000 workers were indirectly exposed. Officials said there was little risk that users of the finished products made with acrylonitrile were in danger. The emergency action was touched off when E. I. Du Pont de Nemours & Co. conducted a survey of a group of workers at its plant in Camden, South Carolina, and found that the incidence of cancer among those exposed to acrylonitrile for a long period of time was nearly three times the "expected" rate. The emergency standards permitted a worker to be exposed to only 2 parts per million of air in an eight-hour period. The previous standard set before the carcinogenic effects of the chemical were understood was 20 parts per million.[10] *See also* Vinyl Chloride.

ACTINOMYCETES. An organism that can be best characterized as falling somewhere between a bacterium and a fungus. Various streptomyces species are included in this category. When injected into rats, they were found to induce tumors.[11] *See also* Actinomycin C and Actinomycin D.

ACTINOMYCIN C. *Sanamycin.* A family of antibiotics produced by streptomyces. Active against *E. coli* and other bacteria and fungi infections. It is also used to treat tumors and as an immunosuppressive agent. It has been shown to cause tumors when given intravenously to rats.[12] However, a NIOSH review gives it a negative determination for carcinogenicity.[13]

ACTINOMYCIN D. *Dactinomycin.* Employed in biology as an inhibitor of DNA-directed RNA synthesis and as an antitumor agent, it has produced sarcomas at the site of injections and invasive mesothelioma (a rare form of cancer) in rats injected repeatedly with doses of only a few tenths of a milligram.[14] NIOSH gives it a positive determination for carcinogenicity in animals.[15] *See also* Actinomycetes and Actinomycin C.

ADENINE 1-OXIDE. White odorless powder with a salty taste. It occurs in RNA and DNA and in many coenzymes. Derived by extraction from tea, uric acid, and yeast RNA, it is used in medicine and in biochemical research. It caused tumors when injected under the skin of rats.[16]

ADRIAMYCIN. *Adriaicine, adriblastina.* Isolated from cultures of streptomyces, it is used to treat tumors and to prevent recurrence. It has been found to be a potent carcinogen and causes tumors in hamsters, rats, mice, dogs, and rabbits when administered intravenously.[17]

AEROSOLS. The first aerosol patent was actually issued in 1899 but was not used until 1940, when insecticides were first packaged in self-dispensing gas-pressurized containers. Freon, the most commonly used group among aerosol gases, is a lung irritant, central nervous system depressant, and in high concentrations can cause coma. In addition to Freon, hair sprays contain PVP (*See* polyvinyl pyrrolinone) or shellac. PVP is believed to cause cancer. In addition, thesaurosis, a condition in which there are foreign bodies in the lung, has been found in persons subjected to repeated inhalation of hair sprays. In powder products (*see* Talc) the inhalation of powder or its component silicones can damage the lungs. In 1972 the Society of Cosmetic Chemists reported that powder aerosols evidence a high particle retention in the lungs and profound pulmonary effects. Tests showed large powder particles in 23 separate areas of the lungs.

In 1974, Dr. F. S. Rowland, professor of chemistry at the University of California, Irvine campus, and Dr. Mario J. Molina, a University of California research associate, reported in *Nature,* the international scientific journal published in England, that man-made chemicals used extensively in aerosol spray cans and refrigeration units pose a threat to the fragile layer of stratospheric ozone that shields the earth from much of the sun's ultraviolet radiation. The result could be a great increase in skin cancers. In 1974 the FDA proposed a warning label to be affixed to an estimated one billion aerosol spray cans containing certain fluorocarbon propellants deemed dangerous to public health and the environment: "Warning: contains a chlorofluorocarbon that may harm the public health and environment by reducing ozone in the upper atmosphere." In December 1977 the government announced a ban on the manufacture of nearly all aerosol products containing chlorofluorocarbons because of fears that they were damaging the earth's ozone layer *(see).* The ban affected 97 to 98 percent of all aerosols using chlorofluorocarbons as propellants, including deodorants, hair sprays, household cleaners, and some pesticides. Most of the products are available with mechanical sprayers or other propellants such as carbon dioxide or hydrocarbons *(see).* Sales were down 40 percent in the three years prior to the ban. Exempt from the ban are contraceptive vaginal foams, drugs used in inhalation therapy, certain electrical cleaning sprays, aircraft maintenance products, and some insecticides. The action did not affect chlorofluorocarbons used as coolants in refrigerators and air-conditioners, or in the production of plastic foams. But the federal agency is considering regulations for these nonaerosol uses. The government ordered a ban on interstate shipment of nonessential aerosol products on April 15, 1979. In the vast majority of cases aerosols are unnecessary. They are also more expensive. Do not buy aerosols when other methods of application are available.

2 AF. *See* 2-Acetylaminofluourene.

AFLATOXINS. These are the best-studied members of a class of compounds called "mycotoxins" (toxins formed by molds). An outbreak in 1960 in England of Turkey X disease, an acute liver condition, was traced to peanut meal contaminated with the mold, which occurred after improper harvesting and storage. There is no known way to remove the mold once it occurs in meal. Peanut oils, however, are free of mold because of the alkaline treatment they receive during processing.

The effect on humans of aflatoxins, and of mycotoxins in general, has been difficult to demonstrate because as moldy food is not aesthetically pleasing for human consumption, it often ends up in animal feed (milk currently on the market contains aflatoxins because cows are sometimes fed moldy grain). Scattered incidents of human poisoning by mycotoxins have occurred, generally under special conditions, such as starvation or war.

A single dose of 5 milligrams per kilogram of body weight has induced tumors in rats. The marked differences in geographical distribution of liver cancer in humans has long suggested the presence of some common factor. In areas of Africa where there is a high incidence of liver cancer, aflatoxin contamination is common. The FDA has had informal standards for peanut aflatoxin for a decade. Similar regulations are planned for other affected commodities. Aflatoxin Bl is one of the most potent cancer-causing agents known in animal testing. Levels as low as one part per billion produced liver cancer in rats. Previous experiments showed a 100 percent incidence in rats on a lifetime diet containing 15 times that amount of aflatoxin Bl.

In addition to liver cancer, aflatoxins have been implicated in the formation of tumors of the stomach, kidney, and some other tissues. Aflatoxin Bl appears to be the most potent liver-cancer inducer known. In the northwestern part of the United States, rainbow trout died of liver-cancer, believed due to aflatoxin, but there was no evidence of a relationship between the outbreak and human cancer. Since aflatoxin is a mycotoxin, it has been recommended that other mycotoxins be investigated for cancer-causing abilities, such as patulin *(see)*, penicillic acid *(see)*, zearalenone, sterigmatocystin, leukoskyrin, and others.[18,19,20]

Make sure the nuts you eat are fresh. Dr. William Wardell, director of the Center for the Study of Drug Development, University of Rochester School of Medicine, speaking at a symposium on Public Issues and Private Medicine, December 6, 1978, in Philadelphia, pointed out that "when a batch of peanuts is imported containing aflatoxin levels that are too high for us to eat, the current method of control is to dilute the contaminated batch with a clean batch to bring the level down to acceptable proportions."

AGENT ORANGE. A defoliant that was used in heavy quantities in Vietnam to denude jungle areas and expose enemy hiding places, it is currently being used in lesser amounts throughout the United States to kill poisonous weeds in cattle pasturelands and farm-crop areas and to contain roadside weeds and brush and forest growth. A mixture of the phenol-related compounds 2,4-D and 2,4,5-T, it contains a trace impurity, dioxin *(see)*, a highly toxic substance.

Many veterans exposed to Agent Orange in Vietnam, as well as others who have come into contact with the herbicide, have complained of symptoms ranging from headaches, numbness, and other neurological problems to psychological changes, skin problems, liver imbalances, intestinal disorders, and cancer. It has also been suspected of causing human birth defects. John Bederka, Ph.D., chief of the section of toxicology, University of Illinois Hospital, Chicago, is coordinating a study to determine the human health effects of Agent Orange. The program includes a study of a Wisconsin farm accidently sprayed with the herbicide in 1971, and a computerized study of Vietnam veterans exposed to the pesticide and their wives. The Illinois researcher is attempting to determine whether veterans exposed to the herbicide are fathering deformed children. If so, it will be the only nongenetic case in which a male has been shown to cause such defects. The farmer's wife suffered two miscarriages after the accidental spraying. Changes also took place in some of the farm animals. Pigs and chickens were born deformed, cows gave bitter milk, and hens laid soft-shelled eggs. The farmer also reported finding dead birds and snakes and dwarf skunks in the area. Dr. Bederka has warned that the public should not purchase any substance containing 2,4,5-T for household use—many weed-control agents sold for yards and gardens contain it. He says that any product containing 2,4,5-T also contains dioxin, and he feels that this poses a grave hazard to the health of persons who use or come in contact with the product.[21]

In February 1979 the EPA ordered an emergency ban on most uses of 2,4,5-T and Silvex (both contain dioxin). It was the first emergency ban ever evoked by the EPA, which halted use of an estimated 7 million pounds of the compound scheduled for use in spring spraying of forests, pasturelands, and power-line rights-of-way. The EPA ban was based on studies conducted in Oregon showing that women in areas sprayed by the herbicides had increased incidences of miscarriages; on laboratory reports showing that animals had suffered birth defects, miscarriages, and tumors after exposure to dioxin-containing herbicides; and on the explosion-generated chemical cloud of herbicide that occurred in Seveso, Italy, in 1976, causing many ailments among the population. The EPA said its ban would prohibit the use of herbicides on forests, pastures, and rights-of-way but not on rangelands or rice fields because, according to an agency spokesman, the human exposure was not significant in the latter case.[22]

AIRCRAFT ENGINES. Spectrofluorescent methods of analysis have shown that soot and exhaust products of airplane engines, both piston and turbine, contain benzopyrene *(see)*. A modern engine releases from 2 to 10 milligrams of benzopyrene per minute into the atmosphere. Extracts of airplane engine soot applied to the skin of mice induced malignant tumors in almost all the animals treated. The ground within airports is polluted with benzopyrene; the level of pollution diminishes in proportion to the distance from the runway. The concentration of carcinogenic polycyclic hydrocarbons *(see)* in aircraft exhaust is dependent on the working regime of the engine and on the character of fuel combustion. A big modern airport receives or sends out an average of one plane every four minutes. Thus about 4 milligrams of benzopyrene per minute, or nearly 2 kilograms per year, would be discharged. This amount is less than that discharged in an automobile parking lot in a big city, since one automobile engine discharges about 10 milligrams per minute. One automobile can discharge over one kilogram of benzopyrene in a year. And the release of automobile discharge takes place within the zone of human inhalation, whereas benzopyrene discharge from planes occurs at a height that ensures its degradation (decomposition) by the sun's rays and ozone, although the amount of degradation of the latter is likely to decrease in the case of ultrasonic aviation.[23]

AIRPLANES. *See* Aircraft Engines.

AIR POLLUTION. Polluted air affects the health of human beings and of animals and plants. Emitted pollutants are diluted in the atmosphere and swept away by winds, except during an inversion (when surface air cannot rise). Then, for a period that varies from a few hours to a week or more, pollutants are trapped and the dilution process is impeded. When an inversion persists for a week or more, pollution increases substantially, and there is an accompanying increase in the death rate. Scientists are convinced that air pollution is very definitely a factor contributing to the three major types of diseases that cause sickness and death in our country—heart disease, lung and respiratory diseases, and cancer. Research has shown that air pollution will accelerate the advance of disease in those persons already afflicted, and earlier death is a real probability. Studies have shown that air pollution can actually be hazardous to people who live 50 or 100 miles away from the pollution source. This is because some common pollutants while moving through the atmosphere are transformed by chemical reactions with sunlight into more hazardous pollutants, such as photochemical oxidants that attack the lungs and respiratory system. Sulfur oxides aggravate asthma, lung and heart diseases, and the lung function of children. The amount of suspended particles in the air is related to injury to the surfaces of the respiratory system, that is, to the linings of the lung and throat. Chemicals carried into the lungs by particulates may cause cancer to develop on the lung lining. Carbon monoxide is harmful to persons who have lung disease, anemia, or cerebral-vascular disease. Photochemical oxidants may cause respiratory irritation and even changes in lung function. Nitrogen oxides in high concentrations can be fatal, and in lower concentrations they can cause acute bronchitis and pneumonia.

Air pollution accounts for a doubling of the bronchitis mortality rate for urban as compared to rural areas. In 1958 the rate of death from lung cancer was 1.56 times as high in the urban areas as in the rural areas. Stomach cancer is significantly related to a deposit index and a smoke index. The mortality rate due to stomach cancer is more than twice as great in areas of high pollution as in areas of low pollution. The mortality rate of all cancers is 25 percent higher in polluted areas than in areas of relatively clean air. Cigarette smoke and automotive exhaust, the most common environmental air aggressors, are composed of gases, liquid, and solid aerosols. Personal pollution from smoke is the main cause of respiratory cancer. Municipal incinerators are major sources of several toxic elements in the air of many cities. Refuse incineration can account for major portions of zinc, cadmium, antimony, and possibly silver, tin, and indium observed in airborne particles. Many of the toxic elements from incinerators are associated with predominantly small particles that easily can be inhaled into the lungs, where these poisonous elements can be dissolved in body fluids and transported about the body.

Air pollution appears to have greater adverse impact on men than on women in age groups under 65. For people older than 65, however, the effects are approximately the same on both sexes. This suggests the possibility of relatively higher exposure levels at work for men compared to exposure levels experienced by women.

The impact of air pollution on humans generally increases with age. This indicates either that the ability of the human body to fight off the effects decreases with age or that air pollution stress has a cumulative effect on health.

It has been estimated that 25 percent of the deaths from lung cancer could be saved by a 50 percent reduction in air pollution.[24,25,26,27]

AIRPORTS. *See* Aircraft Engines.

ALANINE. Colorless crystals derived from protein. Believed to be a nonessential amino acid, it is used in microbiological research and as a dietary supplement in the L and DL forms. The FDA has asked for supplementary information.[28] It is now Generally Recognized As Safe for addition to food. (see GRAS List) It caused cancer of the skin in mice, and tumors when injected into their abdomens.[29]

ALANINE,3-(p-(BIS(2-CHLOROETHYL)AMINO)PENYL)-,L-. *See* Melphalan.

ALCOHOLIC BEVERAGES. Consumption of alcoholic beverages entails an increased risk of developing cancer of the mouth, larynx, pharynx, and esophagus, according to the International Agency for Research on Cancer of the World Health Organization. The evidence is that the increase in cancer of the esophagus is proportional to the amount of ethanol consumed. In all four cancer sites the role of tobacco is also important, and the ill effects of these two factors—drinking alcoholic beverages and smoking tobacco—tend to multiply when they act together. The mechanisms that cause alcohol in beverages to produce cancer in humans is not known but may vary among cancer sites. On the basis of animal experiments, WHO reports say that ethanol itself cannot be said to be a carcinogen. But, it may act as a cocarcinogen by enhancing the role of other cancer-causing agents. Ethanol is an excellent solvent for chemicals that are themselves cancer-causing agents, such as polycylic hydrocarbons and nitrosamines *(see* both*)* The presence of these chemicals has been detected in some commonly consumed alcoholic beverages drunk in areas where esophageal cancer is common.[30]

ALCOPHOBIN. *See* Disulfiram.

ALDOMYCIN. *See* Nitrofurazone.

ALDRIN. A pesticide introduced in 1950. Two of its major uses have been foliage application on cotton plants and soil application for cornfields. Smaller amounts were used in food products. Registration of products containing aldrin were canceled in 1974, but the compound was selected for cancer testing because data regarding its carcinogenicity were controversial and because there was a potential for long-term human exposure to residues, especially in foods. In one study reported in 1978 by the NCI, purified technical grade aldrin was fed to Osborne-Mendel rats and B6C3F1 mice for 80 weeks. Aldrin caused liver cancer in male mice, but in female mice the increases in liver cancer could not be related to treatment. In rats, aldrin could not clearly be associated with liver tumors.[31]

ALKALOIDS. *See* Anticancer Drugs.

ALKYLATING AGENTS. Introduced with increasing frequency, these agents are used as industrial intermediates *(see)* in the creation of inorganic substances, as organic solvents, and also as chemotherapeutic agents. Examples of chemicals belonging to this group are the nitrogen and sulfur mustards *(see)*, epoxides, ethylenimines *(see)*, alkyl sulfates, and sulfones. They have been found to be carcinogenic in animals and, in some cases, humans.[32] *See also* Anticancer Drugs.

ALLYLAMIDE. *2-Propenylamine.* A colorless to light yellow liquid; strong ammoniacal odor; attacks rubber and cork. The fumes are strongly irritating to eyes and skin. It is used as a pharmaceutical intermediate *(see)* and in organic synthesis.

ALLYL CHLORIDE. *3-Chloropropene.* A chemical intermediate *(see)* used in manufacturing other compounds, it was given by stomach tube to rats and mice for 78 weeks. It was carcinogenic in mice, causing low rates of stomach cancer in both sexes. The test was inconclusive in rats because of early mortality.[33]

AMEBAN. *Carbarsone, arsanilic acid, N-carbamoyl, Ambarsone, N-carbamoylarsanilic acid.* A white powder used as an intestinal amebicide and to combat vaginal infections due to trichomonas. When given in oral doses to rats in doses of 5,000 milligrams per kilogram of body weight, it caused cancer.[34]

AMES TEST. *See* Introduction, page 7.

AMINES. A class of organic compounds derived from ammonia. They are basic in nature—synthetic derivatives of ammonium chloride, a salt that occurs naturally. Quaternary ammonium compounds used in detergents are examples.

AMINO ACIDS. Certain amino-acid deficiencies appear to have tumor-suppressing action. Amino-acids are the building blocks of proteins. There are about 20 important ones. Eight amino acids are called "essential" because the body cannot synthesize them and they must be obtained ready-made from protein foods. The amino acids of protein foods are separated by digestion and go into a general pool from which the body takes the ones it needs to synthesize its own personal proteins. A diet deficient in cystine (a nonessential amino acid found in Keratin and urine) was reported to inhibit the induction of leukemia in DBA mice. Spontaneous mammary carcinoma in C3H female mice was inhibited by lysine-deficient or cystine-deficient diets (lysine is an essential amino acid isolated from casein, fibrin, or blood, and is necessary for growth and tissue synthesis).

This tumor-suppressing action may be due to the effect on the body's immune system. Cell-mediated immunity, that is the defense against invaders maintained within the cell, is believed to be a major barrier against cancer. The other type of natural immunity, "humoral," involves the body's ability to manufacture antibodies against invaders. The theory is that the manufacture of antibodies against a tumor may increase the chance of tumor development by protecting the tumor from the cell's immune defenses. Studies indicate that certain amino-acid deficiencies may be able to correct this situation by leaving cell-mediated immunity intact while at the same time depressing antibody production. The inhibitory effect of low-protein diets on certain types of tumors may also be explained by this mechanism. In addition, severe protein deficiency can limit the amount of tumors developed or the area of the body where tumors develop by altering the metabolism of the carcinogenic agent.[35]

2-AMINOANTHRAQUINONE. An intermediate *(see)* used in the manufacture of dyes, it was fed to rats and mice for 78 to 80 weeks. It caused liver cancers in male rats and in mice of both sexes and lymphomas in female mice. The study did not provide evidence for carcinogenicity of 2-aminoanthraquinone in female rats. *See also* anthraquinone.[36]

p-AMINOBIPHENYL (PAB). *p-biphenylamine.* Prepared from diazoaminobenzene, it was used as an antioxidant in the rubber industry in the 1940s and 1950s. It is now sometimes used to detect sulfates and as an experimental carcinogen. In July 1978 the Monsanto Company reported that 14 of its employees had died of bladder cancer between 1953 and 1973 because they had been involved with the manufacture of PAB more than 30 years before. Monsanto said that since it halted production of the chemical in 1955, more than 100 employees had developed bladder tumors.[37]

AMINOTRIAZOLE. *3-Amino-1,2,4-triazole; amitrole.* This was the herbicide and plant-growth regulator that caused the removal of cranberries from American tables one Thanksgiving in the 1960s. Rats were fed 100 parts per million (ppm) aminotriazole continuously for two years in their diets, and thyroid cancers were produced in 4 of the 26. Scientists point out that cabbages, turnips, peas, beans, strawberries, and milk contain natural and related chemicals. Rutabagas (Swedish turnips) naturally contain up to 200 ppm of a thyroid-cancer inducer, L-5-vinyl-2-thiooxazolidine; one serving of these turnips may contain 100 times as much thyroid-cancer inducing activity as cranberries badly contaminated with aminotriazole.[38,39]

AMITRAZ. *Baam.* A pesticide used on pears in Washington, Utah, Oregon, Michigan, New York, and Pennsylvania since 1975 on an emergency basis to control an aphidlike insect called pear psylla. It is claimed that there is no effective alternative pesticide available to control the pear psylla, which is capable of damaging both the fruit and the trees. The EPA claims that without amitraz the economic losses to growers could be as high as $33 million for three years. On January 15, 1979, the EPA proposed to approve the pesticide on the condition that certain restrictions be imposed "to reduce potential risks to human health." They said that amitraz could be used on pears for four years, pending completion of additional laboratory tests by the manufacturer. The proposal follows a full-scale review of the risk versus benefits of using the pesticide on pears. There is some evidence that it may cause tumors in laboratory animals and therefore might present "a small risk of cancer to humans." As a result, EPA would require application only by trained users wearing protective clothing. To reduce residue levels on the fruit before it is marketed, EPA would require longer time periods from the time a crop is sprayed to the time it is harvested. Amitraz is distributed in this country by Upjohn of Kalamazoo, Michigan. It is estimated that about 120,000 pounds of it might be used on pears each year. Under the proposal, EPA would not allow use of amitraz on apples to control mites, as requested by the distributor.[40]

AMMONIA. Obtained by blowing steam through incandescent coke, ammonia is extremely toxic when inhaled in concentrated vapors and is irritating to the eyes and mucous membranes. It is used in permanent wave lotions and hair bleaches, in the manufacture of detergents, and in cleaning preparations. It is also used in the manufacture of explosives and synthetic fabrics. It has been shown to produce cancer of the skin in humans in doses of 1,000 milligrams per kilogram of body weight.[41]

AMMONIUM. *4- p- (Dimethylamino)- alpha- (2- hydroxy-3, 6- disulfo-1- naphthyl) Benzylidene)-2,5-cyclohexadien-1-ylidene), dimethyl, hydroxide, inner salt, sodium salt. See* Greens.

AMMONIUM. *Ethyl 4-(p-(ethyl(m-sulfobenzyl) amino)-alpha-phenyl-benzylidene) 2,5-cyclohexadien-1-ylidene) (m-sulfobenzyl)-hydroxide, inner salt, sodium salt. See* Greens.

27

AMMONIUM. *Ethyl 4-(p-(ethyl (p-sulfobenzyl) amino)-alpha-(o-sulfophenyl) benzylidene)-2,5-cyclohexadien-1-ylidene) (m-sulfobenzyl)-hydroxide, inner salt, diammonium salt.* See Blues.

AMMONIUM. *Ethyl 4-(p-(ethyl(m-sulfobenzyl) amino-alpha-(p-sulfophenyl) benzylidene) 2,5-cylohexadien-1-ylidene) (m-sulfobenzyl) hydroxide, inner salt, disodium salt.* See Blues.

AMMONIUM. *Ethyl 4-(p-(ethyl(m-sulfobenzyl) amino-alpha-(p-sulfophenyl) benzylidene)-2,5-cyclohexadien-l-ylidene) (m-sulfobenzyl)-hydroxide, inner salt, disodium salt.* See Greens.

AMOSITE. *See* Asbestos.

ANABASINE, 1-NITROSO. *Neonicotine.* A naturally occurring alkaloid, it is a colorless liquid that darkens on exposure to air. It is extracted from *Anabasis aphylla* and *Nicotiana glauca* and is toxic when ingested, inhaled, or absorbed through the skin. It is used as an insecticide.[42] Caused cancer in rats when administered orally in doses of 8,550 milligrams per kilogram of body weight.[43]

4-ANDROSTENE-3,17-DIONE. *Androst-4-ene-3,17-dione.* Derived from the female hormone progesterone *(see)*, it is used as a medicine. Caused tumors when injected subcutaneously in mice.[44]

ANESTHESIA. Since 1967, when a Russian study cited evidence that the female anesthesiologists under observation had a higher incidence of abortions and children with congenital malformations than did the control-group women, a controversy has raged about the risk of anesthesia to operating room personnel. In 1974, Dr. Thomas Corbett of the Veterans Administration Hospital in Ann Arbor, Michigan, revealed a cancer rate three times higher than expected in operating room personnel. He said in his paper that an estimated 20 million anesthetics are administered to patients each year in the 25,000 operating rooms throughout the United States. Approximately 50,000 operating room personnel are exposed daily to low concentrations of anesthetic gases that permeate the operating room throughout the administration of inhalation anesthesia. In his study, sponsored by the American Society of Anesthesiologists, with the financial support of NIOSH, 50,000 operating room professionals were surveyed, with 24,000 unexposed medical and nursing professionals as controls. The frequency of cancer was 1.3 to 2 times greater among exposed women—the highest risk was shown to be among women physician-anesthetists, followed by nurse anesthetists.[45] In 1977 another report in the *Journal of the American Medical Association* described a 17-year review of deaths among anesthesiologists conducted by the American Cancer Society. It showed that anesthesiologists tended to live longer than general practitioners and the rest of the population, and that their causes of death were about the same as those of the general population. In particular, deaths from cancer were no higher among them than among other physicians or the general population.[46]

ANESTHESIOLOGISTS. *See* Anesthesia.

ANGELICA LACTONE. *2-Pentenoic acid, 4-hydroxy-, gamma-lactone.* It is distilled from levulinic acid derived from starch or sugar. It is used in flavorings and has been shown to cause tumors in rats when injected under the skin in doses of 2,600 milligrams per kilogram of body weight.[47]

ANILINE. A colorless to brown liquid that darkens with age. Slightly soluble in water, it is one of the most commonly used of the organic bases, the parent substance for many dyes and drugs. It is derived from nitrobenzene or chlorobenzene and is toxic when ingested, inhaled, or absorbed through the skin. It is an allergen (it induces allergies). It is used as a rubber accelerator to speed vulcanization and antioxidant (retards aging), and as an intermediate *(see);* it is also used in dyes, photographic chemicals, the manufacture of urethane foams, pharmaceuticals, explosives, petroleum refining, diphenylamine (chemical used in dyes), phenolics (resins used in laminated and adhesive products); herbicides, and fungicides. It caused cancer in mice when injected under the skin and in rats when administered orally and under the skin. It also caused tumors.[48]

ANILINE DYES. A synonym for coal-tar *(see)* dyes, it refers to a large class of synthetic dyes made from intermediates *(see)* based upon or made from aniline. Most are somewhat toxic and irritating to eyes, skin, and mucous membranes but are generally much less toxic than the aniline itself. These dyes caused tumors in animals whose skins were painted with them.[49]

ANILINE HYDROCHLORIDE. An intermediate *(see)* in the manufacture of dyes, it was fed to rats and mice for 103 weeks. It caused a variety of cancers in male and female rats but did not produce cancer in mice. *See also* Aniline and Aniline Dyes.

o-ANISIDINE, N-METHYL-4-(PHENYLAZO)-. Yellowish liquid derived from 2-nitroanisole, a substance used in the manufacture of azo dyes *(see).* A skin irritant and sensitizer, it can be absorbed through the skin.[50] It caused cancer in rats when given orally and in rats when painted on the skin.[51]

ANTABUSE. *See* Disulfiram.

ANTHOPHYLLITE. *See* Asbestos.

ANTHRACENE. *Green oil.* Derived from a coal-tar fraction, it consists of yellow crystals with blue fluorescence. Used in the dyes alizarin, phenanthrene, carbazole, and anthraquinone; in calico printing; and in organic research. Caused cancer when injected subcutaneously and into the abdomen in rats and mice.[52]

2-ANTHRACENESULFONIC ACID. *1-Amino-9,10-dihydro-4-(m-(2-hydroxyethyl) sulfonyl) anilino; 9,10-dioxo-,hydrogen sulfate (ester); disodium salt. See* Blues.

ANTHRALIN. An odorless, tasteless, yellow powder derived from anthraquinone *(see),* it has been used for many years in the treatment of the skin condition, psoriasis. It has been found to be a potent tumor-promoting agent when applied to mouse skin, which is a substance that does not itself induce malignancy but increases the potency of the agents that cause cancer. It has not been found to have any deleterious effect upon humans at the levels used clinically, although when administered in high doses, it has been found to be irritating to human skin. A property that anthralin has in common with other tumor-promoting agents is its compatibility with fats and with water. Such molecules would exert much influence at the point where a fatty material comes into contact with water. Since cell walls are composed largely of fat-containing material, the presence of a tumor-promoting chemical might modify the ability of the cell wall to fend off cancer-causing agents.[53]

ANTHRANILIC ACID. An aromatic amine *(see)* that occurs as a metabolite (metabolic waste) of the amino acid tryptophan, it is used commercially as an intermediate *(see)* in dye manufacture, drugs, perfumes, and pharmaceuticals. Certain tryptophan metabolites, including anthranilic acid, have been found in abnormally high concentrations in the urine of bladder-cancer victims and in persons with a high risk of getting cancer, such as cigarette smokers or patients with parasitic bilharzial bladder infections. It has been suggested that people with abnormal tryptophan metabolism may be at risk for bladder cancer. Under test conditions, anthranilic acid was not carcinogenic in rats or mice.[54]

ANTHRAQUINONE. *Anthracine; 9,10-dihydro-9;10-dioxo.* Produced from anthracene or benzene, it is an important starting material for vat dyes. Consisting of light yellow needles, it has a low systemic toxicity but may cause skin irritation and sensitization.[55] It is also used as an organic inhibitor to prevent growth of cells and as a repellent to protect seeds from being eaten by birds. Caused tumors when given orally to rats in doses of 72 milligrams per kilogram of body weight.[56]

2-ANTHROL. *1-(Phenylazo)-, benzeneazo-2-anthrol.* Used in the manufacture of dyes, it causes cancer in mice when injected under the skin in doses of 25 milligrams per kilogram of body weight.[57] *See also* Anthracene.

ANTICANCER DRUGS. Chemotherapy or drug treatment of cancer had its historic origin in nitrogen mustard compounds *(see)* developed for warfare in World War II. Investigators found that war gases might reduce the numbers of malignant cells in certain cancers such as leukemia and lymphomas. Early research produced distinct beneficial effects in Hodgkin's disease *(see)*. Some 40 anticancer agents are now available in the United States for use in standard medical practice. These drugs attack cancers through a variety of mechanisms:

- *Alkylating agents* inhibit cell growth by cross-linking molecules of DNA (deoxyribonucleic acid), the genetic material that controls cell function and reproduction.

30

- *Antimetabolites* block the formation of DNA or other cell components by inhibiting essential enzymes. Many antimetabolites interfere with the formation of protein by incorporating themselves into the cell's DNA and inhibiting the growth and development of malignant cells.
- *Alkaloids* hinder cell division, or mitosis.
- *Hormones* can either suppress or speed up growth of cells in tissues and target organs and so can be manipulated to prevent the cancer cells from multiplying.
- *Enzymes,* at least one enzyme, acts by starving leukemia cells and sparing normal ones.

Most anticancer agents are powerful drugs that also affect normal tissues in varying ways, producing undesirable but usually manageable side effects. In addition, evidence is building up that some drugs used in treating cancers may themselves cause cancer years later. This comes mainly from long-term follow-up of the increasing number of cancer patients successfully treated with these drugs for an initial cancer condition. Alkylating agents, for example, used against cancers of the ovary and breast, have been associated with the development of leukemia in a small number of long-term survivors. The clinical problem is to measure the carcinogenic risk of these drugs in order to decide whether the risk is worth taking for the patient's well-being. The anticancer drugs' potential for causing second cancers is certainly not clear-cut. In most of the studies with cancer patients to date, second cancers have occurred chiefly in patients treated with radiation as well as drugs. Radiation *(see)* is known to be capable of causing cancer at the high doses used in cancer treatment. It is possible that second cancers are part of the natural history of the first cancer and appear after the patient has survived the initial attack. It is believed that cancer patients in general, even before or without drug treatment, have a rather high potential for second cancers. Further, some of the life-threatening noncancer diseases that are treated with these same powerful drugs are thought to predispose patients to later cancers.

Many new anticancer compounds, some of them similar to drugs currently in use, are in various stages of testing and development. The cancer-causing possibilities of these new chemical compounds must be assessed to help provide data for medical decision making. Anticancer agents undergoing NCI tests include: acronycine, 5-azacytidine, beta-TGDR, emitine, IPD, and estradiol mustard.[58] *See also* Cytoxin, Imuran, Melphalan, and Methotrexate.

ANTITHYROID COMPOUNDS. Thiourea has been detected in the seeds of certain plants in the genus *Laburnum.* Thiourea is an antithyroid compound that has produced thyroid tumors, cancers, benign and malignant liver tumors, and tumors of the eyelid and tear-duct gland in rats upon administration in the diet of only 1 to 0.1 percent. Another antithyroid compound (-)-5-vinyl-2 thiooxazolidine is derived from a substance in turnips, kale, cabbage, and rapeseed. Rats fed a diet containing 45 percent rapeseed have developed thyroid tumors.[59]

APPLE JUICE. *See* **Patulin.**

ARAMITE. *Sulfurous acid, 2-(p-t-butylphenoxy)-1-methyethyl-2-chlorethyl ester, Acaracide, Ortho-Mite.* Liquid practically insoluble in water. Can be mixed with many organic solvents. Used as an insecticide for plants. In undiluted form it may cause skin irritation. Large doses may cause central nervous system depression.[60] Caused cancer when given orally to mice in doses of 130 milligrams and to dogs in doses of 35 milligrams per kilogram of body weight.[61]

AROCLOR. *Biphenylechlore.* A polychlorinated biphenyl (PCB) used as a heat transfer agent, it was given in feed to rats from 104 to 105 weeks. According to the National Institutes of Health Office of Cancer Communications, aroclor was not carcinogenic to the rats under test conditions, although previous reports showed that it caused tumors when given orally to mice.[62] There is an OSHA standard for it pertaining to both air and skin to protect workers. *See also* PCBs.

AROMATIC AMINE COMPOUNDS. Derived from aniline *(see)*. Examples are benzidine and aminophenols.

AROMATIC AMINES. Compounds derived from benzene, naphthalene, and raw anthracene. Many of them have similar effects on the body but vary greatly in toxicity. All the liquids in the group are irritants. The vapors are irritating and can lead to lung and kidney damage. Among the compounds associated with bladder cancer in workers are 1-NA, 2-NA, benzidine, 4-aminobiphenyl, magenta, and auramine. Although their name implies distinctive odors, these chemicals may be difficult to detect by smell; odor cannot be depended upon to warn of their presense. Exposure to aromatic amines can occur not only in industrial environments but also through the air, foodstuffs, plastics, and drinking water.[63]

AROMATIC COMPOUNDS. Any organic compound, such as benzene. The vast majority are obtained from petroleum and coal tar. They are called aromatic because of the strong but not unpleasant odor of the chemicals.

AROMATIC NITRO COMPOUNDS. Derivatives of nitrobenze *(see)*.

ARSENIC ACID. *Calcium salt.* Caused tumors in hamsters when administered in doses of 753 milligrams per kilogram of body weight[64] and there is an OSHA standard for it pertaining to worker exposure to arsenic in the air. *See also* Arsenic Compounds.

ARSENIC COMPOUNDS. Arsenic is an element that occurs throughout the universe and is highly toxic in most forms. Its compounds are used in hair tonics and hair dyes and have been employed in the treatment of spirochetal infections, blood disorders, and skin diseases. (Fowler's solution, or potassium arsenite, for instance, has been used to treat leukemia and skin problems.) Ingestion causes nausea, vomiting, and death. Chronic poisoning can result in pigmentation of the skin and kidney and liver damage. In hair tonic and dyes it may cause contact dermatitis. The acceptable amount of arsenic in colors is 0.0002 percent. Arsenic can also cause the skin to be sensitive to light and break out in a rash or to swell. At the 1976 meeting of the American Chemical Society it was reported that arsenic was found in a variety of fruit-related foodstuffs—especially domestic wines and fruit juices—and often exceeded the safe allowable level established by the U.S. Public Health Service for drinking water, sometimes by a factor greater than 20. The report containing a history of a chronic alcoholic with arsenic poisoning was made. Some domestic wines, selected at random, contained more than 200 micrograms of arsenic per liter, and some fruit juices contained 100 micrograms per liter. The U.S. Public Health Service's maximum allowed limit for arsenic in drinking water is 50 micrograms per liter and the safe level is 10 micrograms. Foreign wines tested contained considerably less arsenic. Arsenic is not a cumulative poison in a strict sense since it is eliminated from the body in about one to six weeks. However, it is known that even medicine containing arsenic used topically can cause skin cancer 20 years after treatment. Low levels of arsenic ingestion in wine have been reported to cause a higher incidence of cancer and cancer mortality. The source of the arsenic in wine may be from two arsenicals, sodium arsenate and lead arsenate, whose use is permitted in vineyards during some phases of the growing season.[65]

A 1974 follow-up study conducted by the Dow and Allied Chemical companies in a Midland, Michigan, arsenic plant closed since 1956 showed that about a third of the former workers died from cancer. In another plant, of 27 exposed to arsenic at work, 19 died from cancer. Lung and lymphatic cancer rates were found to be six and seven times higher than expected for male workers.[66] An estimated 1.5 million American workers and countless consumers are exposed to arsenic, which is used in the manufacture of metal alloys, ceramics, dyes, drugs, glass; in garden and farm pesticides; as a defoliant during cotton harvesting; as a growth stimulant for livestock and poultry; as a wood treatment to prevent rot; and for the control of sludge in lubricating oils. High rates of lung cancer have also been found among both men and women in two Montana cities with copper mining and smelting facilities. The best explanation seems to be that the airborne arsenic, which the men are exposed to on the job, has also polluted the air in the community, contributing to a rise in lung cancer among women.[67] The 'incubation period for arsenic is believed to be 11 to 15 years. Target organs are the bladder, skin, lung, vulva, eyelids, face, neck, and larynx. Read the labels of pesticides, ceramic clays, and other products to see if they contain arsenic. If they do, do not buy them, or if you must buy them, exercise extreme caution when using them.

ARSENIC TRIOXIDE. *Crude arsenic, white arsenic, arsenious acid, ar-*

senious oxide, arsenious anhydride. A white, odorless, tasteless powder. It is slightly soluble in water, soluble in acids, soluble in glycerin. Highly toxic when ingested or inhaled. it may be carcinogenic. It is used in pigments, ceramic enamels, aniline colors; as a decolorizing agent in glass; in insecticides, rodenticides, herbicides, sheep and cattle dip; as both a hide and wood preservative; and in the preparation of other arsenic compounds.

ARSENIOUS ACID, POTASSIUM SALT. *Fowler's solution, potassium arsenate.* Caused tumors of the skin in mice when administered in doses of 291 milligrams per kilogram of body weight.[68] *See also* Arsenic Compounds.

ARSINE, DIPHENYCHLORO-. *Sneezing gas.* Caused skin tumors in mice when applied in doses of 33 milligrams per kilogram of body weight.[69]

ASARONE. *See* Calamus.

ASBESTOS. *Actinolite, amosite, anthophyllite, crocidolite, chrysotile, and tremolite.* These naturally occurring fibrous silicates classified as "asbestos" are now believed to be the most important cancer-causing agents in the workplace. There has been a thousandfold increase in output of asbestos during the past 60 years, and although it has been known for more than half a century that persons who inhaled large amounts of it in the course of their work sometimes developed disabling or fatal fibrosis of the lungs, it has only been within the last 30 years that it has been found to cause cancer. It is estimated that as many as 3,000 different products in daily use throughout the world contain some asbestos. The total world production each year is approximately 4 million tons. Canada accounts for about 30 percent of the total and the United States for about 3 percent. Asbestos is used in so many products because it inhibits combustion, is acid resistant, and has great tensile strength and light weight.

The very word *asbestos* comes from the Greek, meaning "inextinguishable."

The first suggestion that it could cause cancer was raised in 1935 by two physicians who noticed a correlation between asbestosis, a condition caused by fibers remaining in the lung, and lung cancer. The link was definitely established around 1960 when Mt. Sinai School of Medicine researchers found that asbestos was the cause of mesothelioma, a rare and always fatal cancer of the membranes surrounding the lungs and lining of the abdominal cavity. Cancer of the stomach has also been found among American insulation workers and among the Japanese who like to eat rice coated with talc, a substance usually contaminated with asbestos. Asbestos has also been linked with cancer of the larynx, and a study by the American Cancer Society showed that asbestos workers who smoke may be 92 times more likely than the average nonsmoker to develop lung cancer. Even relatively brief exposure can increase the risk of cancer 20 to 40 years later. Employees at the Johns-Manville Corporation plants were informed in June 1978 that they would no longer be able to smoke at asbestos manufacturing facilities.[70] In the same month, EPA announced a broadening of their asbestos regulations instituted in 1973. The rules were extended to cover all friable materials (those that can be easily broken up, pulverized, or reduced to powder) that contain asbestos. The regulations require that when buildings are being demolished or renovated, asbestos materials be wetted and removed before wrecking begins, that pipes and other items coated with asbestos cannot be dropped or thrown to the ground, and that in buildings higher than 50 feet, asbestos debris must be lowered to the ground in dust-tight chutes or containers. Some materials containing more than one percent asbestos are permitted in spraying operations, however. Examples of these materials or products, in which the hazardous amount of asbestos is encapsulated in a binder of asphaltlike or resinous compounds, are waterproofing for exposed insulation, automobile undercoating, and some coatings used in industrial maintenance. No acceptable asbestos-free substitutes for these materials are available, the agency said, and the fact that they are encapsulated will make it unlikely that the asbestos will remain airborne. Asbestos has been found in the air we breathe. An estimated 158,000 pounds of this mineral is released from automobile brake linings (see Auto Brakes) every year, and thousands of schools and other buildings have been constructed with asbestos insulation and flameproofing.

Despite this ubiquitous presence, there is no alarm over the general health of the public. The government attempts to lessen exposure of the general public and industrial workers by regulations reducing permissible amounts of airborne asbestos in the workplace. Some industries are installing exhaust ventilation systems and providing employees with protective equipment. All told, about 11 million workers have been exposed to asbestos since the early years of World War II: most of the workers affected have been those assigned to work areas where asbestos was used to insulate boilers, steam pipes, hot-water pipes, and nuclear reactors.[71] Dr. Irving Selikoff of Mt. Sinai School of Medicine, one of the world's leading experts on asbestos, says that a worker could be exposed heavily to asbestos for one day and develop cancer much later in life as a result, because his lungs continue to be exposed to the asbestos fibers deposited there. Altogether, 2.5 million Americans are now working in trades involving asbestos, including asbestos mining and processing, insulation work, building demolition, and brake-clutch repair.[72] Families of asbestos workers also run a risk of lung disease. One investigation is monitoring more than 600 wives and children of men who worked in a Paterson, New Jersey, asbestos factory before it closed in 1954.[73] In the study, one-third of the relatives have been found to have asbestosis. The clothes the men brought home carried fatal dust. The modern home has asbestos from roof to basement—asbestos roofing or roof tiles, gutters, rainwater pipes, ceiling and floor tiles. The tiles, even if polished, are subject to wear and tear and presumably the liberation of asbestos. The instances of pleural disease, one of them mesothelioma, have been found in workers who sanded asbestos floor tiles. Central-heating furnaces and pipes insulated by asbestos are common. Insulation of electrical equipment in the home, such as electric irons and stoves, is almost always compounded with asbestos. Ironing-board covers are made from the substance. The use of asbestos-containing spray on fireproofing compounds in high-rise buildings has been banned in the United States. There has been a question about asbestos-containing filter materials releasing asbestos fibers in potentially hazardous quantities into liquors, beers, wines, soft drinks, and other liquids. Manufacturers claim that the filters release only minute amounts of microscopic-sized asbestos fibers and that the filters save the public from bad-tasting and potentially harmful contaminants in their drinks. In 1972, after fibers were found in British beer, the World Health Organization looked into the matter and found "no evidence of an increased risk of cancer resulting from asbestos fibers present in water, beverages, food or in the fluids used to administer drugs."

The incubation period for asbestos-caused cancer is from 4 to 50 years. It primarily appears in the lung, pleural cavity, gastrointestinal tract, ovary, skin, liver, and larynx.[74]

Avoid asbestos whenever possible. Do not use it in do-it-yourself projects unless you are protected. When repairing walls at home, buy premixed spackling, jointing, and patching compounds if possible. Products without asbestos are available. Use a damp cloth to smooth compounds before they set, instead of sanding them after they harden. When raising dust is unavoidable, wear a mask. If you work on your car and change your brakes, vacuum up loose asbestos from brake linings. If you have old and frayed insulating materials in your home, protect yourself from fibers that may break loose. Ironing-board covers and floor tiles may contain asbestos. Repair frayed or torn items.

If you or your child has attended a school with asbestos ceilings, have your lungs checked and NEVER smoke. If you have been exposed to asbestos and you smoke, you greatly increase your chances of getting cancer.[75]

ASPHALT. *Mineral pitch, bitumen.* Found naturally and also produced by distillation of crude petroleum, hot asphalt can cause burns, and the fumes are highly irritating to the eyes and skin. Asphalt can cause skin cancer.[76]

ATHLETICS. A relationship may exist between participation in college athletics and cancer mortality. Body size also may have a linear relationship. Evidence is now on record suggesting that major athletes may die more often from neoplasms than nonathletes. Experiments in animals have suggested that exercise alters the response to cancer. No such study has been performed for humans. However, Dr. Anthony P. Polednak of the Argonne National Laboratories compared the cancer mortality experience of 8,393 college men exposed and not exposed to physical exercise and training as young adults. Death certificates showed that major athletes (lettermen) died significantly more often from neoplasms than nonathletes. Mean age at death from tumors was significantly lower in major athletes than in minor and nonathletes.[77]

ATOMIC BOMB. The people of Hiroshima and Nagasaki who survived exposure to the two prototype atomic bombs have been carefully studied during the past 25 years by the Atomic Bomb Casualty Commission. The information leaves no doubt that a single exposure at high doses produces leukemia in man. Also increased was the incidence of cancer of the lung, breast, and thyroid.[78]

ATRAZINE. One of the most widely used pesticides in the United States, it reacts under acidic conditions such as those found in the stomach, to form a potential carcinogen. It is used as a weed-control agent for corn and for noncrop and industrial sites. Found in drinking water supplies in Iowa and Louisiana, atrazine reacts with nitrite *(see)* to form N-nitrosoatrazine, a suspected carcinogen. Sodium nitrite is used as a meat preservative and may also be present in acid soils because of the large amounts of nitrite fertilizers used.[79]

AURAMINE. Yellow dye for paper, textiles, leather. Also used as an antiseptic and fungicide. Those involved in the manufacture and use of dyestuffs, as well as workers in rubber and paint plants, risk getting cancer of the bladder and pancreas. The incubation period is from 12 to 30 years.[80] *See also* Aniline.

AUTO BRAKES. Studies with an electron microscope—an instrument that has 10,000 times the resolution of ordinary instruments—have shown that automobile brakes give off a dust containing filaments of deformed "chrysotile" asbestos, a type of asbestos that many researchers consider a health hazard. According to public health officials, these fibers may not be particularly dangerous to the average consumer because when you drive a car, you breathe in only small amounts of the brake-drum dust. However, there may be a real risk factor for workers such as brake repairmen, who use compressed air to blow asbestos fibers from the brakes. The researchers believe that the asbestos in brake-drum dust may be more of a health hazard than the ordinary chrysotile form because much of it is further deformed, and deformation in asbestos fibers might have a significant role in causing lung disease or cancer.[81]

AZACYCLOPROPANE. *See* Ethylenimine.

5-AZACYTIDINE. Experimental chemotherapeutic agent against cancer, it was found to cause lung tumors in mice.[82]

AZIRANE. *See* Ethylenimine.

AZIRIDINE. *See* Ethylenimine.

AZIRINO. *See* Mitomycin C.

AZOBENZENE. Derived from nitrobenzene, these orange and red leaflets have produced liver injury in rats. It is used in the manufacture of dyes and rubber chemicals and as a fumigant and acaricide. It caused tumors in rats when injected under the skin in doses of 17 milligrams per kilogram of body weight.[83] A NIOSH review found it a positive animal carcinogen.[84]

AZO DYES. A large category of colorings used in both food and cosmetics, these dyes are characterized by the way they combine with nitrogen. They are made from diazonium compounds and phenol *(see)* and usually contain a mild acid such as citric or tartaric acid. Among the foods in which they are used are "penny" candies, caramels and chews, Life Savers, fruit drops, filled chocolates (but not pure chocolates); soft drinks, fruit drinks, and ades; jellies, jams, marmalades; stewed-fruit sauces; fruit gelatins; fruit yogurts; ice cream; pie fillings, puddings (vanilla, butterscotch, and chocolate puddings), caramel custard, whips, dessert sauces (such as vanilla and cream in powdered form); bakery goods (except plain rolls); crackers, cheese puffs, chips; cake and cookie mixes, waffle/pancake mixes; macaroni and spaghetti (certain brands); mayonnaise, salad dressings, catsup (certain brands), mustard, ready-made salads with dressings; remoulade, bearnaise, and hollandaise sauces, as well as sauces such as curry, fish, onion, tomato, and white cream; mashed rutabagas, purees; packaged soups, and some canned soups; canned anchovies, herring, sardines, fish balls, caviar, cleaned shellfish.

Azo dyes can cause allergic reactions, particularly hives. But as far back as 1906 an azo dye, scarlet red, was found to cause tumors in rabbits in Germany. In 1924 it was reported to cause liver tumors in mice. In 1934 Tomizu Yoshida, professor of pathology at Tokyo University, Japan, reported liver cancers in rats that ingested azo compounds in their diet. Azo dyes have since been found carcinogenic in a wide variety of experiments worldwide, but they are still used in our food and cosmetics.

AZOTHIOPRINE. *See* Imuran.

AZOXYBENZENE. Prepared from nitrobenzene, it is a pale yellow compound used in organic synthesis. It caused cancer in rats when injected under the skin in doses of only 4 milligrams per kilogram of body weight.[85]

BAAM. *See* Amitraz.

BACON. Meat from the back and sides of the hog that has been salted, smoked, and colored with nitrites *(see)*. In 1977 the U.S. Department of Agriculture began an effort to make processors reduce the amount of these chemicals used because research reports showed that crisply fried bacon that had been processed with nitrites contained nitrosamines. Nitrosamines (formed when nitrites combine with naturally occurring amines) are known to be powerful cancer-causing agents in animals. Processors had been using 150 parts per million of nitrite to cure bacon and the USDA issued a temporary order to cut the amount to 120 parts. Processors are now required to keep nitrosamine formations to under 10 parts per billion. They can add 550 ppm of sodium erythrobate or sodium ascorbate, vitamin C derivatives that serve to block nitrosamine formations. There are researchers who believe, however, that nitrites should not be used at all in bacon processing, and some manufacturers are experimenting with other methods of curing to eliminate the chemical.

BACTERIA. Ethionine, a metabolite of several bacteria, including *E. coli,* is toxic in several rodent species and causes changes in the liver, pancreas, and other tissue that result in a high incidence of liver cancer. There is much to be learned about it.

BARBERS. *See* Hair Coloring.

BARBITURATES. *Phenobarbital, barbinol, hypnogen, phenobarbitone, somonal.* Prepared from barbituric acid, barbiturates are used as a medical hypnotic and in the manufacture of dyes and plastics. Barbiturates have been shown to cause tumors when applied to the skin of mice in doses of 480 milligrams per kilogram of body weight.[86] Furthermore, researchers at the University of Notre Dame's Lobund Laboratory have found evidence that barbiturates accelerate the growth and spread of tumors. Aged germ-free rats with prostate and breast cancer were fed sodium barbiturate and phenobarbital in their drinking water. When they were examined later, it was discovered that the rate of growth of their tumors and the rate of spread was significantly greater than in drug-free control rats.[87]

BARBITURIC ACID. *Malonylurea; pyrimidinetrione; 2, 4, 6-tri-oxohexanhydro pyrimidine.* Consists of white crystals that are efflorescent, odorless, slightly soluble in water and alcohol, and soluble in ether. It reacts with metals to form salts. Used in the preparation of barbiturates and dyes, and as a polymerization catalyst. It is toxic and habit forming. *See also* Barbiturates for other hazards.

BEAUTICIANS. *See* Hair Coloring.

BEEF. There is substantial geographic evidence that beef consumption is a key factor in bowel cancer. In 1973, for instance, investigators from the NCI Epidemiologic Pathology Unit of the Carcinogenesis Program reported that bowel-cancer incidence in the United States is higher in the North than in the South, higher in urban areas than in rural areas, and correlates with beef consumption statistics: southerners and the rural population get most of their animal protein from pork and chicken, while northerners and city dwellers are generally beef-eaters. The Scots eat 19 percent more beef than the English and also have a 19 percent higher mortality rate from bowel cancer. New Zealand and Uruguay are also particularly high in beef consumption, and New Zealand has the highest reported national incidence rate for bowel cancer, while Uruguay's rate, as projected from mortality data, is even higher. In Hawaii, Japanese immigrants were studied. The rate of cancer of the colon was much lower in those who adhered to the traditional Japanese diet based on fish than in those who adopted the beef-rich American diet.

Dr. Ernest Wynder, longtime cancer researcher and president of the American Health Foundation, believes it may not be the beef, or even meat, but rather the total intake of fat. There are others who believe that chemicals added to feed to fatten the cattle might be at fault. In any event, there seems to be a definite correlation between the amount of beef eaten and the rate of bowel cancer.[88,89]

BENZANILIDE, 4'-PHENYL-. Artificial essential oil of almond that occurs in kernels of bitter almond made from benzyl chloride and lime or by oxidation of toluene. Caused tumors when injected into the abdomen of rats in doses of 540 milligrams per kilogram of body weight.[90]

BENZANTHRACENE (a). *1,2-Benzanthracene; napthanthracene.* A greenish yellow liquid found in coal tar. It caused cancer in mice when given orally (4 milligrams per kilogram of body weight), applied to the skin (240 milligrams per kilogram), and injected into the abdomen (8 milligrams per kilogram). It caused cancer when applied to the skin of hamsters (2 milligrams per kilogram of body weight), when injected under the skin of guinea pigs (30 milligrams per kilogram of body weight), and when given intravenously to dogs (21 milligrams per kilogram of body weight).[91]

BENZENE. For more than a century scientists have known that benzene is a powerful bone-marrow poison, causing such conditions as aplastic anemia. In the past several decades evidence has been mounting that it also causes leukemia. The first case of "benzene leukemia" was identified in 1928 in a worker heavily exposed to the solvent, and yet it is thirteenth on the list of most highly produced chemicals in the United States. Derived from toluene or gasoline, it is used in the manufacture of detergents, nylon, dyes; as an antiknock in gasoline; in artificial leather, airplane fuel dope, varnish, lacquer, and as a solvent for waxes, resins, and oils. Once used to treat leukemia, polycythemia, and malignant lymphomas, it is acutely toxic when ingested or inhaled; it causes irritation of the mucous membranes, restlessness, excitement, and depression; death may follow from respiratory failure. It has a chronic effect on bone marrow, destroying the marrow's ability to produce blood cells.

The Consumer Product Safety Commission voted unanimously in February 1978 to ban the use of benzene in the manufacture of many household products. The commission took the action in response to a petition filed by the Consumer Health Research Group, an organization affiliated with consumer advocate Ralph Nader. Earlier in the year OSHA and the EPA both cited benzene as a threat to public health. Dr. Sidney Wolfe, director of the

Consumer Health Research Group, said the ban was inadequate and that allowing products with benzene to remain on the shelves was unconscionable. On February 2, 1978, OSHA ordered a 90 percent cutback in worker exposure to benzene. However, on June 27, 1978, it relaxed part of the restrictions, saying that trace amounts of benzene in liquid mixtures would be exempted from the permanent standard for three years. The rule change came during a court fight launched against the standard by the oil industry and several large chemical rubber and steel companies. They contended that the standard is unnecessarily strict and economically unfeasible to meet. The safety agency said that the key changes in the standard exempts liquids containing 0.5 percent or less benzene until 1981, when the exemption would apply to liquids with 0.1 percent or less benzene.

In the meantime, the Consumer Product Safety Commission reported that its tests showed that persons exposed for five minutes to a common paint remover would inhale a mean concentration in the air of 130 parts per million of benzene—more than 43 times the exposure currently permitted by federal occupational exposure standards. In one study it was reported that 576,000 persons a year may be exposed to benzene vapors from paint removers and as many as 591,000 to vapors from rubber cement. Those most highly exposed are workers in rubber-cement plants, explosive industries, and distilleries. Also at risk are those who work with dyes or paints. The incubation period is three to five years.[92,93,94]

BENZENESULFONIC ACID. *Reazol yellow G, Acid leather orange I, Dye orange no. 1, FD & C orange I, napthol orange, tertracid orange I.* It was delisted as a food coloring when children were made ill by eating Halloween candy made with it. Caused tumors when applied to the skin of mice in doses of 460 milligrams per kilogram of body weight and when injected subcutaneously in rats at the rate of 9,400 milligram doses per kilogram of body weight.[95]

BENZIDINE. *Fast corinth base B, p-diaminodiphenyl, 2-amino-diphenyl, C.I. azoic diazo component 112, p-p'-bianiline, benzidine dihydrochloride, benzidine sulfate, and 4-4'diaminobiphenyl.* White or slightly reddish compound usually found as crystals or a crystalline powder, it is a potent carcinogen. Millions of pounds of benzidine are produced in the United States each year and are used mainly in the production of aniline dyes and in the manufacture of rubber and plastics. It is also used in printing inks, in the fireproofing of textiles, and in chemical and biological laboratories, including hospital labs. Probably the most widespread use of benzidine today is in the laboratory test for occult blood (blood in excrement or secretion not clearly evident to the naked eye). A kit to test the amount of chlorine in swimming pools contains a benzidine compound.

Benzidine or its metabolites have been found in the urine of production workers and production-area maintenance men in plants that either produce or use benzidine. It induces bladder tumors. Although the development of tumors is related more to the amount of exposure, thoroughness of personal hygiene may also be important. Bladder tumors are slow in developing, usually taking 15 to 20 years, and may not appear until years after the workers were initially exposed to the carcinogen. While benzidine can enter the body through the lungs or mouth, the major pathway is apparently absorption through the skin. OSHA has strict standards for protection of workers involved in the manufacture, production, packaging, release, handling, or storage of any material containing more than one-tenth of one percent of benzidine.

Benzidine was termed carcinogenic by the World Health Organization in 1968, and England has discouraged its use as have other European countries. The Italians have introduced substitutes for benzidine dyes. They are good, but somewhat more expensive. It is still in use in the United States. Those most highly exposed are dyestuff manufacturers and users, rubber workers, paint manufacturers, and gas station workers. The incubation period is from three to five years.[96,97,98]

BENZIDINE, 3,3'-DIMETHOXY-. *Acetamine diazo black RD, blue base NB, diazo fast blue B., blue B. salt, etc.* A NIOSH review determined this to be a positive animal carcinogen, and it is now subject for a hazard review by NIOSH.[99] See also Benzidine.

BENZO (a) PYRENE, BENZOPYRENE, BENZPYRENE, BaP. One of the most widely studied cancer-causing agents in the environment, this polycyclic hydrocarbon is a component of soot, cigarette smoke, and city air. Although it has been recognized as a cause of cancer for at least 200 years, its relevance as a cancer-causing agent in air pollution has been investigated for only 25 years. Domestic coal fires have been shown to be significant sources, and smaller amounts come from industrial sources and from motor vehicles. There is evidence that the concentration of benzopyrene in large towns in Britain has decreased by a factor of ten during the past few decades, as a result of changes in heating methods and smoke control. Roofers and waterproofers who work with hot pitch and asphalt are exposed to far greater amounts of BaP than even heavy cigarette smokers who live in urban areas. Studies conducted by the American Cancer Society and the Mount Sinai School of Medicine in New York City showed that among 6,000 members of the United States Tile and Composition Roofers, Damp and Waterproof Workers Association, those exposed to BaP regularly for 20 years or more have significantly higher death rates from lung cancer, as well as from cancers of the mouth and lip, throat, larynx, and esophagus. The scientists maintained that it is difficult to pin the blame solely on BaP since fumes from hot pitch contain a number of other substances. Also, many of the roofers smoked, and it is possible that the very high rate of lung cancer after 20 years was due to a combination of the BaP and cigarette smoking.

The first direct observation of cancer caused by BaP in live animals was presented on September 1, 1977, at the meeting of the American Chemical Society in Chicago. When BaP was applied to the skin of live mice, it penetrated the skin cells and underwent transformation to a much more potent carcinogen that attacked the genetic material of the cell.[100]

Benzopyrene has been listed by the EPA as an official air pollutant. The agency believes that a 50 percent reduction of it in urban air might reduce the lung-cancer rate by 20 percent. The automobile emissions of benzopyrene are small but hazardous because they are highly localized. According to one study, in some suburbs they may contribute as much as 42 percent to the overall benzopyrene level. This substance has been found to cause tumors and/or cancer when given orally, subcutaneously, or by inhalation to mice, hamsters, ducks, frogs or when applied to their skin or injected into their abdomens.[101,102,103]

BENZO (b) NAPHTHO (2,3-d). *Pyrido (3′,2:5,6); chrysene; thiophen; (1,2-F) quinoline.* Found in coal tar, coal gas, and benzene, the liquid smells like benzene. Like benzene, it is used as a solvent, but is suitable for use at lower and higher temperatures. It is employed in the manufacture of resins, dyes, and drugs. It caused tumors when injected under the skin of mice in doses of 72 milligrams per kilogram of body weight.[104]

p-BENZOQUINONE. Yellow crystals with an irritating odor derived from aniline *(see)*. Toxic when inhaled. Strong irritant to the skin and mucous membranes. Used in the manufacture of dyes and fungicides, it caused tumors when applied to the skin of mice in doses of 2,000 milligrams per kilogram of body weight and caused cancer in mice when injected intravenously into the abdomen and intravenously into the rat.[105,106]

BENZOTHIAZOLE. Yellow liquid with an unpleasant odor. Slightly soluble in water. May be toxic when ingested. Used as a rubber accelerator to speed vulcanization. Causes cancer in rats when administered orally in doses of 540 milligrams per kilogram of body weight.[107]

BENZOYL PEROXIDE. *Dibenzyl peroxide.* White crystalline solids with the taste and smell of benzaldehyde. Flammable and explosive, it is used as a bleaching agent in flour, fats, oils, and waxes. It is also used as a polymerization catalyst and a drying agent for unsaturated oils. Used in drugs and cosmetics, in the manufacture of acetate yarns, in the production of cheese, and for embossing vinyl flooring. It caused tumors when applied in doses of 25 milligrams per kilogram to the skin of mice. It can cause pulmonary problems when inhaled by humans in amounts of 12 milligrams per 3 parts of air. There is an OSHA standard for it pertaining to the air in the workplace.[108]

BENZYLAMINE, N-METHYL-N-NITROSO-. Light amber liquid that is stongly alkaline and is derived from benzyl chloride and amino acids. Used as a chemical intermediate *(see)* for dyes, pharmaceuticals, and polymers. Highly irritating to the skin and mucous membranes.[109] It caused

43

cancer when given orally to rats in doses of 142 milligrams per kilogram of body weight.[110]

BENZYL CHLORIDE A colorless liquid with a pungent odor that causes eye tearing. Derived by passing chlorine over boiling toluene, it is intensely irritating to the eyes and skin. It is used as an intermediate *(see)* and in benzyl compounds, synthetic tannins, perfumes, pharmaceuticals; in the manufacture of photographic developer, gasoline gum inhibitors, penicillin precursors, and quaternary ammonium compounds.[111] There is an OSHA standard for it pertaining to air in the workplace. It caused tumors in rats when injected under the skin in doses of 50 milligrams per kilogram of body weight.[112] A NIOSH review reported it to be a carcinogen.[113]

BERTRANDITE. A NIOSH review found it a positive carcinogen for animals.[114] *See also* Beryllium.

BERYL. A natural silicate of beryllium and ammonium. *See also* Beryllium.

BERYLLIUM. A hard brittle gray white metal, it is soluble in acid and resistant to oxidation. Found chiefly in South Africa, Rhodesia, Brazil, Argentina, and India. Principal sources in the United States are Colorado, Maine, New Hampshire, and South Dakota. A rocket-fuel additive, it is used in space technology and in nuclear reactors. Beryllium is used to harden alloys, and exposure of workers to this element occurs during this operation and also when the ores are processed. It causes lung, skin, liver, and kidney disease; however, the effects on the lungs are the most prominent and disabling. The skin may be inflamed or ulcerated by beryllium dust entering open sores, and the ulcers will not heal until the metal is removed. Granulomas, little lumps under the skin, may develop. Under a microscope, these look the same as the lung inflammations observed in beryllium lung disease and are thought to be an allergic response. The liver may also develop granulomas. Standard patch tests can be negative even in advanced cases, and the only sure test is study of tissue removed from the affected area.

Acute berylliosis is a severe, pneumonialike lung inflammation that can occur after brief, intensive exposure or prolonged exposure to low concentrations. The typical symptoms are cough with phlegm that can be bloody, severe shortness of breath, and weight loss over a period of a few weeks. The chest X-rays may be normal initially, even though the worker is seriously ill. The lung inflammation may be severe enough to block oxygen transfer into the blood. The disease is frequently fatal, and those who recover may have sustained permanent damage to the lungs. Chronic berylliosis may develop after one year or even up to 20 years of exposure. At first the symptoms may be mild, slowly progressing to a more severe and disabling illness in which chronic inflammation makes the lungs stiff and unable to transfer oxygen to the bloodstream. The heart is affected by years of straining to breathe.

Results of recent epidemiological studies indicate an increased risk of lung cancer mortality among persons exposed to the metal. Using data from Social Security Administration files, it was discovered by researchers that workers occupationally exposed to beryllium at two production facilities (Kawecki Berylco Industries, Inc., in Pennsylvania, and Brush Wellman, Inc., in Ohio) had an excess incidence of lung cancer. These cases and others turned up by NIOSH showed that exposure of these workers was short and that beryllium is carcinogenic. Not all researchers agree, and there is a great deal of current controversy.[115] Beryllium has been used by American industry since 1931.

BERYLLIUM FLUORIDE. A hygroscopic solid. Readily soluble in water and sparingly soluble in alcohol. It is highly toxic when inhaled or ingested. It has a tolerance level of 2.5 milligrams per cubic meter of air. It is used in the production of beryllium metal by reduction with magnesium metal.

BERYLLIUM OXIDE. White powder used as a ceramic material. It is undamaged by nuclear radiation and transparent to microwaves. It is highly toxic when inhaled. Used in electron tubes, transistor mountings, high-temperature reactor systems, and as an additive to glass, ceramics, and plastics. Caused cancer when injected or implanted in rabbits in doses of 10 to 500 milligrams per kilogram of body weight and caused tumors when injected under the skin of pigs in doses of 7 milligrams per kilogram of body weight.[116] There is an OSHA standard pertaining to air for beryllium oxide.

BERYLLIUM SULFATE. Colorless crystals. Soluble in water and insoluble in alcohol. It is highly toxic when inhaled or ingested.

BETA-NAPHTHYLAMINE. *See* 2-NA.

BETA-PROPIOLACTONE (BPL). *Betaprone, 2-oxetanone, propiolactone, B-lactone hydrocrylic acid, 3-Hydroxypropionic acid lactone, etc.* A colorless, highly poisonous liquid, it was used until recently as a chemical intermediate *(see)* in the production of acrylic plastics. In 1972 at least 50 million pounds of BPL were produced in the United States. However, its major producer, which was also the major user, has been reconstructing both its plant and its procedures to eliminate BPL. This substance is also used to sterilize certain vaccines (such as rabies vaccine for humans). However, the amount of BPL used in these instances is small in comparison to the amount used in the production of acrylates. Since BPL is the cause of many forms of tumors in a wide variety of animal species, it is assumed to be carcinogenic for humans as well. OSHA has a carcinogen standard for any substance containing more than one percent of beta-propiolactone.[117]

BETEL NUTS. Grown in India, Ceylon, Malaysia, the leaves are used medicinally as a counterirritant, for example, orally for coughs. (It was once employed as a treatment for diphtheria.) The betel nut is the fruit of the betel palm. When dried and chewed, it mildly stimulates the nervous system, and it is estimated that 200 million people around the world chew betel nuts. The FDA does not allow the importation and interstate sale of betel nuts because it has been shown that chewing the nut may cause cancer. To back up its restrictions, the FDA cites studies indicating that there is a high incidence among betel-nut users of cancer of the mouth and esophagus.[118]

BFV. *See* Formaldehyde.

BILE ACIDS. Secreted by the liver to aid in fat metabolism and to retard putrefaction, bile acids are a by-product of cholesterol as well. Studies have shown that people on high-fat diets have more bile acids than average, as do colon-cancer victims. It may be that bile acids are carcinogens themselves, or cancer-promoting agents. Americans whose diet is high in animal fats have higher bile acids in their stool than Finns whose diet is high in dairy fat. The Finns also eat more fiber, which reduces the amount of bile acids in the stool. *See also* Diet and Fiber.

BIPHENYL, 4-NITRO-. *See* 4-Nitrobiphenyl.

4-BIPHENYLAMINE. *p-Aminobiphenyl.* Prepared from diazoaminobenzene, it is used in the detection of sulfates and as a carcinogen in cancer research. It can cause bladder tumors in humans;[119] cancer when administered orally to rats, mice, and dogs; cancer when injected subcutaneously in mice; and tumors when given orally to rabbits. There is an OSHA standard for it.[120]

BIRTH-CONTROL PILL. *See* The Pill.

BIS (CHLOROMETHYL) ETHER (BCME). *Chloro (chloromethoxy) methane, sym-dichloromethyl ether.* A colorless liquid with a suffocating odor that may be one of the most dangerous carcinogens in the workplace. Usually present to some degree in chloromethyl methyl ether, but it is also used as an alkylating agent in its own right. BCME is found in chemical plants during the production of ion-exchange resins: these resins then go into products that soften water or remove specific impurities from solutions (such as those that desalinate brackish water) and that decolor and clarify food, beverages, and chemicals. BCME is an intermediate *(see)* in the production and is not present in the final product, according to OSHA. After use, BCME can be destroyed chemically by water and strong caustics. It causes cancer in mice after inhalation, skin contact, or injection under the skin. It causes cancer in rats that breathe it or have it injected under the skin. Workers exposed to BCME itself, or as a contaminant of chloromethyl methyl ether (CMME), show a greatly increased frequency of lung cancer. Exposed workers in one study suffered seven times the number of lung cancers as the general population—most of them from "cat-cell" carcinoma of the lung, a form of cancer extremely rare in the general population and usually found in uranium miners exposed to ionizing radiation and workers exposed to alkylating agents. All workers in one study died of lung cancer within 20 months of diagnosis.

Most of the lung-cancer victims smoked cigarettes, which indicates that cigarette smoke may have promoted the effect of the carcinogen, as in the case of asbestos workers *(see)*. The evidence, however, against BCME is strong, because the disease struck nonsmokers as well as smokers, and it also occurred at a younger age and was a different type of lung cancer from that usually caused by smoking.

NIOSH findings of a high lung-cancer risk among BCME workers are supported by other studies, such as a Philadelphia chemical plant investigation that showed workers had eight times the rate of lung cancer as people not exposed to BCME. Researchers from the Institute of Environmental Medicine at New York University recently studied 1,800 workers exposed for at least five years to CCME, which is usually contaminated with 2 to 8 percent of BCME. These workers died from lung cancer at a rate of two and a half times that of a control group.

The extent of the BCME hazard became dramatically apparent when it was reported that the vapors of hydrochloric acid and formaldehyde, two chemicals found together in many industrial plants, could combine spontaneously to form BCME. In a survey of various workplaces, NIOSH found that small concentrations of BCME were forming in the textile industry. The institute is now checking to see whether BCME is forming in other places, such as biological and chemical laboratories, insect-rearing laboratories, particle-board plants, and paper-manufacturing plants where hydrochloric acid and formaldehyde are commonly found together. In light of the BCME discovery, NIOSH experts warn that these two chemicals should not be used in the same plant except under very well-controlled conditions. OSHA has strict standards involving the manufacturing, processing, repackaging, releasing, handling, or storage of any substance containing more than one-tenth of one percent of bis-chloromethyl ether (BCME).[121,122]

BIURET, 1-ETHYL-1-NITROSO-. *Allophanamide, carbamylurea.* Derived from urea by heat. Used in analytical chemistry. Caused cancer in rats when given orally in 25 milligram doses per kilogram of body weight.[123]

BLACK GOLD. *See* Magnetite.

BLACK IRON OXIDE. *See* Magnetite.

BLACK OXIDE. *See* Magnetite.

BLADDER CANCER. A form of cancer known to be associated with chemical carcinogens and strongly correlated with cigarette smoking. There are approximately 32,000 new cases each year and about 16,000 deaths. Symptoms include persistent pain or discomfort in the small of the back, blood in the urine (bright red or smoky or pink), burning on urination and frequent urination, fever of unknown origin. Because these symptoms could be signs of other diseases as well, medical evaluation is needed to determine their cause. This form of cancer is more frequent in people who have congenital abnormalities of these organs. Urinalysis will detect blood in the urine as well as the presence of infection. An X-ray using a dye is employed in diagnosis. The incidence of bladder and kidney cancers has been related to chemical exposure.

Two classes of chemicals have been associated with the disease—naphthylamines and benzidines *(see both)*. Workers who risk bladder cancer from overexposure to these chemicals include those producing coal-tar products and working with aromatic amines; asphalt, coal tar, and pitch workers; gas stokers; still cleaners; dyestuff users; rubber workers; textile dyers; paint manufacturers; and leather and shoe workers. The occurrence of cancer of the urinary tract, therefore, may be prevented by avoiding occupational exposure to such agents. The tropical disease schistosoma *(see)* is also associated with increased bladder cancer. Cigarette smoking, which leads to the presence of chemicals in the urinary tract, is also considered a cause of bladder cancer. A simple urinalysis can pinpoint underlying irritations and the presence of cancer. Diagnosed early, bladder cancer can be cured.[124]

BLUE. (The following blues have the same derivation: acid blue 9, acid sky blue A, acilan turquoise blue AE, A. F. blue no. 1, brilliant blue, calcoid blue EG, C. I. acid blue 9, C. I. food blue, FD & C blue no. 1, peacock blue X = 1756, xylene blue VSG). *Ammonium, ethyl (4-(p-(ethyl (p-sulfobenzyl) amino)-alpha-(o sulfophenyl) benzylidene) 2,5-cyclohexadien-1-ylidene) (a-sulfobenzyl-, hydroxide, inner salt, diammonium salt.* Caused tumors in rats when injected under the skin.[125] *See also* FD & C Blue No. 1.

BLUE BASE NB. *See* Benzidine and Benzidine, 3,3'-Dimethoxy-.

BONE CANCER. Believed to be caused by ionizing radiation. People working with radium must guard against overexposure.

BONE-MARROW CANCER. Cancer agents considered to cause it include benzene and ionizing radiation. Those who work with benzene, explosives, and rubber cement as well as distillers, dye users, painters, and radiologists must all take special precautions on the job.

BORIC ACID. An antiseptic with bactericidal and fungicidal properties, it is used in baby powders, bath powders, eye creams, after-shave lotions, soaps, and skin fresheners. It is still widely used despite repeated warnings from the American Medical Association of possible toxicity. Severe poisonings have followed both ingestion and topical application to abraded skin.[126] When given intravaginally to mice, it caused tumors in doses of 8 milligrams per kilogram of body weight.[127]

BRACKEN FERN. *Pteridium aquilinum.* Bracken fern is used as human food in greens or salads in New Zealand, in the United States, and especially in Japan. It has been known for a long time to damage bone marrow and the intestinal mucosa and to induce polyps in urinary bladder mucosa in cattle fed the fern. It can produce tumors in many sites in many animals. Cattle raised in mountainous, wooded wastelands develop cancer traced to the fern.[128]

BRAN. Lack of fiber *(see)* in the diet has been linked with cancer of the colon. J. S. Cummings of the Medical Research Council, Dunn Nutrition Unit in Cambridge, England, and his team added bran, cabbage, carrots, apples, and guar gum to the diets of 10 healthy volunteers. Bran produced the most robust bowel movements by far, followed by guar, with carrots, cabbages, and apples producing comparably lesser benefits. Thus, cereals appear to be much more effective than vegetables and fruits as colon cancer *(see)* defenses. Their studies suggest that those persons who produce fewer bowel movements probably need to consume more fiber to combat colon cancer than those who produce ample bowel movements. Still another finding: those fibers that produce the best bowel movements are especially rich in chemicals that retain water well.[129] *See also* Fiber and Colorectal Cancer.

BREAST CANCER. Breast cancer is the major cause of cancer deaths among women in the United States. If you are a woman who had your first child before you were 20 years old, your chances of getting breast cancer have been reduced by 50 percent from the national average of 7 out of 100 women. If you live in the country, your chances are reduced a little more. No definite cause of breast cancer has been identified, but clues are found in epidemiological studies. Japanese women, for example, rarely get breast cancer. Is it their diet? Their genes? What is it in our environment that may cause the disease?

The incidence of breast cancer among women 40 to 50 years old is increasing. Whether the disease is latent and therefore goes undetected, or the cancer is appearing earlier, is not known. It is now believed, however, that breast cancer before 50 years and breast cancer after menopause (usually after 50 years) are almost two different diseases taking two separate courses. Insuring the discovery of breast cancer at the earliest stage requires monthly self-examination by the woman herself, in addition to annual checkups by her physician. Once a cancer is discovered there are two approaches to treatment. One is to remove the entire breast plus the lymph glands in the armpit (the so-called auxiliary nodes). The other is lumpectomy, the removal of the lump for diagnostic purposes while leaving the breast intact and treating it with radiation. Both methods are associated with complications, and there are sufficient unknowns so that it is not possible to say that one is clearly superior to the other.[130]

As to what causes breast cancer, there are only clues and theories. There is some evidence of a viral etiology: although a human B-type virus has been found in the milk of women who because of family history face a greater risk of getting breast cancer, it does not offer sufficient proof that a virus is the cause of the disease.[131,132] However, the evidence is strong enough to caution these women against breast-feeding their children, especially infant girls. In thinking about the etiology of breast cancer and weighing the various possibilities, scientists continue to place considerable emphasis on the roles that heredity and hormones play. They tend to favor the view that an excess of hormones has a carcinogenic effect. Estrogen and prolactin *(see both)*. have been implicated in the etiology of breast cancer in animals and, by analogy, in women. Results also show that the amounts of androsterone and etiocholanolone excreted by women who eventually develop cancer are significantly lower than those excreted by women who do not. In addition to finding these low levels of androgen hormones in women who subsequently develop cancer, it has been found that young women with benign breast disease, a condition also correlated with later development of cancer, have low hormone levels. Genetics, too, may be a factor: it has been suggested that heredity plays an important role in the early onset of multiple breast tumors, but not in the late onset of a single tumor.[133,134,135,136] *See also* Estrogen, Mammography, and Fat.

BRILLIANT BLUE. *See* FD & C No. 1.

BRILLIANT FAST OIL YELLOW. *See* Aniline.

BRILLIANT OIL ORANGE Y BASE. *See* Phenylenediamine.

BRILLIANT OIL YELLOW. *See* Aniline.

BRILLIANT PONCEAU. *See* 1,3-Napthalenedisulfonic Acid.

BRILLIANT RED B. *See* Naphthalene.

BROWN OXIDES OF IRON. *See* Magnetite.

B-TGdR. *Beta-2'-deoxy-6-thioguanosine monohydrate.* An experimental anticancer drug that was given by abdominal injection to rats and mice for 52 weeks. According to the NCI, it caused cancer of the ear canal in male rats and may have been a cause of ear-canal cancer in female rats. In mice, determination of carcinogenic potential could not be made because of poor survival in both control animals and those given the test compound. A growing body of evidence indicates that some drugs used in treating cancers may themselves cause cancer years later. This comes mainly from a long-term follow-up of the increasing number of cancer patients treated effectively. The benefits from use of anticancer drugs in the treatment of life-threatening diseases are considered to outweigh the possible risk of new cancers developing in a small proportion of long-term survivors. Nevertheless, B-TGdR and other compounds are being studied for carcinogenic activity so that drugs with less cancer-causing potential may be used in cancer treatment whenever the opportunity exists.[137]

BUSULPHAN. In a two-year study of anticancer chemotherapy following removal of all visible lung cancer, 4 cases of leukemia occurred among 243 patients treated with busulphan compared to none among 243 patients treated with cyclophosphamide and none among 249 given a placebo. None of the 4 had received radiotherapy or anticancer drugs other than busulphan, and all 4 were among 19 patients who developed depression of all elements of the blood-forming cells (pancytopenia) while receiving busulphan. Their therapy with busulphan occurred five to eight years before leukemia was diagnosed.[138]

BUTADIENE OXIDE. Produced from petroleum gases, it is used in the manufacture of synthetic rubber. Severely irritating, it can cause delayed irritation of eyes and swelling of lids. Repeated skin exposure causes cancer in animals, as well as severe blood damage.[139]

BUTANE. *Methylsulfonal, bioxiran, dl-butadiene dioxide.* Butane is a natural gas that occurs in petroleum and in refinery cracking products. It is the raw material for motor fuels and is used in the manufacture of synthetic rubber. It may be narcotic in high concentrations. It caused tumors when injected under the skin of mice in 1,900 milligram doses per kilogram of body weight, when injected into the abdomen of rats 38 milligram doses per kilogram, and when inhaled by mice in doses of 3,400 milligrams per kilogram of body weight.[140] It has been determined by NIOSH to be an animal carcinogen.[141]

1,4-BUTANEDIOL DIMETHYLSULFONATE. Causes tumors when injected under the skin and given intravenously to mice 48 milligram doses per kilogram of body weight.[142] *See also* Busulphan.

BUTTER YELLOW. *p-Dimethylamino azobenzene.* It was used in foods until it was found to cause cancer. Its yellow crystals are used in organic research and to cause cancer in experimental animals. *See also* Aniline.

BUTYLAMINE, N-ETHYL-N-NITROSO-. *Ethyl-n-butylnitrosamine.* Flammable, toxic liquid used as an intermediate *(see)* for rubber chemicals, emulsifying agents, insecticides, and pharmaceuticals. It caused cancer in rats when given orally in doses of 380 milligrams per kilogram of body weight and intravenously in doses of 1,000 milligrams per kilogram. It also caused cancer in mice when given orally in 2,360 milligram doses per kilogram of body weight.[143]

BUTYRIC ACID. *4(p-Bis) (2-chloroethyl) (aminophenyl)-.* A colorless liquid, it occurs as a glyceride in animal milk fats. A strong irritant to skin, it is used in the manufacture of butyrate esters for perfume and flavor ingredients, and in pharmaceutical agents, disinfectants, and for sweetening gasoline. It caused tumors when applied to the skin of mice in 108 milligram doses per kilogram of body weight and cancer when injected into the abdomen of mice in 18 milligram doses per kilogram of body weight.[144] A NIOSH review has determined it is a positive animal carcinogen.[145]

BUTYRIN,TRI. *See* Tributyrin.

BUTYROLACTONE. *2(3H)-Furnone (Dihydro-); 1,2-butanolide; butyric acid; 4-hydroxy-gamma-lactone.* Derived from ethylene chlorhydrin, it is an oily liquid used as an intermediate *(see)* in the manufacture of polyvinylpyrrolidone. It is a solvent for plastics. Caused tumors when applied to the skin of mice in 49 milligram doses per kilogram of body weight.[146]

CADMIUM. A naturally occurring metal that is used to control mold and also diseases that attack home lawns, golf-course turfs, and other grasses. It is also used in electroplating processes, the manufacture of rubber tires, and the solder employed in plumbing. However, less than 0.1 percent of the annual United States consumption of 12 million pounds of cadmium is used in pesticides—most of it is used in industry. An estimated 100,000 workers in the United States are exposed to this metal that is employed not only in the electroplating and rubber industries but also in the manufacture of nickel-cadmium batteries, brazing-soldering alloys, pigments, and chemicals that act as stabilizers in plastics. Other sources of human exposure are cigarette smoke, air pollution, drinking water, and sludge.[147] Most cadmium gets into sewage-treatment plants as part of the discharge from electroplating processes, from disintegration of rubber tires on streets, and from solder in plumbing. Some of the one million tons of sludge dumped yearly on farmland contains large amounts of cadmium. One EPA study of sewage-treatment plants in the nation's 26 largest cities found that two-thirds of their daily sludge production contained potentially hazardous levels of cadmium. No one knows how much cadmium is picked up by plants when the sludge is applied to land, how much is transmitted to fruit and vegetables, and how much leaches out of landfills. Cadmium in drinking water has been correlated with cancer of the pharynx, esophagus, intestine, larynx, lung, and bladder.[148]

A study of 300 men who had worked at least two years in a cadmium smelter revealed that these workers had significantly higher death rates from all forms of cancer, especially of the lung and prostate gland. Lung cancer occurred at more than twice the expected rate, and as with many other occupational cancers, the risk of developing the disease increased in relation to the length of elapsed time after initial exposure to the metal.[149] Cadmium is also believed to cause mutations: this conclusion is based upon findings of chromosomal and DNA damage resulting from the presence of cadmium in the blood of workers and in bacteria. In addition, exposure to home-lawn-treatment products containing cadmium may be dangerous to women of child-bearing age.

CADMIUM CHLORIDE. Caused tumors when injected under the skin in rats and when administered intravenously. It also caused cancer in mice when it was injected under the skin.[150] A NIOSH review determined that it is a positive animal carcinogen.[151] *See also* Cadmium.

CADMIUM OXIDE. Causes cancer when injected under the skin in rats at 90 milligrams per kilogram of body weight.[152] *See also* Cadmium.

CADMIUM SULFATE. Caused cancer in rats when injected under the skin in doses of 2 milligrams per kilogram of body weight.[153] A NIOSH review found it carcinogenic to animals.[154] *See also* Cadmium.

CADMIUM SULFIDE. *Aurora yellow, cadmium golden, cadmium yellow, C.I. pigment orange 20, C.I. pigment yellow 37.* Caused cancer in rats when injected under the skin in 90 milligram doses per kilogram of body weight.[155] A NIOSH review determined that it is an animal carcinogen.[156] *See also* Cadmium.

CALAMUS. *Sweet flag.* An aromatic flavoring from the dried root of a plant grown in Europe, North America, West Asia, Burma, and Ceylon. Used in bitters, vermouth, root beer, spice flavorings for beverages, candy, baked goods, ice cream, and cordials. The oil is used in chocolate, fruit, Benedictine, Chartreuse, nut, root beer, sarsaparilla, spice, ginger ale, vanilla, wintergreen, birch beer, flavorings for beverages, ice cream, ices, candy, baked goods, gelatin desserts, puddings, and liquors. Calamus has been used against intestinal gas and as a vermifuge (an agent causing expulsion of intestinal worms). Rats fed up to 5,000 parts per million for up to two years showed a dose-related formation of malignant tumors of the small intestine. At present calamus is not allowed as a flavor ingredient in American food, although it is still used in Germany and some other countries.[157]

CARBAMIC ACID, ETHYL ESTER. Carbamic acid is not known in the free state but only in the form of its salts that occur in the blood and urine of mammals. It is used in sedatives. It is carcinogenic when given orally or subcutaneously to rats and mice.[158] Determined as an animal carcinogen by a NIOSH review. Now being considered for a NIOSH hazard review.

CARBANILIC ACID. *m-Chloro- isopropyl ester.* Known only in the form of its salts and esters. A herbicide. Caused tumors when given orally to mice in 600 milligram doses per kilogram of body weight.[159] A herbicide candidate for review by EPA for carcinogenesis. *See also* Aromatic Amines.

CARBOLIC ACID. *See* Phenol.

CARBONIC ACID. *Diethyl ester, cyclic vinylene ester, ethyl carbonate.* A liquid with a pleasant ethereal odor that is a solvent for nitrocellulose and is used in the manufacture of radio tubes. It is also used to fix rare earths to cathodes. It caused cancer when injected under the skin in doses of 1,760 milligrams per kilogram of body weight.[160]

CARBON TETRACHLORIDE. *Tetrachloromethane, perchloromethane.* Colorless, clear, nonflammable, heavy liquid obtained from carbon disulfide and chlorine. It is used as a fire extinguisher; for cleaning clothing; for rendering benzene nonflammable; as a drying agent for wet spark plugs in automobiles; as a solvent for oils, fats, lacquers, varnishes, rubber waxes, resins; for extracting oil from flower seeds; for exterminating insects; as a solvent; and for starting material in the manufacture of many organic compounds used to kill hookworm and tapeworm. It is poisonous by inhalation, ingestion, or skin absorption. Acute poisoning causes nausea, diarrhea, headache, stupor, kidney damage and can be fatal. Chronic poisoning involves liver damage but can also cause kidney injury. When it is absorbed through the skin it can cause a defatting action.[161] It has caused cancer in rats, mice, and hamsters when given orally, subcutaneously, or rectally.[162] Currently being tested for carcinogenesis by the NCI and selected for priority attention by the EPA.[163]

CARBOWAX. *See* Polyethylene Glycol Monostearate.

CARBOXYMETHYLCELLULOSE. *Sodium.* Made from cotton by-products, it occurs as a white powder or in granules. A synthetic gum used in bath preparations, beauty masks, dentifrices, hair-grooming aids, hand creams, rouge, shampoos, and shaving creams, it is also used as an emulsifier; as a stabilizer in ice cream, beverages, and other foods; medicinally as a laxative or antacid; and as a foaming agent. It has been shown to cause cancer in animals when ingested. Its toxicity on the skin is unknown.[164]

CARCINOMA IN SITU. *See* Precancerous conditions.

CARRAGEENAN. *Carrageenin, chondrus extract.* An Irish moss derivative, it absorbs water easily, has a seaweedlike odor and a gluey, salty taste. It is used as a stabilizer and emulsifier in chocolate products, chocolate-flavored drinks, chocolate milk, gassed cream (pressure-dispensed whipped), syrup for frozen products, confections, evaporated milk, cheese spreads, cheese foods, ice cream, frozen custard, sherberts, ices, French dressing, artificially sweetened jellies and jam. Carrageenan is completely soluble in hot water and is not coagulated by acids. It is an extract of Irish moss, and along with any combination of two or more salts—ammonium, calcium, potassium, or sodium—it is used in beverages, baked goods, puddings, and syrups. It is also used as a demulcent to soothe mucous-membrane irritation. The use of Irish moss in food and medicine has been known in India for hundreds of years. Its use in the United States began in 1935, but it really became common during World War II as a replacement for Japanese gelatin (agar-agar). Sodium carrageenan is on the FDA list for further study. Carrageenan stimulated the formation of fibrous tissue when subcutaneously injected into the guinea pig. When a single dose of it dissolved in saline was injected into the subcutaneous tissues of rats, it caused sarcomas after approximately two years. Its cancer-causing ability may be that of a foreign body irritant, because upon administration to rats and mice at high levels in their diet it did not appear to induce tumors, although survival of the animals for this period was not good. Its use as a food additive and as a treatment for gastric ulcers is being restudied.[165]

CATS. Periodically, there is a scare about cats transmitting feline leukemia to humans. Human embryonic cells are highly susceptible to infection with feline leukemia and sarcoma viruses in laboratory cultures. Feline leukemia and sarcoma are caused by C-type RNA viruses similar to those that cause the naturally occurring leukemia and sarcomas in mice and chickens. Researchers from NCI reported in *Science* that it is conceivable that human cells that are quite susceptible to infection in vitro (in cultures) may have some degree of susceptibility in vivo (in a living organism), such as when the virus is introduced subcutaneously through a bite or scratch of a cat who may or may not have exhibited clinical symptoms of leukemia. Although there is no evidence to implicate feline leukemia and sarcoma in human cancer, further studies are necessary to rule out the spread of cancer by this mode.[166] In the meantime, scientists at Washington State University have been working to develop a vaccine to protect cats against feline leukemia virus.[167]

CB RADIOS.   *See* Electromagnetic Radiation.

CELLULOSE.   *Carboxymethyl ether, ammonium salt, carboxymethyl cellulose.* Made from a cotton by-product, it occurs as a white powder or granules. It is used as a stabilizer in ice cream, beverages, confections, baked goods, icings, toppings, chocolate milk, chocolate-flavored beverages, gassed cream (pressure dispensed), syrups for frozen products, variegated mixtures, cheese spreads, and certain cheeses. Cellulose is also used in French dressing, artificially sweetened jellies and preserves, gelling ingredients, mix-it-yourself powdered drinks, and baby foods. It is used medicinally as a laxative and antacid, and in pharmaceuticals for preparing suspensions. It caused tumors when injected subcutaneously in rats in doses of 12 milligrams per kilogram of body weight.[168]

CERVICAL CANCER.   This disease has its origins in adolescence and its serious consequences in later years. The woman who delays her first sexual experience beyond age 20, certainly age 17, significantly reduces her chances of getting cancer of the cervix. In studies in 1962 and again in 1967, dramatic evidence that first intercourse at an early age was what distinguished more than 400 cervical cancer patients from a like number of cancer-free women. Early intercourse seems to be the important factor increasing risk of the disease. Also contributing to a woman's chances of contracting the disease was the number of different sexual partners. (Scientists have repeatedly found this type of disease almost nonexistent among virgins and Catholic nuns and of significantly low frequency among Jewish women.) Other circumstances popularly associated with cervical cancer, such as frequency of intercourse, pregnancy and delivery, and noncircumcision of male partners, had little or no significance. It has been speculated that a DNA virus could be the agent, passed from a male to an adolescent female, initiating the changes resulting in cancer. The rapid cellular growth and change that distinguish a younger woman's tissues from those of an older woman increase the chance that such a virus might become incorporated into a cell or cells.

It appears that cervical cancer develops an average of 30 years after the early sexual contact. A physician would be well-advised to counsel frequent Pap-smear tests for women whom he knows to have had early sexual experience, married early, and particularly those who have had multiple partners. In 1968 it was found that 83 percent of a population of women with cervical cancer showed evidence of having been exposed to a herpes virus, type 2 *(see)*, which causes an infection characterized by blisters. Cold sores are a herpes infection. Every woman (of any age) who is no longer a virgin should see her physician regularly and should request Pap smears. —Sharp conization, in which a piece of the cervix is removed, has the maximum diagnostic value and in certain instances may have a temporary, possibly even permanent, therapeutic effect. Chemotherapy has not proved particularly valuable in the treatment of this disease. The best results appear to occur when it is possible to remove all tumor tissue.[169,170] *See also* Circumcision.

CHARCOAL BROILING. Cancer-causing agents can be formed in charcoal-broiled food according to the NCI. It is safer to boil or poach food than to charcoal broil it. It is believed that at least two kinds of substances are formed in broiling: one is related to the tar in cigarette-smoke condensate and is produced when the surface of the food is charred; the other factor involves the breakdown of some amino acids in protein.[171] *See also* Hamburger.

CHEMISTS. Chemists and chemical engineers are more likely to die of cancer than nonchemists, according to a Swedish study described in the June 28, 1976, issue of *Chemical and Engineering News*, and also according to NCI epidemiologists. The study from Sweden also cited figures showing that the death rate from cancer among 517 chemical engineers, 408 of whom were exposed to chemicals in jobs after graduation, was almost twice as high as among the general Swedish population. Of 58 graduates who had died by the end of 1974, 22 died of cancer, and all but one of these 22 had an occupational exposure to chemicals. In contrast, only 13 cancer deaths would be expected among a similar group drawn from the general population. Malignant lymphomas were the causes of 6 of the 22 deaths, significantly more than the 1.7 deaths from this cause that would be expected in a group of this size drawn from the general population. Three deaths in the group were attributed to Hodgkin's disease, fully 10 times the expected rate. Cancer of the kidney and bladder were also higher than expected.

The NCI conducted a statistical study involving deceased members of the American Chemical Society; it showed a proportion of cancer deaths significantly higher than expected, and nearly half the "excess deaths" were from malignant lymphoma and carcinoma of the pancreas. In this study, in the group of chemists 20 to 64 years of age, there were 444 deaths from cancer, as compared to the 354 expected on the basis of comparison with the control group. The difference is highly significant. The 250 cancer deaths among male chemists over the age of 64 also exceeded expectations. These studies show that the excess of cancer deaths among chemists and chemical engineers appears to be linked to actual work with chemicals in factories and laboratories.[172,173]

CHLORAL HYDRATE. A bitter, colorless crystalline compound formed by treating chloral (a caustic liquid) with water. It is used as a rubefacient (a substance causing redness to the skin) to help stimulate the scalp in hair tonics and dandruff preparations. It penetrates the skin and has a pungent odor. It is also used in the manufacture of DDT. Chloral hydrate can cause gastric disturbances and skin eruptions. When given orally it produces sleep and is narcotic. A lethal dose for man is a 10 milligram dose per kilogram of body weight. It caused tumors when painted on the skin of mice in 960 milligram doses per kilogram of body weight.[174]

CHLORAMBUCIL. *See* Leukeran.

CHLORAMPHENICOL. A broad-spectrum antibiotic originally isolated from *Streptomyces venezuelae*. It is effective against a number of staph and other bacterial infections resistant to other antibiotics. Once widely prescribed, it is now recommended for use only in the case of serious infection when less potentially dangerous drugs are ineffective. There have been reports of serious and fatal blood dyscrasias (abnormalities), such as aplastic anemia terminating in leukemia.[175]

CHLORDANE. An organochlorine pesticide, it was introduced in 1945 and was among the first to be developed for insect control. Because of its persistence in the environment, most of its uses were suspended by order of the EPA in 1975. Several specified uses are still permitted, including pest control on pineapple, strawberries, and Florida citrus crops; it can also be used to remedy a number of other pest-control problems that plague certain areas of the United States. Chlordane and heptachlor were once used at the rate of 14 to 16 million pounds per year. Current legal usage (mostly for termite control) accounts for 6 to 8 million pounds per year. Chlordane causes cancer of the liver in mice. It is less toxic than other similar pesticides, but acute exposure has the effect of stimulating the central nervous system. It has also been implicated in acute blood dyscrasias (abnormalities), such as aplastic anemia. It is said to be absorbed through the skin. It has been found to be mutagenic. Eventually, it will probably be banned entirely.[176]

CHLORDIMEFORM. A major cotton insecticide taken off the market in 1976 by its producers as a possible "health threat," it was introduced in 1978 under new restrictions to minimize human exposure to the compound. The chemical is used to control destructive bollworms and budworms throughout the Cotton Belt. The pesticide may be used only on cotton and not on other crops, such as fruits, vegetables, and nuts, as it was in the past.

It may be applied only from aircraft operated by applicator-pilots who have been certified or trained in the safe handling and application of the pesticide both by the state and by chlordimeform's producers. Applicators must wear a respirator. Persons handling the pesticide—loading it onto planes for application, or cleaning equipment that contained it—must wear a respirator and protective clothing, including a rubberized suit, boots, and neoprene gloves. Farmers and farm workers must stay out of the treated fields for one day, unless wearing protective clothing. Bollworm and budworm caterpillars do an estimated $113 million worth of damage to cotton each year. Chlordimeform was introduced in 1968, but in September 1976 its producers stopped the sale of the pesticide and recalled existing stocks because preliminary test results indicated that it caused malignant tumors in mice. Whether chlordimeform will continue to be available depends on further studies of these tests by the EPA.[177]

CHLORINATED HYDROCARBONS. Hydrocarbons in which one or more of the hydrogen atoms have been replaced by chlorine *(see)*. Many members of the group have been shown to cause cancer in animals and some of them to cause cancer in humans. Among the designated carcinogens: chloroform, vinyl chloride, bis chloromethyl ether, trichloroethylene, aldrin, chlordane, dieldrin, heptachlor, lindane, methoxychlor, toxaphene, terpene polychlorinates, and carbon tetrachloride *(see all)*. Concern about the potential hazard of certain chlorinated hydrocarbons is based on their ubiquity; their persistence in the environment; their capacity to accumulate in living organisms, including humans and the human fetus; and the experimental evidence of a potential carcinogenic effect.[178]

CHLORINE. A nonmetallic element, a diatomic gas that is heavy, noncombustible, greenish yellow, and has a pungent, irritating odor. In liquid form it is a clear amber color with an irritating odor. It does not occur in a free state but as a component of the mineral halite (rock salt). Toxic and irritating to the skin and lungs, it has a tolerance level of one part per million in air. It is used in the manufacture of carbon tetrachloride and trichloroethylene *(see both);* in water purification; in shrink-proofing wool; in flame retardant compounds; and in processing fish, vegetables, and fruit. The chlorine used to kill bacteria in drinking water often contains carcinogenic carbon tetrachloride, a contaminant formed during the production process. Therefore, according to the EPA, carbon tetrachloride has been inadvertently added to drinking water in Philadelphia and many other cities.[179] Chlorination has also been found to sometimes form undesirable "ring" compounds in water, such as toluene, xylene, and the suspected carcinogen, styrene—they have been observed in both the drinking-water and waste-water plants in the midwest.[180]

CHLOROACETONE. *Chloropropanone.* It is used in the manufacture of couplers for photography, as an enzyme inactivator, an intermediate *(see)* in perfumes, as an antioxidant in drugs, in insecticides, and in the manufacture of vinyl compounds. It is intensely irritating to the eyes, skin, and mucous membranes.[181] Chloroacetone has caused tumors when painted on the skin of mice.[182]

CHLOROBENZILATE. *Benzilic acid; 4,4'-dichloro-; ethyl ester; acaraben; dichlorobenzilate; kop-mite.* Viscuos yellow liquid used as an acaricide to kill spiders and mites. It is a synergist for DDT. A NIOSH review found it to be a positive carcinogen for animals. Tested by NCI for cancer-causing properties, it was found to cause liver cancer in mice.[183,184] The test did not provide convincing evidence of carcinogenicity in rats, however. The EPA then completed a review of this pesticide used to control mites on oranges, grapefruit, and other citrus. EPA decided to allow continued use of chlorobenzilate on citrus in Florida, Texas, Arizona, and California but with certain restrictions to reduce possible risks to applicators. Noncitrus uses on almonds, apples, melons, cherries, cotton, pears, walnuts, ornamentals, and trees will be canceled.

EPA's review began in May 1976 based on data showing the pesticide caused tumors in mice. The data was confirmed, indicating the pesticide may pose a cancer risk to humans. However, restrictions on uses of the pesticide will limit applicators' exposure to reduce the potential risks of cancer and possible testicular effects. Companies registered to manufacture and sell the chemical will be required to collect data over an 18-month period on field-applicator exposure and on residues on citrus, citrus by-products, and meat and milk from cattle fed on citrus by-products. In addition, the manufacturers are now required to submit test data on possible testicular effects of chlorobenzilate on laboratory animals. If results of these studies indicate that exposure is higher or risk greater than currently estimated, the EPA will reassess the continued use of chlorobenzilate.

Chlorobenzilate is currently used in Florida, Texas, and California because it kills citrus mites without harming beneficial insects. Loss of chlorobenzilate would result in increased use of other pesticides, some more hazardous than chlorobenzilate. The EPA said that without chlorobenzilate the four states would have to spend an additional $28 to $57 million a year for other pesticides. This decision completed the EPA's full-scale risk/benefit review of this pesticide under the Rebuttable Presumption against Registration (RPAR) provisions of federal pesticide regulations.[185]

CHLOROETHENE. *See* Vinyl Chloride.

CHLOROFORM. *Trichloromethane.* Chloroform in the United States is used mostly for manufacturing fluorocarbons for refrigerants, aerosol propellants, and plastics. It is also used for purifying antibiotics, as an industrial solvent, in photographic processing, in industrial dry cleaning, and in dyes, drugs, and salves. It was banned from toothpastes, cough medicines, and mouthwashes in 1976. Chloroform has been found to cause liver and kidney cancers in test animals. The most frequent finding was liver cancer, which killed most male and female mice given the compound orally. High incidences of kidney tumors, predominantly cancerous, occurred in male rats at both high and low dosages of chloroform and in some female rats at high dosages. Thyroid tumors also appeared in some female rats. The tests were part of a continuing NCI program to screen chemicals for cancer-causing activity in animals under specific conditions. NIOSH estimates that 80,000 workers in pharmaceutical plants, chemical plants for the synthesis of other compounds, and other related industries are potentially exposed to chloroform, and it has drawn up occupational standards for the chemical.[186]

CHLOROPICRIN. Developed as a tear gas and currently used as an agricultural fumigant in stored grain and soil, it was given orally by stomach tube to rats and mice for 78 weeks. According to the NCI, the test did not give conclusive evidence for carcinogenicity in mice. In rats, the test was inadequate because of the short survival time of dosed animals. Chloropicrin is highly toxic when inhaled and is a strong irritant. Since its toxicity resembles chlorine *(see)*, it is still considered a possible carcinogen.[187]

CHLOROPRENE. Introduced by Du Pont in 1931, it is used mainly in the manufacture of neoprene (synthetic rubber). For years scientists have known that chloroprene can act as a central nervous system depressant and can harm the lungs, liver, and kidney, but they had never associated it with cancer. When reports about linking vinyl chloride and cancer surfaced, researchers began to take a closer look at other chemicals, including chloroprene, that are similar in structure. Du Pont reviewed the health records and death certificates of its employees who had worked with chloroprene and found that the number of lung cancers had increased in recent years. A survey of foreign scientific literature turned up two reports from the Soviet Union that linked exposure to chloroprene with unusually high rates of lung and skin cancer. The incidence of cancer increased with the length of the time workers had been exposed. In view of the Soviet findings, Du Pont and NIOSH have started detailed investigations of the causes of deaths among all people who ever worked with chloroprene. Du Pont also started long-term studies to determine if chloroprene causes cancer in animals.[188]

CHLORPROMAZINE. It is a frequently prescribed tranquilizer, and when given to females in large doses, it encourages lactation and moderate breast engorgement. It also causes skin pigmentation and a decrease in the production of white blood cells. It may form the powerful cancer-causing agents nitrosamines *(see)* when mixed with nitrites in the stomach. Chlorpromazines are potent stimulators of prolactin *(see),* which has been shown to encourage the growth of breast cancers in some cases.[189]

CHOLEIC ACID. *Apocholic acid, deoxycholic acid.* It occurs in the bile of man, oxen, sheep, dogs, goats, and rabbits. It is used medically as a choleretic to increase the flow of bile. When injected under the skin of mice in high doses of 1475 milligrams per kilogram of body weight, it caused tumors.

CHOLEST-5-EN-3-BETA-OL. *See* Cholesterol.

CHOLESTEROL. A fat soluble, crystalline, fatty alcohol that occurs in all animal fats and oils, nervous tissue, egg yolk, and blood. It is used commercially as an emulsifier and lubricant in cosmetics. It is important in metabolism but has been implicated as a contributing factor to hardening of the arteries and cardiovascular disease. While high cholesterol in the blood may contribute to heart disease, low cholesterol levels have been reported in some experiments to contribute to cancer. During an epidemiological study of an entire community, Tecumseh, Michigan, mortality rates among parents of persons with varying concentrations of serum cholesterol were compared. Higher cancer mortality rates among mothers tended to be associated with low levels of serum cholesterol among their sons and daughters (on the other hand, a lower mortality rate from coronary heart disease was observed in the parents of these same offspring). This association between cancer and cholesterol was more likely to be present when the mother's death from cancer occurred relatively early in life.[190] In another study, a comparison of cancer experience in four clinical trials of serum-cholesterol-lowering diets revealed that there seemed to be no greater risk of cancer with such diets.[191] Cancer and cholesterol are also being intensively studied at the Jackson Laboratory in Woods Hole, Massachusetts. The cholesterol in question is not the kind eaten with food, but the sterol that is produced by the body's cells. Investigators found abnormal amounts of cholesterol were present in several different types of tumors. The precise cholesterol-cancer connection is not yet clear.[192]

The hypothesis that cholesterol may play a role in tumor formation has been advanced for several reasons. One is because of the association between coronary artery disease and neoplasms, including breast cancer, leukemia, and colon and rectal cancer. It has been suggested that cholesterol may be the common causative factor in these diseases. In one study, the administration of cholesterol-lowering drugs was followed by cancer remission. However, there are contradictory studies. One study reported that the serum-cholesterol level was significantly lower in patients with colon cancer than it was in the control group.

CHROANALINE. A food-packaging adhesive banned in 1969 as a carcinogen by the FDA. It was the second time that the Delaney Amendment (*see* Introduction, page 10) was invoked.

CHROME GREEN. *See* Chromium.

CHROME LEMON. *See* Chromic Acid.

CHROME ORANGE. *See* Chromium.

CHROME YELLOW. *See* Chromic Acid.

CHROMIC ACID. *Chromium trioxide, chromic anhydride.* It consists of dark purplish red crystals that are soluble in water, alcohol, and mineral acids. It is highly toxic and corrosive to the skin. The tolerance level (as CrO_3) is 0.1 milligram per cubic meter of air, according to an OSHA standard. A powerful oxidizing agent, it may explode on contact with reducing agents and may ignite on contact with organic metals. It is used in chemicals (chromates, oxidizing agents, catalysts), in chromium plating, as an intermediate *(see),* in medicine as a topical antiseptic and astringent, and in process engraving, anodizing, ceramic glazes, colored glass, metal cleaning, inks, tanning, paints, and as a textile mordant. Its carcinogenic determination, according to OSHA, is "indefinite."[193]

CHROMITE. *Iron chromate.* A natural oxide of ferrous iron and chromium *(see),* it sometimes is combined with magnesium and aluminum. It usually occurs with magnesium and is iron black to brownish black. It is found in Russia, South Africa, Rhodesia, the Philippines, Cuba, and Turkey. It is the only commercial source of chromium and its compounds. It caused tumors when injected into mice in doses of 400 milligrams per kilogram of body weight.[194] A NIOSH review determined it to be a positive animal carcinogen.[195]

CHROMIUM. Occurs in the earth's crust. Chromium oxide is used for green eye shadow and greenish mascara. Inhalation of chromium dust can cause irritation and ulceration. Ingestion results in violent gastrointestinal upsets. Application to the skin may result in violent allergic reactions. Chromium can cause injury to the skin, the nasal membrane, and less frequently the voice box and the lungs. The most serious effect of chromium is lung cancer, which may develop 20 to 30 years after exposure. One study has shown that the death rate from lung cancer for exposed workers is 29 times that for average members of the population.[196] Among workers at risk are acetylene and aniline workers, bleachers, glass and pottery workers, battery makers, and linoleum workers. The incubation period is estimated to be 15 to 25 years.

CHRYSENE. Crystals from distillation of coal tar used in organic synthesis. Official tolerance is 0.2 milligrams per meter of cubic air. It caused cancer in mice when injected under or applied to the skin.[197] A NIOSH review determined it is a positive animal carcinogen and has selected it for hazard review. EPA has selected it for priority attention as a toxic pollutant.[198]

CHRYSOTILE. A form of asbestos used in paving roads, playgrounds, and parking lots throughout the United States. Dr. Arthur L. Frank and his colleagues reported to an American Lung Association meeting, May 15, 1978, that they had performed what they believed was the first demonstration of significant biological activity of this quarried material. In text-tube experiments they demonstrated damage to mouse macrophagelike cells (scavenger cells in the lung and other organs) caused by the chrysotile found in the rocks. Crushed rock that did not contain the chrysotile did no damage to the mouse cells.[199]

In a study reported in *Occupational Medicine* in 1977, Dr. W. Weiss of the Division of Occupational Medicine, Hahnemann Medical College, Philadelphia, reported a 30-year historical mortality study of 264 men who had worked for at least a year with chrysotile. Follow-up was 94 percent complete. Two men had died of asbestosis. The overall mortality was the same as the comparison group. For asbestos-related diseases the differences in work duration had no effect on mortality, and in fact, the men exposed to chrysotile alone had a better mortality rate than the comparison group.[200]

C.I. VAT YELLOW 4. A dyestuff used in wool, silk, and synthetic fibers; as a paper pigment; and by the armed services as a smoke screen and signaling agent. It was given in feed to rats for 104 weeks and to mice for 106 weeks. It was a cause of lymphomas in male mice but was not found carcinogenic for rats or female mice under the test conditions.[201]

CINNAMYL ANTHRANILATE. A reddish yellow powder with a fruity taste that is used as a synthetic flavoring. It is used in cherry, grape, honey, and vanilla flavorings for beverages, ice cream, ices, candy, baked goods, gelatin desserts, and chewing gum. In experiments testing for cancer-causing agents, cinnamyl anthranilate was the only one of 41 additives that caused lung tumors in mice. The anthranilic-acid structure may be suspected as the source of activity because of the reported induction of bladder tumors in mice by compounds similar in structure to this coal-tar derivative.[202]

CIRCUMCISION. Cancer of the penis is almost unknown among Jews. Cancer of the penis accounts for about 2 percent of all cancers among Mohammedans and about 15 percent of all cancer among Chinese. Jewish boys are circumcised in the first few days of life, Mohammedan boys between the ages of 3 and 15; the Chinese do not practice circumcision. Circumcision prevents the accumulation of irritating secretions beneath the foreskin of the penis. Statistics have also shown that women whose husbands are circumcised are less likely to develop cancer of the cervix than women with uncircumcised mates.[203]

CITRUS RED NO. 2. *Monoazo.* Used only for coloring orange skins that are *not* intended for processing and that meet minimum maturity standards established by or under laws of the states in which the oranges are grown. Oranges colored with citrus red no. 2 are not supposed to bear more than 2 parts per million of the color additive calculated on the weight of the whole fruit. Citrus red no. 2 toxicity is far from determined, although, theoretically, consumers would not ingest the dye because they peel the orange before eating. If ingested in quantity, the 2-naphthol constituent of the dye can cause eye-lens clouding, kidney damage, vomiting, and circulatory collapse. Application to the skin can cause peeling, and deaths have been reported after application to the skin.[204] When it was given orally to mice in 365 milligram doses per kilogram of body weight, it caused cancer, as it also did when injected in 80 milligram doses per kilogram of body weight in mice.[205]

CLAVACIN. *See* Patulen.

CLOCKS. *See* Radioluminescent Paint.

CLUSTERS. An alarm was sounded in the spring of 1978 when the town of Rutherford, New Jersey, reported a higher than average incidence of cancers, particularly among children at one school. Dr. Glyn Caldwell, chief of the National Center for Disease Control's cancer branch, said that such clusters are not that unusual. "Clusters are only an indication of increased incidence in a given area and a given time." Investigations of the air, water, and other environmental factors in Rutherford, as in other reported "cluster" areas, failed to produce any cause for the 16 blood-related cancers. Since 80 to 90 percent of cancers are thought to be environmentally caused, epidemiologists will keep looking at geographic patterns to try and find clues to causes.

COAL TAR. *Soot.* The by-products in the destruction of coal include benzene, toluene, naphthalene, anthracene, xylene, and other aromatic hydrocarbons *(see);* phenol, cresol, and other compounds; ammonia, pyridine, and some other organic bases; and thiophene. Coal-tar products are usually black, thick liquids or semisolids with a characteristic odor. They serve as raw materials for plastics, and for solvents, dyes, drugs, and other organic chemicals. The crude or refined products or fractions are also used in waterproofing, paints, pipe coating, roads, roofing, insulation, pesticides, sealants, and medicines. The association with cancer of products from the incomplete combustion of fuels can be traced back more than 200 years to the original observation of Percival Pott. He noted the occurrence of scrotal cancer among chimney sweeps. Through the years, the realization of the cancer-causing potential of coal-tar products slowly evolved. In 1933, benzopyrene *(see)* was identified as a potent carcinogen. Anthracene has been found to cause cancer in workers, but there is a question as to whether the disease is caused by pure anthracene or by the impurities found with it. Coal-tar creosotes are complex mixtures of more than 160 chemicals, and after years of exposure to them workers may develop skin cancer.[206] Any product derived from coal tar must be suspect as far as cancer is concerned, including dyes, creosotes, and asphalt.[207]

COBALT. Cobalt is a metal occurring in the earth's crust. It is gray, hard, and magnetic. It is prescribed for people as a mineral supplement in doses of one milligram per day. An overdose can produce an overproduction of red blood cells, plus toxic symptoms in the gastrointestinal tract. It is generally recognized as safe by the FDA as a food additive. It caused sarcomas at the site of injection in rats and mice.[208,209]

CO-CARCINOGENS. Agents that act synergistically with one or more cancer-causing agents to produce a cancer. They may promote the growth of tumors after the initial action of a weak carcinogen, which without help might not be able to overcome the body's defenses. Examples of co-carcinogens are croton oil *(see)* and latex from the plants of the Euphorbiaceae family. Co-carcinogens greatly increase the cancer-causing ability of coal tar when painted on mouse skin.[210]

COKE. The residue of the destructive distillation of bituminous coal, petroleum, and coal-tar pitch. The principal type is produced by heating bituminous coal in chemical recovery—one ton of coal yielding about 0.7 tons of coke. It is used in the manufacture of aluminum, pig iron, phosphorous, silicon carbide, and calcium carbide. An extensive study of 58,000 men employed at seven Pittsburgh-area steel plants showed that working on or near coke ovens is one of the most dangerous jobs in industry. The discovery was made that full-time topside oven workers with five or more years' exposure were almost 11 times as likely to get lung cancer as are other steel workers. For side-oven workers the risk is two and a half times as great.[211] It is estimated that 20,000 people work in coke ovens in the United States. Coke-oven workers die of lung cancer at a rate of 1.7 to 20 times that of other steel workers, depending on the type and length of employment in the coke ovens. Death rates from both kidney and prostate cancer were also shown to be significantly elevated among United States coke-oven workers. Increased mortality from cancer of the skin, including the scrotum, has been demonstrated among British coke-oven and other workers exposed to the product of coal carbonization.[212] The University of Pittsburgh School of Public Health and NIOSH found that all coke-plant workers, not just those on the ovens, have a higher rate of cancer than do other steel workers. Nonoven workers have less lung cancer but more digestive system cancers, particularly of the colon and pancreas. They also have cancers of the mouth and throat.

COLCHICINE. Poisonous yellow crystalline alkaloid extracted from the seed of meadow saffron. It is used experimentally to create new plant varieties and medicinally to treat acute gout and rheumatism. Its precise pharmacologic action in gout is not known. However, it is thought to decrease the lactic-acid production by the cells, thereby decreasing urate-crystal deposition and the subsequent inflammatory response. Prolonged administration may cause bone-marrow depression and aplastic anemia. It has caused tumors when applied to the skin of mice in doses of 144 milligrams per kilogram of body weight.[213]

COLON. The colon is the middle and longest section of the intestine; it joins the rectum and small intestine.

COLORECTAL (COLON) CANCER. The large intestine and its lower end, the rectum, are involved in the commonest form of internal cancer in the United States. Only lung cancer kills more men, only breast cancer kills more women. Each year, according to the NCI, 100,000 Americans are attacked by it. Half of that number die annually from the disease. If symptoms are mild, and early symptoms (gas, constipation) are usually mild, people tend to see a druggist instead of a physician. Tumors of the colon are common. Although the majority are not malignant, cancers develop more frequently in the colon than in other parts of the intestinal tract. Precisely why this is so is not known. Leading theories hold that it is a combination of heredity and diet. No one directly inherits colorectal cancer, but it frequently occurs in families with a high incidence of cancer in various sites. Ulcerative colitis is also frequently associated with subsequent cancer, 5 to 10 times more than in the general population. There is now evidence indicating that fat-rich diets may be linked to colorectal cancers. Studies have shown that in countries such as Japan, where the people eat mostly fish and vegetables, and in certain groups such as the Seventh-Day Adventists, who eat no meat, the incidence of the disease is much lower than in countries and groups where the diet is high in fats. Researchers do not recommend that meat and other fat-rich foods be eliminated but that high amounts be avoided and well-balanced nutritional meals be consumed. Colorectal cancer does not occur more frequently in people of a particular sex, ethnic group, or socioeconomic class, but it does increase sharply in incidence among those over 40, and continues to rise twofold in each succeeding decade. It can also appear in younger people, although rarely, in the teens and twenties.[214]

CONGENITAL DEFECTS. Certain cancers have been associated with congenital defects. Here is a chart published by the Biometry Branch of the NCI. *See also* Heredity and Genetics.

CONGENITAL DEFECT	CANCER
Down's, Bloom's, and Fanconi's syndromes	leukemia
certain phakomatoses (multiple hereditary tumors)	glioma, medulloblastoma
congenital hemihypertrophy (muscular increase in size of one side of the face or body)	Wilm's tumor, primary liver tumor, and neoplasia of the covering of the adrenal gland.
aniridia (absence of the iris)	gonadoblastoma

immunologic disorders (ataxia,   lymphoma
telangiectasia, Wiscott-Aldrich syndrome, agammaglobulinemia, and
Chédiak-Higashi syndrome.

CONTRACEPTIVES. The U.S. Center for Disease Control reported in
1978 that for every 100,000 women using oral contraceptives, 4 die each
year. Fewer than one woman per 100,000 using intrauterine devices dies,
and 4 women in 100,000 who have abortions die. For every 100,000 women
who undergo surgical sterilization, 16 die. Twenty-three women die from
events related to pregnancy and childbirth for every 100,000 births. *See also*
The Pill and Estrogen.

COSMETICS. The General Accounting Office Survey of Cosmetics was
presented to Congress February 3, 1978: it revealed more than 100 ingredients used in cosmetics suspected of causing cancer and birth defects. The
report was critical of the FDA for laxity of enforcement of existing federal
cosmetics laws but determined that the law does not provide adequate
powers to the FDA to protect consumers from potential health hazards.[215]
Among the hazards were many coal-tar dyes used in hair-coloring products
(see Hair Coloring*).* The FDA is studying a cancer-causing agent N-
nitrosodiethanolamine (NDELA) after finding this chemical in a number
of widely used cosmetics. NDELA was discovered in 27 of 29 tested skin
creams, body and suntan lotions, shampoos, and other cosmetic products.
The significance is not yet known, but NDELA is considered a "less-
potent" carcinogen.[216]

COUMARIN. Used in perfumes, soaps, and suntan lotions, it has the
odor of new-mown hay and is found in many plants such as the tonka bean
and sweet clover. At one time it was used as a food flavoring but has been
banned by the FDA because it caused liver injury in experimental animals.
It caused skin tumors in mice when applied to the skin in doses of 1,800
milligrams per kilogram of body weight.[217]

CRESLAN. *See* Acrylonitrile.

o-**CRESOL.** Used in hair-grooming preparations and in eye lotions, it is
obtained from coal tar and wood. When used as an antiseptic and disinfectant, it can cause chronic poisoning if absorbed orally or through the skin.
It may also produce digestive disturbances and nervous disorders accom-
panied by fainting, dizziness, mental changes, skin eruptions, jaundice, or
uremic poisoning. It caused cancer when given orally to rats in doses of
1,000 parts per million.[218] *See also* Coal Tar.

CROCIDOLITE. *See* Asbestos.

**CROTONIC ACID, 3-METHYL-, sec-BUTYL 4,6-DINITROPHENYL
ESTER METABOLITES.** *See* Endosulfan.

CROTON OIL. *Tiglium.* Brownish yellow liquid obtained by expressing the seeds of *Croton tiglium.* Croton oil is toxic and a strong skin irritant. Ingestion of small amounts may be fatal. Israeli researchers reported that it is a co-carcinogen, making cancer-causing agents more potent when painted on the skin of mice.[219] Phorbol esters derived from croton oil have been found to be extremely potent tumor promoters, resulting in all animals tested showing tumors; and usually of those tumors, 50 to 60 percent were malignant.[220]

CRUDE OIL. *See* Petroleum.

CUPFERRON. An analytical reagent, it was given in feed to rats and mice for 78 weeks. It proved carcinogenic, producing a variety of cancers in male and female animals of both species.[221]

CYCASIN. Toxic substance from the seeds of *Cycas revoluta.* It occurs in the pulp and husk of the cycad nut, as well as in other parts of the palmlike cycad trees. Many of these species inhabit tropical and subtropical regions and can survive drought and hurricanes. The cycads have provided emergency and staple foods and medicines for natives of these areas for a long time. Native populations have long known of the toxicity of food from this source and that it can cause jaundice hemorrhage and chronic partial paralysis. The toxin is removed from the sliced nut and pit by repeated soaking in many changes of water. The sun-dried and ground starch, and indeed all parts of the plant, often without extraction by water, have been used as food. When fed to rats, the unextracted nuts are highly carcinogenic, especially in the liver and kidney. Tumor induction with cycasin has also been noted in mice, guinea pigs, hamsters, and fish.[222]

CYCLAMATES. *Sodium cyclamate and calcium cyclamate.* These artificial sweetening agents, about 30 times as sweet as refined sugar, were removed from the market September 1, 1969, because they were found to cause bladder cancer in rats. At the time, 175 million Americans were swallowing cyclamates in significant doses in many products, ranging from chewing gum to soft drinks.

CYCLOCHLOROTINE. A fungus. *See* Luteoskyrin.

CYCLOHEXANE. *Hexamethylene, hexanaphthene, hexahydrobenzene.* A colorless, mobile liquid with a pungent odor. Insoluble in water and soluble in alcohol, acetone, benzene. It is flammable, a dangerous fire risk. Moderately toxic when inhaled or applied to skin. It has a tolerance level of 300 parts per million in air. It is used in the manufacture of nylon; as a solvent for cellulose ethers, fats, oils, waxes, bitumens, resins, crude rubber; in extracting essential oils; in chemical synthesis; in paint and varnish remover; in glass substitutes; and its vapor has been used as a lubricant for steel (experimental).

CYCLOHEXANESULFAMIC ACID. *See* Cyclamates.

CYCLOPHOSPHAMIDE. *See* Cytoxan.

CYSTOGEN. *See* Methenamine.

CYTOXAN. *Cyclophosphane.* This is a synthetic antineoplastic drug chemically related to nitrogen mustards. It is a white crystalline powder that is soluble in water. It interferes with the growth of susceptible neoplasms and to some extent certain normal tissues. Secondary malignancies have developed alone or in association with other antineoplastic drugs. These malignancies have most frequently been urinary-bladder cancers and lymph-gland malignancies. Although no definite cause and effect relationship has been established between cytoxan and malignancy (based on available data), before prescribing it, the benefits should be weighed against the risk assessment for the use of the drug.[223]

DDA. *See* Hair Colorings.

DACTINOMYCIN. *See* Actinomycin D.

DANDRUFF SHAMPOO. *See* Selenium.

DAPSONE. A parent chemical of the sulfone drugs, and the major therapeutic agent in this group of drugs for the treatment of leprosy. It was given to some American troops in Vietnam by Army doctors who hoped that it would work as a preventive medicine against a severe form of malaria that was resistent to standard malaria pills. It is also used in combination with X-ray to treat some gynecologic neoplasms. Industrially, it is used as an accelerator to speed the production of epoxy resins. It was chosen for study by the NCI because it has been used for prolonged periods of time by humans. It was found in tests to be carcinogenic for male rats, causing tumors of the spleen and the lining of the abdomen, although it showed no cancer-causing activity in female rats or mice that were tested. A data evaluation expert at the NCI said that the results did not prove that it caused cancer in humans, but merited a follow-up. At least one study in the 1960s of the medical records of about 850 American lepers who took the drug did not show a significant difference in the cancer death rate as against that of the general population.[224,225]

DAUNOMYCIN. An antibiotic of the rhodomycin group. It is isolated from the fermentation of the broths of *Streptomyces peucetius* and used experimentally as an anticancer agent. Caused cancer in rats when given intravenously in 5 milligram doses per kilogram of body weight.[226] Determined by a NIOSH review to be a positive animal carcinogen. Currently being tested by the NCI.[227]

DBCP (DIBROMOCHLOROPROPANE). Used in this country since 1955 to control destructive roundworm in the soil of numerous crops, in home lawns, and in golf-course turf, it is also suspected of being a human cancer agent because it has caused stomach and mammary tumors in laboratory rats and mice. Technical grade DBCP, which is used as an agricultural pesticide, was force-fed to rats and mice for periods between 47 and

78 weeks. According to an NCI report issued in February 1978, DBCP is a stomach carcinogen in rats and mice of both sexes and also is carcinogenic to the mammary gland in female rats. "DBCP poses an imminent hazard to the public and to farmers and other persons that apply it. . . . The DBCP calamity again dramatizes the need for vigilant, responsible regulation of chemical production and use." The EPA is continuing its investigation not only of DBCP's risks but also of its agricultural and economic benefits. Dow Chemical and Shell Chemical, the principal makers of DBCP, voluntarily stopped production last summer following the disclosure that 14 of 27 men who manufactured the pesticide at the Occidental Chemical plant in Lathrop, California, were either sterile or afflicted with decreased sperm counts. Despite this production halt, other firms that formulate DBCP into finished pesticide products may still have some of the compound on hand. The EPA order would prohibit any future sale of these products in the United States unless safeguards and conditions outlined in the order are met.[228,229]

DCDD. *See* 2,7-Dichlorodibenzo-p-Dioxin.

D & C REDS Nos. 10, 11, 12, and 13. Prohibited from all uses in drugs and cosmetics because the FDA determined they could contain carcinogens.

D & C YELLOW NO. 8. *See* Fluorescein.

DDT (DICHLORO-DIPHENYL-TRICHLORO-ETHANE). Though not particularly toxic to humans under ordinary conditions, it is not biodegradable and is ecologically damaging. For that reason it was banned in the United States in 1973, though its export is still permitted. DDT can be used for a few specialized purposes, such as to combat tussock moths and to destroy insect carriers of lethal diseases (malarial mosquitoes and tsetse flies). It is used as an insecticide, especially for tobacco and cotton. There is an indication—though a faint one—that DDT may slow down the growth of one type of cancer. While testing mice there was an indication that DDT may have an inhibitory effect on at least one experimental cancer, ependymoma. In tests with some 5,000 mice it has also been found that when DDT is added to the diet, even at the lowest levels, an increased incidence of tumors in males is observed. These findings reinforce the view that the use of DDT should be avoided where alternate means are practicable.[230,231]

DECANE. *Decyl hydride.* A colorless liquid that is narcotic in high concentrations. It is used in the manufacture of chemicals and also as a solvent and for jet-fuel research. It causes tumors when inhaled or painted on the skin of mice in doses of from 1,040 milligrams per kilogram of body weight to 5,100 milligrams per kilogram.[232]

DECHLORANE. A flame retardant. *See* Mirex for carcinogenicity.

DEGRANOL. *See* Mannomustine.

b-DEOXYTHIOGUANOSINE. A chemotherapeutic agent used experimentally against cancer caused lung tumors in mice.[233]

DEPRO PROVERA. *Methoxyprogesterone acetate, 6(alpha)-preg-4-ene-3, 20-dione, 17-(acetyloxy) 6-methyl.* The FDA refused to approve marketing of a three-month contraceptive injection of this drug that is in use in several countries. It is also used in cancer therapy. Studies have shown that it may cause cervical damage as well as permanent sterility.[234] A derivative of progesterone, it is injected or given orally. It is a white to off-white powder. In inhibits the secretion of pituitary gonadotropin, which in turn prevents ovulation.[235]

DES (DIETHYLSTILBESTROL). *Stilbestrol.* It was reported in medical literature as far back as 1938, by a French researcher, Dr. A. Lacassagne, that stilbestrol, a synthetic estrogen, produced breast cancers in mice. In 1950 Lacassagne provided a summary of the work of other researchers who had also found that stilbestrol caused a variety of tumors in animals.

In the meantime, in the 1940s in the United States, it was discovered that this compound increased fat production in chickens. As a result, pellets of DES were implanted in young chickens to improve the quality of their carcasses. What worked for chickens, it was subsequently discovered, also worked for cattle, and DES was fed to cattle. The use of the pellets was later banned in chickens, but DES is still being added to animal feed. An attempted ban by the FDA was successfully fought by makers and users of DES in the meat industry. They said that the ban was illegal because the FDA did not give them prior notice. The courts agreed, and DES is still being added to our meat. The FDA has stipulated a zero tolerance for the compound after a proper withdrawal period from feed, before the beef goes to market. However, an estimated 100,000 to 150,000 head of cattle containing residues of the hormone are apparently getting to market. OSHA *(see)* levied one of its highest fines ($34,100) in June 1976, when it penalized Dawes Laboratories, a Chicago hormone manufacturer, after male employees exposed to the livestock feed hormone DES complained that their breasts had become enlarged and that they had become impotent. The European Common Market and Sweden have forbidden the use of DES in cattle.

DES was and is used as a drug. It was given in the 1940s through the 1970s to pregnant women in danger of miscarrying and to women after delivery to dry up their milk. Ironically, it was never proven that it did prevent miscarriage. Then in 1966, researchers at Massachusetts General Hospital found a clear-cell adenoma in the vagina of a 15-year-old girl, the first reported case in someone that age. Within three years, a total of seven cancers of that type and an eighth of endometroid vaginal carcinoma had been found. An investigation of these cases found the girls had one thing in common—seven of their mothers were given DES early in pregnancy. An estimated 6 million children were exposed to the estrogen in their mothers' wombs. More than 600 girls from 11 to 25 years old have been found to have lesions due to this prenatal exposure. Abnormalities have also been found in males exposed in Utero. They have cellular changes in their reproductive systems but no cancer as yet. In addition, preliminary reports from the University of Chicago indicate that the mothers who took DES during pregnancy now have an increased risk of breast cancer and to a lesser extent, of cervical and ovarian cancer. During 1976–77 a total of 1,361 mothers were selected for interview—693 DES-exposed and 668 control mothers; 38 DES-exposed and 28 controls had died by the time the interviews were conducted. Twelve DES-exposed and 4 control mothers died of breast cancer. Three DES-exposed mothers and one control died of ovarian cancer. The FDA Obstetrics and Gynecology Advisory Committee, while pointing out that the link is not solid, as yet, between DES and these cancers, advises women who were exposed to the estrogen during pregnancy to have regular breast examinations. In addition, the FDA committee made the following recommendations:

- Indication for use of DES and other estrogens, including combinations with progesterone, be deleted from the labeling so that doctors will not prescribe it.
- The agency will approve use of DES for postcoital use in emergency situations such as rape and incest, if a manufacturer provides a patient labeling and special packagings. To discourage "morning after" use by other women, the FDA has removed from the market the 25 milligram tablets of DES formerly used for this purpose.
- More than 40 years after Lacassagne's correlation of stilbestrol and breast cancer, and more than a decade after the association between DES exposure in utero and cancer, the FDA is still considering removing DES from use in animal feed. The basis of the prohibition is that "illegal residues of the drug continue to be detected in slaughtered animals." 236,237

DEXTRANS. A term applied to polysaccharides produced by bacteria growing on sugar. It is used as a foam stabilizer for beer, in soft-centered confections, and as a substitute for barley malt. It has also been used as a plasma expander for emergency treatment of shock. In November 1977 the FDA approved dextrans as GRAS (Generally Recognized As Safe) for indirect food ingredient uses, but it deleted the substance's listing under GRAS (see) as a direct human food ingredient. Dextrans did not receive an affirmative report as a direct human food ingredient because of insufficient scientific data "upon which to base an approval for direct food use of this substance." The FDA did judge dextrans as safe for indirect food use, such as a constituent of food-packaging materials that are produced at good manufacturing practice levels. Dextrans have been reported to cause cancer in rats, and the Select Committee of the Federation of American Societies for Experimental Biologies in advising on food additives said that further studies were needed to determine whether increased consumption could constitute a dietary hazard.[238]

2,4-DIAMINOANISOLE SULFATE   *4-Methoxy-m-phenylene-diamine.* This chemical coupler used in permanent hair-dye formulations was given in feed to rats and mice for 78 weeks. According to the results, technical-grade 2,4-diaminoanisole sulfate was carcinogenic in both sexes of mice and rats under the test conditions.[239] *See also* Hair Coloring.

DIARYLANILIDE YELLOW.   *Pigment yellow 12.* A member of a family of organic azo *(see)* pigments known as benzidine yellows, it is one of the dyes that may be responsible for the incidence of bladder cancer among dye workers. It is used as an ingredient in industrial paints, most notably the paint applied to lead pencils. It is also an ingredient in printing inks and may sometimes be used to color plastics, rubber, linoleum, floor tiles, textiles, and wallpaper. It was the largest single pigment produced in 1975. There is a risk of exposure to any workers employed in the dye, ink, or paint manufacturing industry (or any company where products containing this pigment are produced) or in facilities where textiles are dyed: among the workers exposed are printers, engravers, lithographers, textile workers, and tailors. Exposure of the general public to diarylanilide yellow is likely due to the large variety of consumer products colored with it. Chronic ingestion over long periods can be from habitually chewing pencils or holding them in the mouth. There has been liver cancer and bladder cancer reported among workers. Tests with experimental animals did not absolutely provide evidence that the pigment was carcinogenic, but there was squamous-cell cancer of the ear in low-dose males, infiltrating duct cancer of the mammary gland in low-dose females, and tumors of the subcutaneous tissues in high-dose females.[240]

DIAZO BLACK.   *See* Benzidine.

DIAZO FAST BLUE B.   *See* Benzidine.

DIBENZ (a,h) ANTHRACENE.   Consists of reddish leaflets derived from acetic acid. It caused cancer and tumors in mice, guinea pigs, pigs, and frogs.[241] *See also* Anthracene.

DIBENZYLINE.   *Phenoxybenzamine hydrochloride.* Chemotherapeutic agent used against tumors of the adrenal gland and its chromaffin cells and in the treatment of vascular diseases and frostbite.[242] Caused lung tumors in mice.[243]

DIBROMOETHANE.   *See* Ethylene Dibromide.

3,3' DICHLOROBENZIDINE (DCB).   *Its salts: 4,4' diamino; 3,3'-dichlorobiphenyl; 4,4' diamine; 0,0'-dichlorobenzidine; and similar names.* A crystalline solid, ranging in color from gray to purple. Found chiefly in the production of pigments for printing inks, textile dyes, plastics, and crayons, particularly yellow pigments. It is, for example, the key component of pigment yellow 13, of which 5.6 million pounds were produced in the United States in 1971. Equal amounts of other yellow pigments were also produced from DCB. Ironically the dyes are prized because they are non-toxic—the DCB is chemically destroyed during their production. DCB is also used as a curing agent in the manufacture of solid urethane plastics. It has caused cancers of the liver, bladder, breasts, and the sites of injection in rats, mice, hamsters, and dogs. However, the usual epidemiologic means of determining its dangers for humans are not available because workers who have been exposed to DCB have either not been in contact with the substance for long periods or have been exposed to it in combination with other carcingogens such as NA beta-napthylamine *(see)* or benzidine *(see).* But since it does cause cancer in four kinds of laboratory animals, and since it has been found in the urine of workers who had minimal exposure to it, DCB, which is readily absorbed through the skin, must be considered carcinogenic for humans.[244] OSHA has strict safety standards for the protection of workers involved in handling, producing, or storing any substance containing more than one percent of DCB and its salts.

2,7-DICHLORODIBENZO-p-DIOXIN (DCDD). This compound, formed as a by-product in the manufacture of chlorophenol and also present as a contaminant in the herbicide 2,4-5-T and the pesticide pentachlorophenol (PCP), was fed to rats for 110 weeks and to mice for 90 weeks. According to the NCI, increased incidences of leukemias, lymphomas, and blood-vessel and liver cancers in male mice were suggestive, but not conclusive, of carcinogenicity of DCDD. The compound was not carcinogenic for female mice or for rats of either sex under the test conditions.[245] *See also* Agent Orange and 2,4,5-T.

1,2-DICHLOROETHANE. *See* Ethylene Dichloride.

DICHLOROMETHANE. *See* Methylene Choride.

DICHLORVOS (DDVP). *Vapona; 2,2-dichlorovinyl dimethylphosphate.* An organophosphate insecticide with contact and vapor action, it has been widely used for control of agricultural, industrial, and domestic pests since the 1950s. DDVP is available in oil solutions, emulsifiable concentrates, and aerosol formulations. It is also impregnated in polyvinyl-chloride-based pellets and strips and blocks for delayed release. It is regularly used as a dewormer, administered orally to swine, dogs, horses, cats, and puppies. Its topical (skin) application has been approved for beef and dairy cattle, goats, sheep, swine, and chickens to control fleas, flies, and mites. It is used in barns, chicken coops, and tomato greenhouses and applied to mushrooms, lettuce, and radishes. Aerosols and strips are used domestically for control of ants, bedbugs, ticks, cockroaches, flies, mosquitoes, silverfish, spiders, and wasps.

According to a report of the American Conference of Government Industrial Hygienists in 1971, exposure to dichlorvos by inhalation of sprays and vapors, from impregnated resins, from skin contact, or orally as a residue should be under 1.0 milligram per cubic meter. The compound was fed to rats and mice for 80 weeks. This report further stated that microscopic studies of the tissues of treated animals and matched and pooled control animals revealed no statistically significant increase in the incidence of tumors attributable to exposure to dichlorvos in either species. Thus under the conditions of the study, dichlorvos was not demonstrated to be carcinogenic. However, there were esophageal tumors in treated mice, but the incidence of overall tumors was within the range normally seen for these test animals. The possible tumorigenicity of dichlorvos is not precluded.[246]

DICHROMIC ACID, DISODIUM SALT. *Sodium bichromate.* Red or reddish orange deliquescent crystals derived from chromic ore by alkaline roasting and subsequent leaching. It is toxic by inhalation and ingestion and is a strong irritant. It is used in chemical processing as a chromic-acid corrosion inhibitor, in the manufacture of pigments, in the tanning of leathers, in electroplating, and as a defoliating agent, catalyst, and wood preservative. Caused tumors when injected into rats.[247] OSHA has a restriction on the amount that may be in the air.

DICYCLOHEXYLAMINE. *Dodecahydrodephenylamine.* It is a colorless liquid with faint amine odor and is combustible. A strong irritant to the skin and mucous membranes, it is used as an intermediate *(see)* in insecticides; in the manufacture of plasticizers, corrosion inhibitors, and rubber chemicals; as a catalyst for paints, varnishes, and inks; and in detergents. Caused cancer when injected under the skin of mice in 2,400 milligram doses per kilogram of body weight.[248]

N,N'-DICYCLOHEXYL THIOUREA. A chemical intermediate *(see)* used in producing other chemicals, it was fed to rats and mice for 104 to 109 weeks. According to a summary of the report given by the NCI, it was not carcinogenic in either mice or rats under the test conditions. Administration of the compound was associated with an increase in numbers of thyroid follicular cells and an increase in tumors of the thyroid in both rats and mice. However, the increases in tumors did not occur at a statistically significant rate in these tests.[249]

DIELDRIN. A chlorinated cyclodiene pesticide, it is also used as a metabolic conversion product of aldrin, another pesticide, but is more effective than aldrin. It is a neurotoxin (a toxin capable of destroying nerve tissue). First introduced by cotton growers in the 1950s, when the chemical was found to be more effective than aldrin *(see)*, dieldrin has also been used as an insecticide on crops, for public health pest control, and for mothproofing woolen goods. Registration for it was canceled in 1974. However, selected federal tests data about its cancer-causing ability were controversial and often inadequate. There was also a potential for long-term human exposure to residues especially in foods. The NCI decided to test dieldrin again. The tests showed that there was a significant increase in the incidence of liver cancers in high-dose male rats and in cancer of the adrenal glands in low-dose female rats. Tumors occurred in the pituitary and thyroid glands in tests but were not clearly related to dieldrin.[250]

DIESEL FUEL.   In 1977 it was estimated that diesel-powered cars made in the United States could claim 25 percent of Detroit's sales by 1985. However, there is some reservation about the safety of the fuel that offers a 25 to 30 percent increase in mileage over gasoline. A study in 1978 by the environmental group Citizens for Clean Air, Inc., argued that the use of diesel engines could cause a cancer epidemic, especially in New York City where the taxi industry was considering putting them into its 11,800 cabs. The group's report to the National Highway Traffic Safety Administration said that known cancer-causing agents that come from diesel exhaust are in a class of compounds called polynuclear aromatic hydrocarbons (PAH). A recent Swiss study on PAH concentrations in roadway soil revealed a very high cancer incidence among people living near highways. About three of ten cars in Switzerland are diesels. The EPA has undertaken a major research program to determine if the exhaust fumes from diesel-burning trucks and buses can cause cancer. Preliminary tests have shown that diesel exhausts caused genetic changes in bacteria and that these mutated bacteria could have cancer-causing capabilities.[251]

DIET.   Statisticians have estimated that eating habits contribute to at least 40 percent of the cancer deaths in the United States. They base their estimates on epidemiological studies. Associations between commonly used foods and cancer are difficult to detect in populations where nearly everyone adheres to the same basic diet. However, studies of populations having widely different food habits have suggested an association between stomach cancer and foods preserved or pickled in salt and between colon cancer and beef and fats. The high incidence of cancer of the pharynx and esophagus among the Swedes and Finns is thought to be related to multiple dietary deficiencies that result in damage to the mucous linings. These changes, in turn, may be precursors of cancer. Iodine deficiency has been related to the development of cancer of the thyroid. Undernourishment has been correlated with cirrhosis of the liver and the subsequent appearance of liver cancer among Africans, Chinese, Japanese, and others. Cancer of the colon is very common in the United States, Britain, and Scotland. In fact, if both sexes are taken together, cancer of the colon is the leading cancer in the United States, affecting more than 100,000 per year. The disease is rare in countries like Poland, Norway, Portugal, and Japan. Heredity is evidently not the causative factor because when natives of these countries move to the United States and adopt our diet, they too show an increased susceptibility to colon cancer.

What are some of the factors in our diet that may cause cancer? There are known cancer-causing agents in our food and water, as this book documents. They may be either deliberately or unintentionally added. There are also naturally occurring carcinogens in food and water. The interaction between the chemicals we eat and drink, inhale, and "paint" on ourselves is mind boggling. Other than a few cases of almost certain cause and effect, such as liver cancer and the aflatoxins *(see)*, and cancer of the mouth and esophagus and betel nuts *(see)*, most of the correlations are difficult to pin down.

Fat, for example, is a prime dietary suspect in cancer. In animals, it has been found to increase the formation of breast, skin, and probably liver cancers, but it did not increase the incidence of sarcomas and primary lung cancers. Epidemiological studies seem to bear out the "fat connection." In countries where little meat and dairy products are eaten, and among vegetarians, breast cancer is rare. A diet high in fats has been linked to prolactin *(see)*, a hormone that has been associated with breast cancer. Studies also show that tumor formation may be affected by the type of fat. Corn oil, for instance, has been found to encourage carcinogenic action more than hydrogenated coconut oil. Experiments with 10 different fats and oils fed to rats at 20 percent of their diet indicated that a diet high in unsaturated fatty acids (usually liquid, double bonded between carbon and hydrogen atoms) enhanced the induction of mammary cancer more than did highly saturated fats (with a single carbon bond). Mice receiving unsaturated corn or safflower oil tended to die with gross tumors at earlier ages than mice fed diets containing more saturated fats. There have been a number of studies involving human diets low in cholesterol (fat). Some have shown a correlation between low-cholesterol diets and a high incidence of cancer. Others have shown the opposite results. Most researchers feel there is a need for controlled retrospective studies before the question of unsaturated versus saturated fats and cancer can be answered.

Another clue to the fat connection is that Finns consume as much dietary fat as we do, but their incidence of colon cancer is much lower. This observation seems to contradict epidemiological and animal experiments that indicate that colon cancer may arise when dietary fats are converted by the liver into bile acids, which in turn act with other dietary components to produce carcinogens. The Finns may have a lower colon-cancer rate because of their greater intake of dietary fiber, and the increased stool bulk that results may act to dilute the levels of fat metabolites associated with cancer formation. Finns get much of their dietary bulk from the large amounts of rye bread they consume with their meals.

Bile acids do seem to be affected by diet. Controlled feeding experiments in animals as well as studies of population groups consuming different diets show that reduction of fat intake results in decreased excretion of fecal bile acids. The dietary regimens compared are high-fat versus low-fat diets; high-meat versus no-meat diets; high-fat, high-meat diets versus vegetarians (including eggs and other dairy products). Those who have more fecal bile acid seem to be at a high risk for cancer of the colon. The effect of dietary fiber on fecal bile acid concentrations involves the bulking effects of fiber, which reduces bile and acid concentrations.

There is also evidence that people who are obese have a greater incidence of cancers of the intestinal tract, liver, gall bladder, and genitourinary tract. Cancer of the uterus is also more frequent in the overweight. In animal experiments, calorie restrictions inhibit the formation of many types of tumors, decreasing the incidence of cancers and delaying the time at which tumors appear. Exceptions to this are liver cancers, which are actually enhanced by caloric restriction, and tumors of the adrenal gland, which are not affected. Several theories exist about why calorie restriction inhibits tumor formation. There is the possibility that it may lead to overactivity of the adrenal and other endocrine glands resulting in an inhibitory effect on the tumor growth. In the case of breast cancer, it may be that it reduces estrogen production. It may also be that the amount of carbohydrates available for the tumor is restricted, inhibiting cell division. Dr. Martin Pine reported in the March 1978 issue of the NCI journal that the survival time of certain leukemic mice could be doubled by restricting their dietary intake of the amino acid phenylalanine. This affect was achieved by stimulating the mice's immune systems against the tumors rather than by starving the tumors. The mice were fed a commercial diet developed for children with phenylketonuria, an inborn inability to dispose of phenylalanine. Such a diet may benefit leukemic patients.

As for the carcinogens in our food, many additives have been banned because they have been found to cause cancer in animals: butter yellow, carbon black, violet 1, reds nos. 4 and 2, sarsaparilla, and cyclamates. There are others which should be banned. Among them are sodium nitrate and saccharin.

In addition to the direct carcinogens in our food, some dietary factors may set the stage for cancer, making us more vulnerable to cancer-causing agents. Among them are dietary deficiencies: vitamin-A deficiency has been associated with the development of tumors of the mouth and salivary glands; magnesium deficiency has been correlated with lymphomas and chronic leukemia; and choline deficiency with cirrhosis and liver cancer. Factors such as intestinal pH (acid balance), motility (movement of food), enzymes, and mucin secretion arc also considered important factors involved in the susceptibility to cancer. Stress, of course, affects pH, motility, and probably the other factors as well.

There is also the possibility, according to recent research reports, that certain elements in food can block carcinogens in the diet. Among the protective agents are believed to be the preservatives BHA and BHT (also suspected carcinogens), vitamin C, vitamin E, and chemicals called indoles (found in plants of the cabbage family), as well as broccoli, brussels sprouts, turnips, cauliflower, and related vegetables. The new work with possible cancer-blocking agents in food is based on the discovery by Dr. Elizabeth Miller and Dr. James Miller more than 30 years ago that chemical carcinogens have to be activated in the body before they can change normal cells to cancer cells. This University of Wisconsin team believes that many so-called carcinogens are "precarcinogens" and must be activated in the body to become carcinogens. The idea of the cancer preventers in the diet is to block the formation of carcinogens. However, researchers are finding some carcinogen "inhibitors" are unpredictable and may make matters worse if they are given at the "wrong time."

The most exciting work being done in the field, as of this writing, concerns a derivative of vitamin A, 13-cis retinoic acid, which seems to prevent cancer in patients highly susceptible to bladder cancer. The compound may also be able to inhibit cancers of the breast, lung, pancreas, colon, and esophagus.

One of the major factors in cancer induction and cancer prevention, obviously, is diet. Cancer of the digestive tract, alone, accounts for 172,000 of the 700,000 new cases of malignant disease that occur in the United States each year, and diet may be responsible for many other forms of cancer. By practicing caution in what we eat, we may also prevent cancer.

The following are some wise dietary choices you should heed in order to reduce exposure to carcinogens:

- Reduce the amount of high-fat beef, lamb, and pork in your diet. When you do eat meat, select lean cuts and trim off visible fat before cooking.
- Drain off all fat that cooks out. Eat more fish and poultry. Substitute skimmed or low-fat milk and cheese for whole-milk products.
- Modify intake of scalding liquids, piping hot foods, and foods that are very spicy.
- Reduce consumption of alcohol to no more than three or four drinks a week.
- Eat more vegetables, whole grains, and fresh fruits.
- Increase your use of cereal fibers.
- Eliminate nitrite-processed meats. If you can't, be sure that you have lettuce, orange juice, or grapefruit juice with the meal.
- Do not use artifical sweeteners known or suspected as carcinogens. They really don't help you lose weight.
- Avoid highly processed foods, especially those with artifical colorings.
- Do not charcoal broil or pan fry your foods. These methods produce carcinogenic residues.
- Restrict your intake of sugar. Read labels carefully because many canned and bottled products are laced with sugar.

DIETHYLAMINE, N-NITROSO-. Derived from ethyl chloride and ammonia. Under heat and pressure it is highly flammable. It is toxic if ingested and is a strong irritant. It is used in rubber chemicals, textiles, as a solvent; in dyes; in resins; in pesticides; as an inhibitor in pharmaceuticals; in petroleum chemicals; and as a corrosion inhibitor in electroplating. It causes cancer in a wide variety of animals including rats, mice, dogs, monkeys, rabbits, pigs, guinea pigs, hamsters, and hens. The dose in rats is 45 milligrams per kilogram of body weight and in dogs is 560 milligrams per kilogram. It takes an oral dose of 18 milligrams per kilogram of body weight to cause cancer in the monkey.[252]

DIETHYLSTIBESTROL. See DES.

DIETHYL SULFATE (DS). *Sulfuric acid, diethyl ester, ethyl sulfate.* Prepared from ethanol and sulfuric acid, it is a colorless, oily liquid with a peppermint odor. It is used chiefly as an ethylating agent and as an accelerator to speed the sulfation of ethylene. It caused cancer when injected under the skin of rats in 50 milligram doses per kilogram of body weight.[253]

N,N'-DIETHYLTHIOUREA. An industrial anticorrosion agent, it was fed to rats and mice for 103 weeks. NCI tests showed that it caused thyroid cancers in male and female rats. The study did not provide evidence for carcinogenicity of the compound in mice.[254]

DILANTIN. This white, odorless chemical that exists in solid or crystalline form is used as an intermediate *(see)* in the manufacture of pharmaceuticals, textiles, lubricants, certain plastics, and epoxy resins. It is also used medically to prevent convulsions. Prolonged use of Dilantin has been associated with lymphoid reactions that resemble Hodgkin's disease. Transformation to malignant lymphoma has occurred in several patients, but the risk is of small magnitude. A further carcinogenic effect *may* be the induction of neuroblastoma in children born to women whose medication included Dilantin throughout pregnancy. Dilantin is transmitted across the placenta and has been associated with a pattern of malformations known as the fetal hydantoin syndrome. As only two cases of children with fetal hydantoin syndrome who have subsequently developed neuroblastoma have been reported, the evidence for this effect of Dilantin is sparse; therefore the Clinical Epidemiological Branch of the NCI has requested that physicians report cases of neuroblastoma associated with maternal Dilantin use.[255]

DILAUROYL PEROXIDE. *See* Lauroyl Peroxide

DIMETHOATE. An organophosphorous insecticide, it has been used since 1956 as an insecticide and as an acaricide to control agricultural crops and ornamental plants. It is also used as a fly spray in animal quarters. It caused tremors and hyperexcitability when fed to animals. However, pathologic evaluation showed no significant increase in tumors associated with the pesticide, and it was concluded that it did not cause cancer in the experimental animals.[256]

3,3'-DIMETHOXYBENZIDINE-4,4'-DIISOCYANATE. An experimental compound scheduled for use in the manufacture of coatings, gaskets, and shock absorbers, it was fed by stomach tube to rats for 22 weeks, followed by administration in feed to both rats and mice for a period totaling 78 weeks. It proved to be carcinogenic in male and female rats, causing skin and uterine cancers, leukemia, and lymphoma. The study did not provide evidence for carcinogenicity of the compound in mice.[257]

4-DIMETHYLAMINOAZOBENZENE. *Solvent yellow 12, fat yellow, oil yellow, cerasine yellow, DMAB, brilliant fast spirit yellow, methyl yellow, aniline/N-dimethyl-p-(phenylazo), etc.* It is a flaky crystal and has long been used as a dye. It appears to have been virtually eliminated since it was formally identified as a carcinogen. It is still used in cancer research laboratories, although in small quantities. It has been shown to induce tumors in many animals, including dogs, and also in trout. It is a suspected human carcinogen. OSHA has a strict work standard for it.[258]

DIMETHYLBENZANTHRACENE. Used in laboratories because a single dose can cause cancer.[259] It is one of the strongest carcinogens known. *See also* Anthracene.

DIMETHYL SULFATE. *Sulfuric acid, dimethyl ester, dimethyl monosulfate, DMS, methyl sulfate.* Colorless liquid derived from fuming sulfuric acid and methyl alcohol. A strong irritant, it can be absorbed by the skin. May be carcinogenic in humans. Induces tumors in animals. Used as a methylating agent for amines and phenols.[260] Caused tumors when injected under the skin of rats in 200 milligram doses per kilogram of body weight.[261] There is an OSHA standard for air and skin.

2,4-DINITROTOLUENE. An ingredient in explosives and an intermediate in dye manufacture. A test conducted by the NCI, whereby 2,4-dinitrotoluene was given in feed to mice and rats for 78 weeks, found that this compound caused benign tumors in male and female rats. However, the benign tumors were not considered a sufficient basis for establishing carcinogenicity. The test produced no evidence of carcinogenicity in the mice.[262]

p-DIOXANE. *1,3,2-Dioxathiolane; 2-2-dioxide, ethylene glycol; cyclic sulfate.* A solvent for cellulose acetate, ethyl cellulose, and benzyl cellulose resins, oils, waxes, and spirit-solvent dyes, and many other organic as well as some inorganic compounds. It may cause central nervous system depression and necrosis (tissue destruction) of the liver and kidneys. May be irritating to the skin, lungs, and mucous membranes.[263] Caused cancer when given orally to rats in doses of 416 milligrams per kilogram of body weight.[264] An OSHA standard sets safe levels for the air and for the skin of workers.

DIOXIN. A highly toxic chlorinated hydrocarbon that occurs as an impurity in the herbicide 2,4,5-T *(see)* and in Silvex. Most chemicals are toxic at the parts per billion level, but dioxin is toxic at levels as low as 5 parts per million. No safe level of dioxin has yet been established. Dioxin attacks the body's immune system and even alters DNA, the genetic information within a cell. One of the weapons used in the Vietnam War was Agent Orange (a mixture of the herbicides 2,4,-D and 2,4,5,-T), which was contaminated with about 3 to 50 parts per million of dioxin. In June 1977 an employee of the Benefits Section of the Veterans Administration Chicago office learned that a Vietnam veteran was dying of cancer. The veteran's wife said he had been exposed to the pesticide in Vietnam. By February 1978 the employee had put together a list of 30 veterans who had symptoms possibly related to dioxin. When no federal officials would listen to her, she went to television-news people. They interviewed ailing veterans and produced a documentary that vividly illustrated the potential cancer time bomb caused by the herbicide used in Vietnam.[265] Meanwhile, relatively high amounts of dioxin have been discovered in the United States in the fat of cattle that graze on pasturelands sprayed with Agent Orange compound to control weeds. These cattle are being used for food.[266] Ironically, dioxin can be removed by extraction with coconut charcoal. Its half-life (the time required for half the amount of a substance to be eliminated) is about a year. *See also* Agent Orange and 2,4,5-T.

DIPHENYLAMINE. It is an aniline *(see)* derivative but is less toxic than aniline. It is toxic, however, when absorbed through the skin. It is used as a rubber antioxidant and accelerator, in solid rocket propellants; in pesticides, dyes, pharmaceuticals, veterinary medicines; for preservation of apples in storage as a stabilizer for nitrocellulose; in the manufacture of dyes; and when topically applied to animals to prevent screwworms. Caused tumors when administered orally to rats in 14 milligram doses per kilogram of body weight.[267,268]

DIPHENYLS. *(Biphenyls).* Characterized by white scales and a pleasant odor, they are derived from passing benzene *(see)* through red-hot iron tubes or by heating bromo and sodium. They are toxic. Used as fungistats in packaging citrus fruit (applied to box or to wrappers) to control plant disease, in the manufacture of benzidine *(see)*, and in dyeing polyesters. The hazards of diphenyls are not really well known. Those that contain chlorine may cause a skin reaction similar to acne. They are of great environmental concern because, like DDT, they are very stable and remain in the environment for a long time. They may have long-lasting effects on birds, fish, and other animals. Scientists have found that they cause cancer in some laboratory animals, and there is concern that they will have the same effect on people.[269]

DIPROPYLAMINE, *N*-NITROSO. An intermediate *(see)* in organic synthesis, it causes tumors when fed to rats in doses of 1,150 milligrams per kilogram of body weight and it causes cancer when injected under the skin in 143 milligram doses per kilogram of body weight.[270]

DIRECT BLACK 38. *Also known as Aizen direct deep black, Atlantic black, benzo deep black, C.I. direct black 38, carbide black, chloramine black, chrome leather black, diacotton deep black, and diamine deep black.* Derived from benzidine, a known human carcinogen, the dye is used in textiles, paper, and leather: it is estimated that 25 percent of the benzidine-derived azo dyes *(see)* are applied to textiles, 40 percent to paper, 15 percent to leather, and the remainder to other diverse materials. Direct black 38 is used for dyeing or staining of wool, silk fibers, rope and matting, hogs hair, cellulose, acetate, nylon, and biological stains.

Cancerous and precancerous liver conditions were found in rats fed these dyes, similar to the damage produced by known liver carcinogens. Degeneration of liver cells was found in mice. Although the dyes tested by the NCI contained less than 4 parts per million residual benzidine when fed to the test animals, greater quantities of benzidine than this initial amount were found in the urine of dosed rats and mice. Preliminary results of NIOSH field studies show that humans working with these same dyes also excrete higher than expected levels of benzidine in their urine. Both laboratory and field studies indicate that these benzidine-derived dyes can be metabolized to benzidine, which is present in the urine of animals and humans. Based on the data from the short-term study, NCI scientists believe a cancer-causing potential exists upon exposure to the benzidine-derived dyes, most likely through the mechanism of metabolic conversion of the dyes to benzidine in the animal system; they suggest minimum exposure of employees to these dyes.[271]

A strong association relating human exposure to benzidine-based dyes with the subsequent development of bladder tumors was presented after a case-control mortality study of 200 bladder-cancer patients in Japan. The patients were found to have been predominantly kimono painters and dyers. The kimono painters had the habit of forming a point on their brushes by drawing the brush between their lips, which is how they ingested the dyes. Several other case-control mortality studies indicate an increased risk of developing bladder cancer in the textile and leather industries, both large users of direct dyes. In Russia, a medical study concerning the early detection of bladder tumors among textile workers using benzidine-derived dyes found an unusual incidence of bladder lesions, some of which were suggested as being of a precancerous nature. The greatest number of such lesions were found in those workers with the highest potential exposure to these dyes.

DIRECT BLUE 6. Also known as *Airedale blue, aizen direct blue, Atlantic blue, belamine blue, benzanil blue, calcomine blue, chrome leather blue, C.I. direct blue 6, diamine blue, diazol blue, fenamin blue, fixanol blue, Kayaku direct blue, Mitsui direct blue, napthtamine blue, Niagara blue, Nippon blue, paramine blue, pontamine blue, and vondacel blue.* Used in dyeing or staining silk, wool, cotton, nylon, leather, paper, biological stains, and writing inks. *See also* Direct Black 38 for cancer-causing effects.

DIRECT BROWN 95. Also known as *aizen primula brown, amanil fast brown, Atlantic fast brown, benzanil supra brown, C.I. direct brown, chloramine fast brown, chrome leather brown, dermafix brown, diazol light brown, fastusol brown, pontamine fast brown, pyrazol fast brown, Sirius brown, Saturn brown, solius light brown, tetramine fast brown, and triantine light brown.* A benzidine-derived dye, used in dyeing or staining silk, cotton, acetate, cellulose, wool, nylon, leather, paper, and certain plastics. *See also* Direct Black 38 for cancer-causing effects.

DISULFIRAM. It is used in the treatment of alcoholics: when a patient who had taken this drug drinks alcohol, he suffers flushing, throbbing head and neck, respiratory difficulty, nausea, copious vomiting, shortness of breath, hyperventilation, palpitations, weakness, vertigo, blurred vision, confusion, and sometimes congestive heart failure and even death. Disulfiram has also been found to decrease the rate at which certain drugs are metabolized and so may increase the blood levels and the possibility of chemical toxicity of drugs given concomitantly. It was discovered that a hazard is also present when people on this drug are exposed to potential carcinogens. Workers taking disulfiram for alcoholism and then exposed to EDB, ethylene dibromide *(see)*, are felt to be in danger. Studies by OSHA in 1977 found that experimental animals exposed to both disulfiram and EDB developed a high rate of malignant tumors. The number of persons receiving disulfiram therapy who are exposed to substantial doses of EDB must be assumed to be small, but the importance of the interaction between the chemicals causing malignant tumors serves as a warning to millions of American workers who are exposed to chemicals both at the workplace and while they are taking prescribed drugs.[273] *See also* Ethylene Dibromide.

2,5-DITHIOBIUREA. A component of photographic chemicals, it was fed to rats and mice for 78 weeks. The test results suggested a carcinogenic effect in female mouse livers but were not statistically significant when compared with the incidences of liver cancer observed in the past in non-dosed animals of this strain. The compound did not prove carcinogenic in male mice or in rats of either sex under NCI test conditions.[274]

D-LACTOSE. *See* Lactose.

DMBA. *See* Dimethylbenzanthracene.

DOCA (DEOXYCORTICOSTERONE ACETATE). *11 Deoxycorticosterone, cortesan, acetate.* An adrenal cortical steroid hormone active in causing the retention of salt and water by the kidney. Derived from adrenal-cortex extract and from other steroids, it has been used as a medicine in adrenocortical insufficiency. Causes cancer when injected under the skin of mice in 480 milligram doses per kilogram of body weight.[275]

DODECANE. *1,2-Epoxy.* This colorless liquid is used as a solvent in organic synthesis and also in jet-fuel research. It caused cancer when inhaled by mice in 150 milligram doses per kilogram of body weight.[276]

DULCIN. *p-Phenetylurea.* White needles or crystals with a taste about 200 times as sweet as sugar. Derived from para-aminophenol. Because it was demonstrated to produce liver cancer in tests and to be toxic in other ways, it was never placed on the market.[277]

DUSTS (TEXTILE INDUSTRY). The dustiest part of the process is the cleaning of raw fibers. Raw wool, for instance, may contain up to 55 percent nonfibrous material. The dust is removed from the wool and raw cotton by beating and crushing it into fine particles that are shaken out and blown or sucked away. Cancers of the tongue, mouth, and throat were found to be common among textile workers in one British study: about three times higher than in the general population.[278]

DYES. Consumers usually do not know what dye is used in a food, cosmetic, or household product, and yet colorings are among the most frequently suspected and proven cancer-causing agents. Most of the artificial colors on the market are coal-tar derivatives; that is, they were originally made from coal tar and are now manufactured from chemicals identical in structure to the original compounds. The United States has banned 12 coal-tar derivative dyes since 1919. The 11 still on the market are also suspect. Five of those banned were found to cause cancer. Most of the coal-tar dyes have been shown to cause cancer in animals. In 1938 Congress exempted coal-tar dyes from the FDA's Food, Drug and Cosmetics Act. While the dyes could not meet safety standards, Congressmen said they should be sold to meet popular demand.

On December 12, 1977, the FDA announced a ban on 5 colorings used in soaps and cosmetics because they contained carcinogens. None of the 5 had been approved for use in food. Four of the dyes were reds nos. 10, 11, 12, and 13; these were used in lipsticks, rouge, face powder, nail polishes, and hand lotions. The fifth, yellow no. 1, was used to color soap. A sixth color, direct blue no. 6 *(see)*, which also had been used in the same cosmetics as the reds, was banned for all uses except as a color in identifying surgical sutures. As studies of dyes continue, more and more are found to be potentially carcinogenic. The problem is that dye workers in particular and the public at large have been exposed to these cancer-causing agents —most of which everyone could well do without—for many years. *See also* Coal Tar, Hair Coloring, Direct Black 38, FD & C Colors, and Azo Dyes.

DYES, HAIR. *See* Hair Coloring.

EDB. *See* Ethylene Dibromide.

EDC. *See* Ethylene Dichloride.

ELECTROMAGNETIC RADIATION. This is a term that includes all kinds of ionizing radiation and nonionizing radiation. The electromagnetic radiation (EMR) emitted by all our uses of electricity may be slowly killing us, much as atomic radiation would. The problem has been growing so rapidly in the last two decades that the skies over our large cities have become literally choked with electromagnetic radiation. Electricity does leak. Wherever it flows through wires, whether high-voltage lines or the wiring in your home, it generates radio-frequency electromagnetic fields that extend far beyond the wire itself. Wherever it flows through complex circuitry, as in your television set or stereo equipment, a wide range of such radio-frequency energies may be emitted. The most common sources of electronic radiation are things run by electric motors. These include such everyday items as automobile motors, elevators, power lawn mowers, electric trains, air-conditioners, washing machines, hair dryers, garbage disposals, and dishwashers.

There is also a danger in microwaves, whose sources include microwave ovens, TV sets, stereo equipment, CB radio transmitters, soldering irons, telephones and their wiring, and electrical wiring. Recent studies show that even small doses of microwave radiation can have lethal and perhaps cumulative effects—each exposure doing a permanent bit of genetic damage to your body's cells. When genetic material is mutilated or destroyed, it does not merely disappear. Damaged organ or brain cells remain, weakening the whole living organism. Furthermore, a study conducted by the CIA indicates that EMR exposure—at a dosage deemed safe by U.S. Public Health Service—can cause chromosome breaks, genetic damage, that is likely to cause mutations in unborn children, abnormal development in young children, and cancer in people of all ages. Other effects of EMR, even at low levels, are altered heartbeat and biorhythms, convulsions and disorientation, and altered chemical composition of the blood.[279,280] *See also* Microwaves.

ELURA. *See* Acrylonitrile.

EMETINE. An anticancer drug and an amebicide used to treat severe amebic intestinal infections of the liver, lungs, brain, skin, and other tissues. Results of a NCI study did not provide sufficient information to determine its carcinogenicity.[281]

EMOTION. There is a modest body of research that links psychological stress and certain emotional characteristics to cancer. Psychological profiles of cancer victims show them to be generally low-gear people, little given to expression of emotion, whose relationships with their parents had been much more cold and remote than those of individuals who developed other diseases. A theory has been put forth that smokers who get cancer have different personalities from the general population of smokers who tend to score high on neuroticism. The more repressed the individual, the fewer cigarettes it took to induce cancer. In other studies, inappropriate coping with anger—usually suppression but sometimes extreme expression—was correlated with the discovery of breast malignancy and lung cancer. Patients with leukemia and Hodgkin's disease were also tested, and it was found that their illness occurred in a setting of emotional distress. In 9 out of 10 cases the disease developed during a time when they felt alone, helpless, and hopeless. It has also been found that cancer specialists, themselves, get more cancer than other doctors. Presumably it is because they establish close interpersonal relationships with their patients and have a tremendous emotional commitment to their work.

Emotions also affect recovery from cancer, according to studies in the field. Among patients successfully operated on for malignant melanoma in stages I and II, those who relapsed tended to minimize the significance of their illness. This supports the theory that repression and denial and the lack of an emotional outlet are related to poor prognosis. It was also discovered that women who expressed a high degree of anger toward not only their disease, but their doctors, lived longer than those who were pliant and cooperative. Doctors found that women who were good at externalizing negative feelings did better, even though that group had, if anything, a poorer prognosis than those who succumbed quickly. Fighters had a better chance. Emotions and hormones are intertwined. Therefore, it is reasonable that emotions could alter hormones and thus alter the course of certain cancers. Of particular interest to psychiatrists is the suspicion cast on the hypothalamus gland in view of its close relationship with central mechanisms concerned with emotions. Its relay-feedback system with all the endocrine glands may during development of cancer endow secretions with a relevance far beyond their immediate effects on the body. In view of the solid relationship between the hypothalamus and ovulation and the mounting clinical and experimental evidence linking ovarian function to mammary tumors, the theory that one's emotional makeup affects cancer makes sense. The immune status of the host appears to be crucial to the outcome of the battle between those forces promoting and those working against the onset of cancer. The probability that carcinogenesis could be affected by psychic factors working via hormones and the immune response is thus very good.[282,283,284]

ENDOMETRIAL CANCER.   Cancer of the uterus. The most common symptom is vaginal bleeding after menopause. The disease can be detected in about two-thirds of the cases by the use of the Pap smear. Another test, the Gravelee, is considered more accurate because it washes out cells from the inside of the uterus. Early cases are highly curable by surgery and radiotherapy. Long-term estrogen therapy has been correlated with the development of endometrial cancer. Supportive data for the estrogen-cancer hypothesis is substantial, and although further analysis is necessary, it is certainly difficult to discount. The incidence of endometrial cancer is higher in young women who fail to ovulate or who have ovarian tumors. It is, however, most common in postmenopausal women. Repeated studies have revealed that women with endometrial cancer appeared to show a greater prevalence for obesity, childlessness, infertility, and dysfunctional bleeding than patients with other neoplasms of the uterus, or with matched controls. These are all conditions in which estrogen may constantly stimulate the uterus without being neutralized by progesterone (see). Progesterone is ordinarily present when the normal cycling woman ovulates. Reports of therapeutic benefit with progestagens in patients with advanced endometrial cancer and evidence of reversibility of adenomatous hyperplasia (a usually benign tumor) and carcinoma in situ of the endometrium (an incipient and symptomless form of cancer) again point up an endocrine trigger. With the advent of better steroid technology, it has already been demonstrated that postmenopausal women with cancer of the endometrium, especially those who are fat, can convert an adrenal steroid, androstenedione, to estrogen, at a greater rate than the controls. Epidemiologic studies have confirmed that estrogen may act as a stimulant to dormant seedlings in the endometrium, perhaps encouraging them to grow into true cancer. Most striking is the finding that women given DES (see) in early pregnancy have adolescent female offspring who now show a high incidence of changes in the cervix and vagina and a small incidence of adenocarcinoma of the vagina. These conditions are almost unknown in adolescent patients without a history of maternal ingestion of estrogen in pregnancy. Furthermore, a small group of young women with Turner's syndrome have recently been found to develop endometrial cancer following estrogen therapy to stimulate growth of their secondary sex characteristics. And recently there have been several reports of women taking sequential oral contraceptives who have developed cancer of the endometrium at a relatively young age, a rare occurrence.

The increased risk of endometrial cancers in women receiving estrogen is related to the duration of estrogen use, progressing from no evidence of risk among those using the hormone for less than 5 years to an 11.5-fold increased risk for those using the hormone for 10 years or more. Strength of medication also affects risk. The relative risk of 1.25 milligram tablets was 12.7 compared with a two- to fourfold risk in users of lesser strength tablets.

Accepting the conclusion that the risk of endometrial cancer is increased by long-term estrogen therapy in postmenopausal women, the following guidelines have been recommended:

• Women who require estrogen to control flushes or atrophic (thinning of tissue) vaginitis (a minority of menopausal women) can be given estrogens safely on a short-term basis under medical supervision.
• The prophylactic use of estrogens for all postmenopausal women to

preserve youth, for cosmetic effect, or for the prevention of coronary disease is without evidence and not justified.

- The use of estrogen for the prevention of osteoporosis (the loss of bony substance resulting in brittleness or softness of the bones), while it may play a role, clearly involves a greater risk than diet or exercise that also play a role.

The current vogue of estrogen therapy to keep postmenopausal women "young" and vigorous is based on a myth that has sadly been dispelled for those women who now have endometrial cancer.[285,286,287]

ENDOMETRIUM. The tissue lining the uterus.

ENDOSULFAN. A crop pesticide. It was given in feed to rats and mice for periods between 74 and 82 weeks. According to a summary of the report, endosulfan was not carcinogenic in female rats and female mice under test conditions. In male rodents of both species conclusions could not be drawn because it caused a high rate of early deaths.[288]

ENU. *Ethyl nitroso-urea. See* Urea, Methyl Nitroso.

EPA. Environmental Protection Agency. *See* Introduction, page 12.

EPICHLOROHYDRIN. A modifier for food starches that the FDA permits to be used up to a level of 0.3 percent in starch. It is also used as a solvent for cosmetic resins and nitrocellulose and in the manufacture of varnishes, lacquers, and cements for celluloid articles. A colorless liquid with an odor resembling chloroform, it is a strong skin irritant. There may be 50,000 workers exposed to epichlorohydrin, according to OSHA. The current agency exposure limit is 5 parts per million during an eight-hour period. NIOSH recommended a limit of 0.5 ppm in 1976.[289] A two-year study of 864 workers who had been exposed to the substance for six months or more before January 1966 showed an increase in the incidence of cancer.[290]

EPOXY RESINS. These substances are made from organic compounds that contain an oxygen atom combined with two other atoms, usually carbons. Epichlorohydrin and ethylene oxide are two widely used epoxides (*see* both). They are used in flame-retardant materials; in surface coatings; on household appliances and gas-storage vessels; in adhesives for metals, glass, and ceramics; in casting metal-forming tools; in the encapsulating of electric parts; in floor surfacing and wall panels; in neutron-shielding materials; in cements and mortars; in nonskid road surfacing; in rigid foams; and for stained-glass windows. According to the Royal Danish School of Pharmacy's report in *Nature,* November 23, 1978, human exposure to epoxy resins must be minimized to "prevent cancer and genetic damage." The investigators found that three aromatic epoxy resins all caused mutations in bacteria tests. Previous studies have shown that simple epoxides also cause mutations are are therefore suspected carcinogens.[291]

ESOPHAGEAL CANCER. Males make up about 70 percent of esophageal cancer victims. More than 90 percent of them either have very poor teeth or false teeth. The majority—75 percent—are big consumers of alcohol and heavy smokers of pipes, cigars, or cigarettes. Also patients who have had a cancer of the mouth—tongue or floor of the mouth, gum or upper pharynx—are likely to have a second cancer in the esophagus. Cancer elsewhere in the gastrointestinal (GI) tract—usually the colon—is also common in combination with esophageal cancer. In addition, esophageal cancer has been found to be very common in certain parts of the world. A vast area of high incidence extends from the Middle East to China and includes Iran, Afghanistan, Soviet Central Asia, parts of Siberia, Mongolia, and northern and western China. In northern and western China incidence of esophageal cancer is remarkably high, as is a similar cancer found in the gullets of the chickens bred in this area. The chicken and human tumors are analogous. The chickens are fed with table scraps, pointing strongly to something common in the peoples' diet. These Chinese eat a dish consisting of chopped willow leaves, sweet potatoes, sesame seeds, turnip greens, and some spices. They boil the dish for a while, and then the vegetables stay in large earthen pots for as long as six months, eventually developing a fungus. The preparation of the dish is highly suspect, especially since Nitrosamines *(see)* were found in the food as well. The *Chinese Medical Journal* said the tests showed that a combination of the nitrosamines and the mold produced precancerous cells in chicken. Chinese party members are working to upgrade water quality and improve food-drying techniques to prevent molds and are discouraging eating of this dish. But because esophageal cancer, like other cancers, has a latency period as long as 30 years, it is not expected that the rate of this cancer will decline in the near future. By manipulating the chickens' diet, they hope to erase gullet cancer soon in chickens, at least.[292,293,294,295]

ESOPHAGUS. The passageway between the throat and the stomach.

ESTRADIOL. *Diogyn, femogen, gynergon, ovocyclin, progynon.* A female sex hormone that occurs in two forms, alpha and beta. Beta estradiol has the greatest physiological activity of any naturally occurring estrogen. The alpha form is relatively inactive. Isolated from human and mare pregnancy urine. Commercial synthesis is from cholesterol or ergosterol. Estradiol mustard is used as a chemotherapeutic agent but has been reported to cause lung tumors in mice.[296]

ESTRIOL. *Destriol, thulol, oestriol.* White, odorless, microcrystalline powder isolated from the human placenta. It is a comparatively weak estrogen, a by-product of estradiol *(see).* There seems to be a protective factor in pregnancy that prevents neoplastic transformation in mammary cells, especially when pregnancy occurs at an early age. This factor may be estriol. The incidence of breast cancer, especially in the postmenopausal age group, is known to be strikingly lower among Japanese and Chinese women living in Asia than it is among blacks and whites living in North America. Second generation Orientals in Hawaii or the mainland United States show an incidence intermediate between that found in the Orient and that of whites. This suggests that in addition to a genetic factor some influence of the environment or life-style must be involved. It has been determined that Oriental women in Asia have a greater amount of estriol in their urine. Whether estriol itself actually exerts a protective effect against malignant transformation of cells, or whether people who have an increased amount in their urine have a lower risk because of some fundamental difference in overall metabolic pattern, remains to be determined. In any case, the apparent correlation of estriol-excretion pattern with breast-cancer risk and the observation that estriol proportion and breast-cancer incidence are subject to concomitant alteration as ethnic groups change their environment emphasize the importance of further investigations of the influence of estriol on induction of breast cancer.[1]

Estriol is said to relieve the symptoms of the menopause without inducing the overproduction of cells, while still having a beneficial effect on cervical mucus and vaginal tissue. Since estriol is a weak estrogen, it apparently does not induce endometrial proliferation of cells or breakthrough bleeding while it modifies menopausal symptoms, according to a study of 52 symptomatic postmenopausal women studied at the Medical College of Georgia. The drug is available in Europe but has not been marketed in the United States because of problems raised by the fact that dosages of estriol required for the relief of menopausal symptoms vary considerably.[297] *See also* Estrogen.

ESTROGEN. Millions of women are taking estrogen, a female hormone, either in oral contraceptives or as a replacement therapy after menopause. The term "estrogen" defines a class of substances that produce estrus or "heat" in animals and that cause the growth of the uterus and cornification of the vaginal epithelium (conversion of vaginal tissue into a horny substance) in many animals and in humans. Estradiol and estrone (*see* both) are the important estrogens produced by women. The use of estrogen during or after menopause has been linked with cancer of the endometrium, the lining of the uterus. Studies have shown that women taking estrogen for menopausal symptoms have roughly 5 to 10 times as great a chance of developing cancer as women who take no estrogens. These findings are supported by the observation that the incidence rates of endometrial cancer have increased sharply since 1969 in eight different areas of the United States with population-based cancer reporting systems, an increase which may be related to the rapidly expanding use of estrogens during the past decade. The risk of uterine cancer increases with the duration of estrogen use and seems to be greater when larger doses are taken. In addition, one study has suggested that use of the menopausal estrogen may increase the risk of breast cancer 10 to 15 years after it is first ingested. Particularly high breast-cancer risk was noted in estrogen users who had benign breast disease. Estrogen use during early pregnancy may seriously harm the offspring as the now infamous case of the DES *(see)* daughters attest. Their mothers took the synthetic estrogen during pregnancy, and years later the daughters developed cancer. Scientists have no direct evidence that oral contraceptives further enhance a DES-exposed daughter's risk of cancer. However, since such enhancement has some basis in theory, DES daughters should choose other methods of birth control. Laboratory studies have shown that when certain animals are given estrogen for long periods, cancers may develop in the breast, cervix, vagina, and liver. Although scientists have no conclusive evidence that cancer is being caused by estrogens taken today, one study has suggested that oral contraceptives have increased the risk of breast cancer in women with benign breast disease (noncancerous nodules or cysts), and other studies have found an increased rate of early cervical cancer in groups of women with noncancerous cervical dysplasia (abnormality).

There is no evidence at present that "natural" estrogens are more or less hazardous than "synthetic" estrogens. What is certain is that through the promise of certain birth control and the hope of "eternal youth," estrogen sales quadrupled in this country between 1962 and 1973 and today are an $80 million per year industry. There is now sufficient evidence to refute the claims that estrogens prevent the progress of arteriosclerosis, and in fact, coronary artery disease may even be accelerated by lipid changes brought about by estrogens. There is also doubt about estrogen preventing or ameliorating osteoporosis (loss of bony substance resulting in brittleness or softness of the bone), and there is no evidence at all that estrogens retard aging. Therefore, before they take estrogens, women should undergo a careful examination to uncover any latent or existing conditions—liver disease, suspicion of early breast or uterine cancer, heart disease—which would preclude this hormone being prescribed. When indicated, estrogens should be taken in as low a dose as possible for as short a time as possible. A woman taking estrogens should be examined every 6 to 12 months for any evidence of side effects. And most important, any abnormal bleeding should be, reported to the doctor immediately. Once the decision is made to discontinue estrogen treatment, it should be reduced gradually to minimize the recurrence of the symptoms that necessitated estrogen use.[298,299,300,301] *See also* The Pill, Progestogen, Hormones, Estradiol, and Estrone.

ESTRONE. A steroid with some estrogenic activity. It consists of small white crystals or white crystalline powder and is odorless, stable in air, insoluble in water, and soluble in alcohol, acetone, dioxane, and in solutions of fixed alkali hydroxide. Used as hormone therapy for menopausal women.

ETHANE,1,1,1-TRICHLORO-2,2-BIS (p-CHLOROPHENYL)-. *See* DDT.

1,2 ETHANEDIOL. *See* Ethylene Glycol.

ETHANOL. *See* Ethyl Alcohol.

ETHANOL,2-HYDRAZING. *See* 2-Hydrazinoethanol.

ETHER, BIS (2-CHLOROMETHYL). *See* Bis (2-Chloromethyl) Ether.

ETHER, CHLOROMETHYL METHYL. *Chloromethyl methyl ether.* Used in resins, it is a known carcinogen. It caused cancer when injected under the skin of mice in doses of 312 milligrams per kilogram of body weight.[302] There is an OSHA standard for it.

ETHER,2,4-DICHLOROPHENYL p-NITROPHENYL-. *See* Nitrofen.

ETHIONINE. Prepared from ethanethiol and acrolein, it is toxic in the liver, pancreas, and other tissues of several rodent species. Chronic feeding of this chemical to rats caused a high incidence of liver cancer among them. Ethionine is the metabolite of several bacteria, including *E. coli* and is in the stomach contents and milk of ruminants.[303] *See also* Bacteria.

ETHYL ALCOHOL. *Absolute ethanol, algrain, ethyl hydrate, grain alcohol.* Contains ethanol, grain alcohol, and neutral spirits. It is used as a solvent in beverages, ices, ice cream, candy, baked goods, liquors, and gelatin desserts. It is rapidly dissolved through the gastric and intestinal mucosa after ingestion. The fatal dose in adults is considered to be one and one-half to two pints of whisky (40 to 55 percent ethyl alcohol). It was approved in 1976 for use in pizza crusts to extend handling and storage life. It causes cancer when inserted in the rectum of mice in doses of 548 milligrams per kilogram of body weight, and it causes tumors when given orally to mice in 2,770 milligram doses per kilogram of body weight.[304]

P,P'-ETHYL-DDD. *See* Perthane.

1-ETHYL-1,2,5,6-DIBENZACRIDINE. *See* Acridine.

ETHYLENEBISDITHIOCARBAMATE. (EBDC). *Manganese (ethylenebis) (dithiocarbamate), Dithane.* An agricultural fungicide based on the salts of ethylene bisdithiocarbamate. Supplied in zinc, magnesium, and sodium forms as a powder. Caused cancer when ingested by rats in doses of 64 milligrams per kilogram of body weight and when injected in 50 milligram doses per kilogram of body weight.[305]

ETHYLENE CHLORO. *See* Vinyl Chloride.

ETHYLENE CHLOROHYDRIN. A colorless liquid with a faint sweet odor that is used as a solvent for cellulose acetate and ethyl cellulose, to activate sprouting of dormant potatoes, and in the manufacture of ethylene oxide and ethylene glycol. It is toxic when ingested or inhaled, and skin absorption may be fatal. It is also a strong irritant. Some major cosmetic manufacturers had to reformulate several shampoos and conditioners because quantities of ethylene chlorohydrin were found in the final mix. The manufacturer of the conditioning agent used in the beauty products ceased production of two ingredients, quaternium 16 and amphoteric 8, because of traces of ethylene chlorohydrin. The dilution of the ingredients probably did away with any danger, but the scientific community has noted that some experiments have suggested ethylene chlorohydrin may be a carcinogen. **ETHYLENEDIAMINETETRAACETATIC ACID (EDTA).** A sequestrant in carbonated beverages, EDTA salts are used in crab meat to promote color retention. It is also used in some dressings. A chelating agent (to bind and precipitate metals in a solution), EDTA may cause errors in a number of laboratory tests including those for calcium, carbon dioxide, nitrogen, and muscular activity. The trisodium salt of EDTA was fed to rats and mice for nearly two years. According to a summary of the report included in the announcement: "Although a variety of tumors occurred among test and control animals of both species, the test did not indicate that any of the tumors observed in the test animals were attributable to EDTA." The tests were part of the NCI's Carcinogenesis Bioassay Program.[306]

ETHYLENE DIBROMIDE (EDB). *1,2-Dibromoethane.* A colorless nonflammable liquid with a sweetish taste, it is widely used as a lead scavenger in leaded fuels. It is also used as a fumigant (insecticide or nematocide), as a synthetic intermediate *(see)*, and it is contained in numerous pesticides. EDB is a severe skin irritant and can produce blistering. Early reports included one death from inadvertent use of EDB as an anesthetic in place of ethylene bromide. Autopsy revealed extensive degeneration of the heart, liver, and kidneys. Another death from ingestion of 4.5 milligrams of EDB in capsule form resulted mainly from kidney and liver damage. Occupational-exposure inhalation has been noted to cause severe eye and throat irritation, headache, depression, and loss of appetite. Volunteers submitting to skin exposure of the forearm demonstrated that EDB is absorbed by skin and causes tissue death, general inflammation, plasma exudation, and allergic sensitization. A serious toxic interaction between inhaled EDB and ingested disulfiram (a chemical in Antabuse and other drugs given to combat alcoholism) caused high death rates in test animals.

EDB was selected for testing by the NCI because of its potential for extensive human exposure. It is produced in large quantities and its principal means of exposure is through inhalation of automobile emissions. Occupational exposures may include gas-station workers, agricultural and grain-storage workers, workers in oil refineries, and those who work in plants producing EDB. EDB is also used as a soil fumigant for a number of food crops, including grains, fruits, and vegetables; and it has been used for disinfecting fruits, vegetables, grains, tobacco, and seeds in storage. It is also used in the manufacture of dyes and drugs.

In the NCI tests, 50 male and 50 female animals of each of 2 rodent species were used. They were fed EDB mixed with corn oil by stomach tube. Although the study was originally scheduled to last 110 weeks for rats and 90 weeks for mice, all groups of dosed animals were terminated early because of excessive death rates. Early development of stomach cancer was a major reason for the deaths. All surviving dosed male rats were sacrificed in week 49, and females in week 61. In mice, the study was terminated in week 78. Stomach cancers occurred in 90 percent of the low-dose male rats, 80 percent of low-dose females, 66 percent of high-dose males, and 58 percent of high-dose females. No stomach cancers were found among control groups. Rats also had increased rates of liver cancers and cancer-related liver nodules, particularly in high-dose females. A blood-vessel cancer, particularly in the spleen, was found in male rats. In mice, stomach cancers were found in 59 percent of high-dose males, 56 percent of high-dose females, 90 percent of low-dose males, and 94 percent of low-dose females. Lung cancers also developed at significant rates in both male and female mice.

In 1973, the latest figures available, 149 million kilograms of EDB were being produced.[307]

ETHYLENE DICHLORIDE (EDC). *1,2-Dichloroethane, ethylene chloride.* Derived from the action of chlorine on ethylene, it is used in the manufacture of vinyl chloride *(see)*; as a solvent for fats, waxes, and resins; as a lead scavenger in antiknock gasolines; in paint, varnish, and finish removers; metal degreasing; soaps and scouring compounds; as a soil and crop fumigant; as a wetting and penetrating agent; in organic synthesis; in ore flotation; and in the making of polyvinyl chloride (PVC) plastic. There is considerable exposure to this compound in the workplace, and it also has been found as a contaminant in water and air. Because EDC is used as a soil and crop fumigant, agricultural workers are exposed to it. The general population may also be exposed through contamination of grain and food, through inhaling gasoline or exhaust fumes, and through contaminated water supplies. EDC also is used as an ingredient in cosmetics and as a food additive. It is highly toxic and potentially lethal when inhaled in large doses. EDC is a colorless, oily liquid with a chloroformlike odor. It is a source chemical from which other chemicals are made. EDC was rated in the *Condensed Chemical Dictionary* as the sixteenth highest-volume chemical produced in 1975. Production is now estimated at about 10 billion pounds annually in the United States and the EPA has projected an increase of 4 percent per year through 1979. According to NIOSH, about 2 million workers are exposed annually in the United States. The EPA estimates about 163 million pounds of EDC were lost into the environment through emissions in 1974. The chemical was detected in 26 percent of the water samples taken near heavily industrialized areas, some samples had as much as 90 parts per billion.

EDC can be highly toxic whether taken into the body by ingestion, inhalation, or skin absorption. Acute poisoning may cause headache, dizziness, feelings of drunkenness, loss of consciousness, internal bleeding, and death. Repeated exposures can bring on nausea, vomiting, stomach pain, irritated mucous membranes, loss of appetite, liver and kidney failure, and possible death. Numerous cases of EDC poisoning, both fatal and nonfatal, have been documented by NIOSH. EDC has been found in human milk and in the exhaled breath of nursing mothers who were exposed to the chemical. In carcinogenesis testing by the NCI, this compound caused stomach cancers, vascularized (bloody) cancers of multiple organs, and cancers beneath the skin in male rats. Female rats exposed to EDC developed mammary cancers—in some high-dose animals as early as the twentieth week of the study. The chemical also caused breast cancers as well as uterine cancers in female mice and respiratory-tract cancers in both male and female mice.[308]

ETHYLENE GLYCOL. *Ethylene dihydrate glycol.* A slightly viscous liquid with a sweet taste, it absorbs twice its weight in water. It is used as an antifreeze and humectant (substance that helps retain moisture), also as a solvent. It is toxic when ingested and causes central nervous system depression, vomiting, and drowsiness, coma, respiratory failure, and kidney damage.[309] Caused tumors when painted on the skin of mice.[310]

ETHYLENE OXIDE. *Epoxyethane oxirane.* The twenty-sixth highest volume chemical produced in the United States, it is a colorless gas at room temperature. Derived from the oxidation of ethylene in air or oxygen with a silver catalyst, it is highly flammable. It is used in the manufacture of ethylene glycol *(see)* and higher alcohols, surfactants, acrylonitrile, ethanolamines, petroleum demulsifiers, fumigants for foodstuffs and textiles, and rocket propellants; and it is also used as an industrial sterilant for medical plastic tubing and to sterilize surgical instruments. In 1978 the EPA placed ethylene oxide's future as a medical sterilant on the benefit-against-risk scale because of its mutagenic properties. Two major reaction products of ethylene oxide, ethylene chlorohydrin and ethylene glycol, both cancer-causing suspects, were found in the sterilized tubing along with the ethylene oxide. The EPA said that the FDA is aware of the local and systemic toxic effects of ethylene oxide but that many products cannot be sterilized by other means without degrading or otherwise damaging them.[311] In the March 16, 1979 issue of the *Journal of the American Medical Association*, two Swedish physicians specializing in Occupational Medicine reported leukemia in workers exposed to ethylene oxide. The three cases of leukemia occurred between 1972 and 1977 among workers in a small technical factory in Sweden where 50 percent ethylene oxide and 50 percent methyl formate had been used since 1968 for sterilizing hospital equipment.

ETHYLENE THIOUREA. *See* ETU.

ETHYLENIMINE (EI). *Azirane, azacyclopropane, aziridine, dimethylenimine, dihydroazirine, etc.* It is a liquid with an intense odor of ammonia that is used in the paper and textile industries for a wide variety of processes, including wet-strength flameproofing, processing fuel oil and lubricants, shrinkproofing, stiffening, and waterproofing. In lesser amounts, it is used in the manufacture of nonpersistent herbicides, and resins, as well as in the production of drugs and rocket and jet fuels. The only known producer in the United States makes about 10 million pounds a year. Ninety percent of this is converted into polyethylenimine and 5 percent is exported. It caused cancer in mice when given orally in 235 milligram doses per kilogram of body weight and in rats when given by injection in 20 milligram doses per kilogram of body weight. It is poisonous and highly flammable. OSHA has standards for workers involved in the processing, handling, release, or storage of substances containing more than one percent ethylenimine.[312]

ETHYLNITROSOUREA. A compound with no commercial uses, it is employed experimentally as a cancer-causing agent. It reacts easily in an animal's body with ingested precurser compounds, and this leads to tumors in animals and their offspring. The mechanism by which it causes tumors remains obscure. When given to young monkeys two or three years after the study began, in 8 of the 13 animals tumors had developed. Then the chemical was given to pregnant monkeys beginning at 30 days gestation, either throughout pregnancy or for a total of 12 injections. Tumors developed in 2 infant monkeys in each category in the first year of postnatal life. One of them had a tumor at birth. Jerry M. Rice, Ph.D., of the Experimental Pathology Branch of the NCI, who conducted the experiments, said that the most striking finding was that all of the tumors seen in the newborn monkeys to date result from transplacental exposure to the carcinogen just following the first month of pregnancy. This is the period at which organogenesis is complete, when teratogens (substances that produce monsters) are most likely to have deleterious effects, and during which pregnancy may not yet be obvious.

Dr. Rice and his colleagues are continuing their observation of the monkeys whose pregnant mothers received ethylnitrosourea to find out if tumors will develop later in their 20-year life-span. The compound is a direct-acting carcinogen, meaning that no enzyme-mediated activation is needed to make it carcinogenic.[313]

ETU 2-IMIDAZOLIDINETHIONE. *Ethylene thiourea.* Cancer-causing ETU, a contaminant and breakdown product of some widely used fungicides, can contaminate plants, whether sprayed onto leaves or mixed in the soil. Readily translocated from roots to leaves, ETU persists for as long as two weeks. For this reason the fungicides called ethylenebisdithiocarbamates (EBDC), important for 30 years, should not be applied to crops two weeks before harvest. Of greater concern may be the subsequent and continuing degradation on crops of longer-lasting parent fungicides to ETU. When ETU is given in large doses it has been shown to be carcinogenic in rats, tumorigenic in mice, and teratogenic (fetus-deforming) in rats and mice. Reports have shown that cooked spinach contained more of the cancer-causing chemical than the corresponding raw spinach: an inadvertent addition to food of a carcinogen caused by the breakdown of remaining fungicide when heated. A heat-caused degradation product of widely used EBDC fungicides, ETU is found 10 to 90 times higher in cooked tomatoes than in raw tomatoes. During cooking, the ETU presumably is formed from residues of the parent fungicides that are present on the food. The amount of ETU formed in the cooked produce varies with the parent fungicide and ultimately depends upon the amount of fungicide residue that remains on the harvested crops. Although the amount of ETU may drop to very low levels in 14 days, that is no reflection of the amount of this carcinogen that may be found in the cooked produce. Moreover, degradation products of unknown toxicity, for instance ethylene thiuram monosulfide, are formed from the EBDC fungicides in the field. ETU does, however, disappear rapidly from plants and soil. Several toxicological studies have shown that ETU was carcinogenic in the thyroid of rats, tumorigenic in the liver of mice, and teratogenic in pregnant rats. Studies have also suggested an effect of ETU on the liver.

EXT. D & C YELLOWS NO. 1, 9, and 10. Prohibited from use in externally applied drugs and cosmetics by the FDA because they could contain carcinogens.

FALLOUT. *See* Radiation.

FALSE MOREL. *See* Mushrooms.

FAMILY CANCERS. Aside from cancers known to be associated with heredity *(see)*, there are certain malignancies that seem to aggregate excessively in families. In one Boston family there were 7 and possibly 10 members who had ovarian cancer. Soft-tissue tumors in siblings during childhood have been found in several families in whom other cancers, especially of the breast in young females, affect close relatives. In addition to the combination of retinoblastoma and osteosarcoma, several other dissimilar types of cancer have been observed in close relatives in several families, for example, glioma (tumor that occurs mainly in the brain, spinal cord, and adrenals), adrenal cortical carcinoma, and either rhabdomyosarcoma (a tumor composed of striated muscle fibers) or osteosarcoma. The same cancers that occur as double primaries may also be distributed individually among family members. When cancers aggregate excessively in families, with or without other disorders, it suggests the possibility of there being some common undetectable factors causing a high risk among members. If doctors can learn what these factors are, then they will ultimately be able to prevent occurrence, or at least provide early detection.[314]

FAST GARNET BASE B. On exposure to the air the needles become red or a reddish crystalline mass. Used in the manufacture of dyes. It is recognized as a cause of malignant tumors of the urinary bladder.[315] *See* also 1–NA (Alpha-Naphthylamine).

FAT. Dietary fat is an important component affecting chemical carcinogenesis. But there is also a link between a high-fat diet and cancer. Findings suggest that the incidence of cancer might be reduced by eating less fat, altering hormonal balances, and eating fiber and vitamin C. Diets high in polyunsaturated fats aimed at reducing cholesterol levels in the blood might conceivably increase the risk of developing cancer of the large bowel. It was also found that the incidence of cancer among men on a diet high in polyunsaturated fat was higher than those men on a conventional diet. However, other trials of the effect of polyunsaturated-fat diets on the incidence of atherosclerotic complications have been negative in regard to an increased incidence of fatal cancer. A study by the American Chemical Society found that unsaturated corn oil increased the potency of a cancer-causing agent in animal studies more than a saturated animal fat did. This study substantiates the fact that fat is an important component of the diet affecting cancer initiation by chemicals. During the last 30 years, studies conducted in various laboratories have demonstrated that rats and mice fed diets containing certain vegetable oils were more prone to develop neoplasms than the animals fed comparable diets containing animal fat or hydrogenated vegetable fats. The latest statistics show that the rate of cancer death is on the rise. Epidemiological studies indicated a linear relationship between the dietary-fat intake and the death rate caused by cancer in breast, prostate, intestine, and skin. Studies have shown that the chemicals formed by oxidation of some of the double bonds in polyunsaturated fats are potent carcinogens. [316,317,318,319,320]

FD & C BLUE NO. 1. *Brilliant blue.* A coal-tar derivative, it is used as a coloring in bottled soft drinks, gelatin desserts, ice cream, ices, dry-drink powders, candy, confections, bakery products, cereals, and puddings. It may cause allergic reactions. It will produce malignant tumors at the site of injection in rats. It is on the FDA permanent list of color additives and is rated 1A for toxicology (completely vegetable).[321]

FD & C BLUE No. 2. *Indigo carmine, indigotine, acid blue E, acid leather blue IC, food blue 2, grape, soluble indigo.* This is a dark blue powder with coppery luster; it is sensitive to light. It is used as a dye in kidney-function tests; as a reagent for the detection of nitrite; in testing milk; and as a coloring in bottled soft drinks, bakery products, cereals, candy, confections, and dry-drink powders. The World Health Organization has given it a toxicology rating of B, meaning available data not entirely sufficient to meet requirements acceptable for food use. It is on the FDA list for provision-approved color additives. Causes cancer when injected under the skin of rats in doses of 10 milligrams per kilogram of body weight.[322]

FD & C COLORS. A color additive is a term to describe any dye, pigment, or other substance capable of coloring a food or drug, or a cosmetic on any part of the human body. In 1900 there were more than 80 dyes used to color food. There were no regulations and the same dye used to color clothes could also be used to color candy. In 1906 the first comprehensive legislation for food colors was passed. When tested, only seven colors were shown to be composed of ingredients that demonstrated no known harmful effects. A voluntary system of certification for batches of color dyes was set up. In 1938 new legislation was passed, superseding the 1906 act. The colors were given numbers instead of chemical names, and every batch used in food had to be certified. There were 15 food colors at the time. In 1950 children were made ill by certain coloring used in candy and popcorn. These incidents led to the delisting of DDC orange no. 1, orange no. 2, and FD & C red no. 32. Since that time, because of experimental evidence of possible harm, red 1, yellows 1, 2, 3, and 4 have also been delisted. Violet 1 was removed in 1973. In 1976 one of the most widely used of all colors was removed because it was found to cause tumors in rats. In 1976, red no. 4, which as of this date was being used only to color maraschino cherries, was banned. Carbon black was also banned at the time because it was shown to contain a cancer-causing agent. Earlier in 1960, scientific investigations were required by law to determine the suitability of all colors in use for permanent listing. Today, orange B, used to color orange skins (limited to 2 parts per million), has been permanently listed. Blue no 1, red no. 3, yellow no. 5, and red no. 40 are permanently listed but without any ppm restrictions. Other food-coloring additives are still on the "temporary list." In 1959 the FDA approved the use of "lakes" (preparing dyes by mixing them with aluminum hydrate, to make them insoluble).

The safety of colors in food is now being questioned by the FDA and regulatory agencies in other countries as well as the World Health Organization. There are inconsistencies in safety data and in the banning of some colors which, in turn, affect international commerce. The FDA has given manufacturers until December 31, 1980, to submit data on the long-term safety of the provisionally listed food colors, yellow no. 6, green no. 3, and blue no. 2. Thereafter, there will probably be no provisionally listed colors. Since most coal tars have proven carcinogenic, there is a real question whether they should be used as cosmetics in our food. The less "colored" food you buy, the better off you are.[323] *See also* Dyes, Coal Tar, and Azo Dyes.

FD & C ORANGE I. *See* Benzenesulfonic Acid.

FD & C RED NO. 2. *Amaranth.* Formerly one of the most widely used food and cosmetic colorings, it was removed from the market by the FDA in January 1976. It is a dark reddish-brown powder that turns bright red when mixed with fluid. A monoazo color (a dye made from diazonium and phenol), it was used in cereals, maraschino cherries, and desserts. The safety of this dye was questioned by American scientists for more than 20 years. Two Russian scientists found that FD & C red no. 2 prevented some pregnancies and caused some stillbirths in rats. The FDA ordered manufacturers using the color to submit data on all food, drug, and cosmetic products containing it. Controversial tests at the FDA's Center for Toxicological Research in Arkansas showed that in high doses red no. 2 caused a statistically significant increase in a variety of cancers in female rats. Red no. 2 was then banned in the United States but not in Canada. *See also* FD & C Colors.

FD & C RED NO. 4. Banned by the FDA in 1974 when it was shown to damage the adrenal glands and bladders of dogs, the agency relented and put in on the provisional list for use in maraschino cherries. It is still in use in some drugs and cosmetics. It is a coal-tar dye. The World Health Organization gives it a rating of IV E, meaning it has been found to be harmful and should not be used in food. It was banned in all foods in 1976 because experiments showed it caused urinary bladder polyps and atrophy of the adrenal glands. It was also banned in orally taken drugs but is still permitted in cosmetics for external use only. *See also* FD & C Colors.

FD & C VIOLET 1. Used as coloring matter in gelatin desserts, ice cream, sherbets, carbonated beverages, dry-drink powders, candy, confections, bakery products, cereals, puddings, and as the dye for the FDA's meat stamp. A Canadian study in 1962 showed it caused cancer in 50 percent of the rats fed the dye in food. The FDA did not consider this valid evidence since the purity of the dye used could not be determined and all records and specimens were lost and thus not available for study. Furthermore, previous and subsequent studies have not confirmed evidence of violet I causing cancer in rats. However, a two-year study with dogs did show noncancerous lesions on the dog's ears after being fed violet 1. The FDA again felt the study was not adequate but that the ear lesions did appear to be dye-related and that perhaps two years was too short a period to determine their eventual outcome. The FDA ruled on October 28, 1971, that violet 1 should remain provisionally listed pending the outcome of a new dog study to be started as soon as possible and to last seven years. The FDA finally banned the use of violet 1 in 1973. The FDA ruled that any mixing of violet 1 with a substance intended for food use will cause the final products to be "adulterated." *See also* FD & C Colors.

FD & C YELLOW NO. 6. *Monoazo, sunset yellow FCF.* A coal-tar dye used as coloring matter in carbonated beverages, gelatin desserts, dry-drink powders, candy and confectionary products that do not contain oils and fats, bakery products, cereals, puddings, and tablets. May cause allergic reactions. It is rated 1A (acceptable in food) by the World Health Organization and is on the FDA provisional list of approved color additives. *See also* FD & C Colors.

FERRIAMICIDE. It is a substitute for another pesticide, mirex, which has been banned because it is suspected of causing cancer. Ferriamicide contains mirex (*see*). Is in limited use in the controlling of fire ants and must be applied by hand to individual fire-ant mounds, although application by utility vehicles or tractors is allowed in parks and cemeteries. Application by airplane is not permitted. Laboratory tests on ferriamicide have shown it to be many times less persistent in the environment than mirex and consequently less toxic to sensitive shrimp, crabs, and crayfish.

Many things are not known about this new pesticide: (1) its immediate effect in people and most wildlife; (2) its potential for long-term hazards to man or the environment; (3) the identity and toxicity of all the products into which it decomposes; and (4) whether it leaves a residue on food crops. The degree of cancer risk is not known; however, it does contain mirex, which is a known carcinogen.[324] An environmental group sued to keep the insecticide from being used to control the stinging fire ant in Mississippi—the ants were accidentally brought into the United States from South America aboard a cargo ship around 1918. They can inflict repeated painful stings on people and livestock.

FERROUS GLUCONATE. *Gluconic acid, iron salt, iron gluconate, ferronicum.* Used for food coloring, it is yellowish gray. It is also used as a flavoring agent and to treat iron-deficiency anemia. It may cause gastrointestinal disturbances.[325] When painted on mouse skin in 2,600 milligram doses per kilogram of body weight, it causes tumors.[326]

FERROUS LACTATE. *Lactate acid, iron (2H) salt, iron lactate.* Greenish white crystals that have a slightly peculiar odor. It is derived from the interaction of calcium lactate with ferrous sulfate, or the direct action of lactic acid on iron filings. It is used as a food additive and dietary supplement. Causes tumors when injected under the skin of mice. [327]

FIBER (DIETARY). If an apple a day keeps the doctor away, is it because of the fiber content? Scientists have suspected that the high intestinal cancer rate in the United States may be linked to the 80 percent decrease of consumption of fiber in the average diet during the past century. Essentially, there are three classes of fiber found in the fruit, leaves, stems, seeds, flowers, and roots of different plants. The first class is the insoluble cellulose found in the plant-cell wall. Some of the other polysaccharides constitute a second class and are also found in the cell wall (hemicellulose and pectic polyerms), in the endosperm of seeds (mucilages), or in the plant's surface (gums). The third class, the lignins, are noncarbohydrates that infiltrate and contribute to the death of the plant cell, which then becomes part of the woody reinforcing plant structure.

Enzymes from a number of the more than 400 kinds of bacteria in the human colon are capable of digesting many components of plant fiber. Doctors have found that the water-holding capacity of some fibers may be helpful in treating colon diseases. The fiber's bile and absorption properties might be used in modifying cholesterol metabolism. Plant fibers are also capable of binding trace metals and bile acids. These properties modify the action of the gut contents. Fibers pass through the gut somewhat like a sponge, probably altering metabolism in the intestine. In fact, researchers at the University of Illinois found in animal research that wheat bran is effective in decreasing exposure to cancer-causing substances at levels often encountered in the human diet. At 100 parts per million of carcinogens, wheat bran prevented 80 percent of the intestinal exposure. Even at 1,200 ppm, it prevented 40 percent exposure. The fibers appear to protect intestinal cells by removing foreign substances, such as carcinogens produced by char-broiling. Increased fiber consumption has been recommended for the relief of some symptoms of diverticular disease, irritable bowel syndrome, and constipation. When the high-fiber content of wheat-bran cereal is cited, it refers to the important part of the wheat kernel retained in the processing of these cereals, the out-layers, or bran, of the kernel. Bran is a highly concentrated source of these indigestible plant-cell materials. Plant cells such as those in bran act like a sponge, absorbing water and holding it. As the bran particles absorb the water in foods, they become softened and in the human gastrointestinal tract serve as dietary "bulk." This dietary bulk has a tendency to decrease intestinal transit time for waste materials. Dr. Denis Burkitt, an epidemiologist, spent many years in Africa studying disease patterns. He observed a low incidence of cancer of the colon, as well as diverticular disease. The stools of the Africans were larger, softer, thus easier to eliminate and passed with considerably more speed than those of typical Westerners. In Britain, Burkitt had observed that stools were small, hard, and difficult to expel, sometimes damaging to the delicate lining of the intestinal tract.[328]

FIBER GLASS. Because of the known danger to the lungs of asbestos, fibrous glass has replaced it in many insulation and fireproofing materials. (Unlike naturally occurring minerals, fibrous glass is a material spun like cotton candy from molten silica sand.) Since commercial production and use of fiber glass in the United States began in 1933, it wasn't until sufficient time had lapsed for job-related cancers to appear. Since various studies had shown that fibrous glass causes cancer in experimental animals and that a large number of fibrous glass workers were retiring on disability because of chronic bronchitis, NIOSH launched a major study of disease and death in the fibrous-glass manufacturing industry. Among 1,448 workers exposed to low levels of airborne glass fibers, there were not excess lung cancer deaths, even 20 years after exposure. However, there was some increased risk of cancer among workers who during the early years of fibrous glass production were involved with a special process that exposed them to glass particles of very small diameter. Since small-diameter fibers have also caused cancer in animals, scientists are still reserving judgment on the safety of fibrous glass.[329] Some researchers look with dismay upon companies that encourage do-it-yourself homeowners to roll out fiber-glass insulation in their enclosed attics. They also point out that there is no warning on the label about possible hazards other than recommending that you wear old clothes.[330]

FIBERS (MICROSCOPIC). Fibers of a certain size are capable of causing cancers in laboratory rats, regardless of the chemical composition of the fibers, according to Dr. Mearl F. Stanton of the NCI's Laboratory of Pathology. Results of tests showed that very fine fibers of asbestos, glass, or sapphire (aluminum oxide) caused a high incidence of lung cancers in animals, while coarse fibers or powdered material of the same compositions only rarely caused cancer. The cancer-causing fibers were between one-half and five microns in diameter and less than 80 microns long (less than one-hundredth as thick as an eyelash and under one-tenth as long). Human mesotheliomas (rare cancers of the membranes lining the lungs and abdomen), occur primarily among persons exposed to asbestos dust. After asbestos fibers have been inhaled into the lung, they often lodge there permanently. Twenty to 40 years later, mesotheliomas or other lung diseases such as asbestosis may develop. Dr. Stanton said that very fine fibrous glass and a sample of fine sapphire caused cancer in more than half the rats tested. None of the rats exposed to two samples of fully pulverized asbestos, nonfibrous aluminum oxide, or two samples of glass with large fibers developed cancer. "We know that asbestos fibers cause cancer in man," Dr. Stanton said. "We have no evidence on whether other kinds of fibers will also prove hazardous. It's rare to find other substances with fibers the same size as asbestos, and few people are known to have been exposed to them. But the results in animals suggest that it would be judicious to avoid inhalation or ingestion of any finely particulate fibrous material."[331] *See also* Asbestos and Fiber Glass.

FISH TUMORS. Are fish tumors to water what canaries were to the mines—early warning devices to humans? It has only been in the last few years that scientists have proven that mollusks and arthropods get cancer. Since invertebrates don't have advanced chordatelike immunity systems—with thymus glands and antibodies—a comparative study of tumor induction in vertebrates and invertebrates may give new insights into the relationship between immunity and cancer.

There is a strong possibility that viruses rather than chemicals may cause some of the lower-animal tumors and that the chemical stress of pollutants may enhance these viruses or cause latent viruses to grow. In addition, parasites may secrete growth-causing fluids that stimulate cellular proliferation. For example, fibrous papillomas (benign tumors) found on the skin of the green sea turtle often contain foreign material such as leeches, barnacles, and plant material. Although there is still much to learn about fish tumors and pollution, it has been determined that most have been found in bottom-feeding fish and filter-feeding mollusks, suggesting that those factors influencing tumor growth accumulate in sediments. Populations of catfish, croakers, salamanders, and other marine animals found in polluted areas often have tumors, while the same species living in a clean environment do not. Scientists have already proven that pollution may be passed along the food chain to people when aquatic organisms accumulate cancer-causing chemicals. Mollusks living in areas polluted with domestic sewage can be reservoirs for disease, and eating mollusks from such areas may cause thyroid and hepatitis. While some shellfish can flush pollutants from their system when placed in clean water, even freezing for weeks will not kill the viruses in crabs. (However humans eat chemicals, germs, and viruses every day when eating beef, eggs, and chicken.)

Pollution certainly seems to play a part in fish tumors. Fish caught in the Fox River on the outskirts of Chicago have almost 16 times as much cancer as do fish caught in Lake of the Woods, Ontario, Canada. In a report published in 1978 in the Annals of the New York Academy of Sciences, Dr. Eric R. Brown details how he compared the cancer rate of six kinds of fish —walleye, northern pike, brown bullhead, catfish, sucker, and carp—in the two kinds of water. Overall, less than half a percent of the fish from Lake of the Woods had cancer, while almost 7 percent of the fish from the Fox River had cancer. The Fox River has heavy population densities along its 170-mile perimeter; it also receives waste from industries along the banks. However, the banks of Lake of the Woods are sparsely inhabited and have little or no industry; it is primarily a vacation area.[332,333] *See also* Water.

FLAGYL. *Metronidazole.* Used to treat common vaginal infections caused by trichomonads and to treat acute amebic dysentery. Men are given it for trichomonas so they will not reinfect their partners. Has been shown to cause cancers, particularly of the lung, in mice, and it is possibly carcinogenic in rats as well.[334] It is not recommended for use except where absolutely necessary.

FLECTOL H. *Poly(1,2-dihydro-2,2,4-trimethylquinoline.* Used as a rubber antioxidant, as a food-packaging adhesive, and for belting and tire carcasses. Caused tumors when given orally to rats in 3,700 milligram doses per kilogram of body weight.[335] The ban of this substance in April 1967 as a food-packaging adhesive marked the first time that the FDA formally invoked the Delaney Amendment (*see* Introduction, page 10.)

FLUOREN-2-AMINE. *See* Fluorene.

FLUORENE. *Fluoren-2-amine, 2-aminofluorene.* Small white crystals that are fluorescent when impure. Soluble in alcohol. It is derived from coal tar and used in resins, insecticides, and dyestuffs. Caused cancer in rats when given orally in doses of 3,200 milligrams per kilogram of body weight and when painted on the skin or injected in doses of from 240 to 160 milligrams per kilogram of body weight. It is carcinogenic to the skin of mice in 11 milligram doses per kilogram.[336]

FLUORENE-2,7 DINITRO. *See* Fluorene.

FLUORENE, 2-NITROSO. *See* Fluorene.

FLUORESCEIN. Orange red crystalline powder that when diluted, turns intensely greenish yellow. It is fluorescent and is derived by heating phthalic anhydride and resorcinol. It is used for dyeing silk and wools, in medicines, and as an indication and reagent for bromine. It is also used as a tracer to locate impurities in wells. Caused tumors when injected subcutaneously in rats.[337]

FLUORIDE. An acid salt used in toothpaste and water to prevent tooth decay. At a House subcommittee hearing on a possible link between fluorides and cancer, the director of the NCI said, "I can state with certainty from the analyses and reviews of the relevant data that no trends in cancer rates can be ascribed to the consumption of water that is artificially or naturally fluoridated." This statement was made to refute allegations made by John Yiamoutiannis, Ph.D., of the National Health Federation, that his studies have shown a correlation between fluoridation and cancer. Fluorides cross the placental barrier and the effects on the fetus are unknown. There is little evidence in the literature that fluorides are associated with cancer.[338]

FOOD. Cancer rates and types vary geographically. Studies of these differences have suggested that various elements of the daily diet may cause as much as 40 percent of the cancers in man. For example, cancer of the colon and rectum is the second most common cancer for both sexes in the United States, Scotland, Canada, and other Westernized countries, striking 100,000 persons a year in the United States. But this disease is relatively rare in countries like Japan, Chile, Portugal, Israel, and among the Bantu of South Africa. Yet studies of migrants have shown that heredity is not responsible. When the Japanese move to Hawaii, for example, they have a higher rate of bowel cancer than those living in Japan. Those who emigrated to California are at a greater risk of developing the disease than those who settled in Hawaii. *See also* Fat, Fiber, Bran, Diet, and Colorectal Cancer.

FORMALDEHYDE. A colorless gas obtained by the oxidation of methyl alcohol and generally used in watery solutions. Vapors are intensely irritating to the mucous membranes. It is used in nail hardeners, nail polish, soap, and hair-growing products. Formaldehyde, generally known as a disinfectant, germicide, fungicide, defoamer, and preservative, is also used in embalming fluid. Ingestion can cause severe abdominal pain, internal bleeding, loss of ability to urinate, vertigo, coma, and death. One ounce taken by mouth causes death within two hours. Skin reactions after exposure to the chemical are very common and can be both irritating and allergy causing. Protects nails from chipping. When injected under the skin of rats in 96 milligram doses per kilogram of body weight, it causes tumors.[340] There is an OSHA standard for formaldehyde in the air of 3 parts per million.

FORMAMIDE. *N-(4-(5-Nitro-2-Furyl)-2-thiazolyl).* Colorless hydroscopic oily liquid derived from ethyl formate and ammonia. Moderately toxic. Solvent, softener, intermediate *(see)* in organic synthesis. Caused tumors in rats, mice, dogs, and hamsters when given orally.[341]

FORMIC ACID. Used as a rubefacient (substance that produces redness) in hair tonics. As a synthetic food flavoring it is colorless, pungent, and highly corrosive. It occurs naturally in apples and other fruits. It is also used as a decalcifier and for dehairing hides; in the dyeing and finishing of textiles and paper; in the manufacture of insecticides and refrigerants; and in solvents for perfumes, lacquers, electroplating, medicines, and brewing. Chronic absorption is known to cause protein in urine. It caused cancer when administered orally in rats, mice, and hamsters in doses of from 31 to 49 milligrams per kilogram of body weight.[342]

FOSTERITE. Trademark for a family of resins. The largest application is a "solventless" varnish for electrical insulations and as a bond for impregnating and laminating asbestos sheets. Rods made of this plastic will carry a beam of light without dispersion, making it possible to bend the beam. It causes tumors when injected into the abdomen of mice in doses of 400 milligrams per kilogram of body weight.[343]

FOWLER'S SOLUTION (POTASSIUM ARSENITE). *See* Arsenic Compounds.

FRUCTOSE. *Fructopyranose, beta-D-.* A sugar occurring naturally in a large number of fruits and honey. It is the sweetest of the foodstuffs. It is also used as a medicine, preservative, common sugar, and to prevent sandiness in ice cream. It caused tumors in mice when injected under the skin in 5,000 milligram doses per kilogram of body weight. [344]

5-FU, (5-FLUOROURACIL). A fluorinated pyrimidine belonging to the category of antimetabolites (a substance that hinders the utilization of a metabolite). It interferes with the synthesis of DNA and to a lesser extent RNA. Since DNA and RNA are essential for cell division and growth, the effect promotes the death of the cell. Cancer cells are most sensitive to it. It is a highly toxic drug and should be used under the supervison of qualified physicians experienced in cancer chemotherapy.[339]

FUCHSIN. *Magenta, C. I. acid violet 19.* An aromatic amine, a mixture of rosaniline and pararosaniline hydrochloride, that is used in the textile and leather industries as a red dye and as a bacterial stain. It is an olive to dark green coarse powder with a bronze luster and a faint odor. It has caused urinary tract cancer in manufacturing workers.[345]

FUNGI. Ergot, the fungus *Claviceps purpurea,* grows on rye and other grasses and has been found to cause neurofibromas of the ears when fed to rats in amounts equaling 5 percent of their diet for two years. About half the animals developed the tumors while none of the control rats did. Stored rice is quite susceptible to contamination by many fungi, especially *Penicillium* and *Aspergillus.* Such contaminated rice, depending on the fungi present, may produce toxic symptoms upon ingestion. Several fungi that grow on rice produce toxins, and much attention has been devoted to metabolites (products of metabolic change) of the *Penicillium* species. Strains of one of them, *P. islandicum* Sopp, have produced liver tumors in rats and mice. Continuous feeding of rats with cereals containing molds produced a wide range of changes in the liver of rats and mice, including liver tumors. Both luteoskyrin and cyclochlorotine fungi are toxic to the liver and produce tumors.[346]

FUNGICIDES. Ethylenethiourea, a toxic degradation product of fungicides widely used in agriculture and food crops, has been found in commercial packages of fungicides in a variety of concentrations. Ethylenethiourea, or ETU (*see* ETU), has been linked with thyroid cancer. Of 18 different commercial formations of ethylenebisdithiocarbamate fungicides, 6 different manufacturers' products all contained ETU. In all 18, concentrations increased under controlled laboratory conditions chosen to approximate climatic storage conditions in warehouses or sheds. Ethylenebisdithiocarbamate has been applied to crops since 1934.[347]

FURACILLIN. *See* Nitrofurazone.

FURACIN. *See* Nitrofurazone.

2-FURALDEHYDE,5-NITRO-SEMICARBAZONE. *See* Nitrofurazone.

4H-FURO(3,2-c)PYRAN-2(6H)-ONE,4-HYDROXY. *See* Patulin.

FYROL FR 2. *See* Tris.

GASOLINE ENGINE EXHAUST TAR. Caused cancer when applied to the skin of mice in 306 milligram doses per kilogram of body weight.[348] *See also* Benzopyrene.

GENETICS. Heredity accounts for some people being more susceptible to cancer than others. In one theory, the inherited mutation does not itself cause cancer but makes the cell more susceptible to insult by cancer-causing agents such as X-rays and chemicals.

GLUTAMIC ACID. *N-(p-)12.4-Diamino-6-pteridinyl (methyl) amino (benzoyl).* *See* Methotrexate.

GOLD. *Burnish gold, shell gold.* Occurring naturally in the earth, it is a soft yellow metal. The pure metal is nontoxic, but some gold salts can cause allergic skin rashes. It has been reported to cause tumors when injected under the skin of mice in 400 milligram doses per kilogram of body weight.[349]

GOUT MEDICINE. *See* Colchicine.

GRAIN ALCOHOL. *See* Ethyl Alcohol.

GRAPHITE. *Black lead.* Obtained by mining, especially in Canada and Ceylon. Usually consists of soft black lustrous scales. Used in lead pencils, stone polish, and as an explosive. It was banned in cosmetics by the FDA in the late 1970s because "it might contain aromatic hydrocarbons, some of which could be carcinogenic."

GRAS LIST. When established by Congress in 1958, this "Generally Recognized As Safe" list contained those substances that had been added to food over a long time and that under conditions of their intended use were generally recognized as safe by qualified scientists. Substances on the list were exempt from premarket clearance. Congress had acted on a very marginal response—on the basis of returns from those scientists sent questionnaires. Approximately 355 out of 900 responded and only about 100 of those responses had substantive comments. Three items were removed from the originally published list.

In recent years, developments in the scientific fields and in consumer awareness brought to light the inadequacies of the testing of food additives and, ironically, the complete lack of testing of the GRAS list. As a result, President Nixon directed the FDA to reevaluate all the items on the list. The in-depth investigation continues at the FDA's testing laboratories at Pine Bluff, Arkansas, a facility once used by the armed forces to develop chemical warfare materials.

GREEN CHROME OXIDE. *See* Chromium.

GREEN OIL. *See* Anthracene.

GREENS. The following greens derived from ammonium salts have been found to cause cancer in animals when given orally or applied to the skin: acidal green, A. F. green no. 1, C. I. food green, FD & C green no. 1, Guinea green, leather green B, sulpho green 2 B, vonacid green L, acid leather green, caocid green S B, wool green S, acid brilliant green B S, FD & C light green no. 2, FD & C green no. 2, aluminum lake, fenazo green, leather green S F, light green F S, light green Lake, light green SFD, acidal light green.[350]

GREEN VITRIOL. *See* Sulfuric Acid and Iron Salt.

GRISEOFULVIN. *Fulcin, fulvicin.* An antibiotic derived from *Penicillium.* Given in large oral doses for human fungi infections, such as ringworm of the scalp and body, athlete's foot, and barber's itch. Griseofulvin was administered prophylactically in Vietnam to military personnel. It can cause hypersensitivity reactions. A diet fed to mice consisting of one percent griseofulvin increased the incidence and size of tumors formed following the application to their skin of a cancer-causing agent, 3-methylcholanthrene. A co-carcinogen *(see)* effect was also noted at 0.01 percent of the antibiotic in the diet, a dose comparable to human doses.[351] Some effects on the white cells of certain patients taking the drug have been reported.[352]

GUANIDINE. *1-Methyl-3-nitro-1-nitroso-.* Found in turnips, mushrooms, corn germ, rice hulls, mussels, and earthworms, it is prepared from guano nitrate. The deliquescent crystals have been used to treat the disease myasthenia gravis. It has been found to cause cancer in rats, mice, dogs, and hamsters when given in small doses either orally, under the skin, or rectally.[353] NIOSH determined it a positive animal carcinogen. NCI has been testing it since 1976.[354]

GUANINE 3-OXIDE. A purine (basic compound found in living matter) constituent of the nucleic acids RNA and DNA. The usual sources are guano, sugar beets, yeast, clover seeds, and fish scales. It has largely been replaced with synthetic pearl or aluminum in cosmetics. It is still used in biochemical research. It caused cancer when injected under the skin of rats in 11 milligram doses per kilogram of body weight.[355]

HABITS. When it comes down to the bottom line, probably the greatest cancer-causing agent in our environment is we, ourselves. How we live and what we do affect, to a large extent, whether or not we will get cancer. Lung cancer is—80 percent of the time—the direct result of smoking. Cancer of the esophagus, throat, and bladder has been linked to drinking alcohol. Early sex has been correlated with cancer of the cervix. Habits are hard to break. The first reports linking tobacco to cancer date back to the 1700s. Yet, even today, despite overwhelming evidence, people still smoke and rationalize about its dangers. Diet has also been linked to cancer. But would Mexicans give up highly spiced food or Japanese forgo talc treated rice in an effort to avoid stomach cancer so prevalent among them? They are no more likely to do so than Americans who would have to forgo high fat diets and highly processed foods to reduce chances of breast cancer and cancer of the colon. Would young girls and middle-aged women stop basking in the sun? No, because they equate a suntan with beauty, they choose to ignore the definite risk link between skin cancer and ultraviolet rays.

HAIR COLORING. More than 33 million Americans use hair coloring in an effort to cover gray or to change their appearance. Permanent hair-coloring products change the color of the hair. They cannot be shampooed away but remain until the hair grows out or is cut off. There are basically three types: natural organics, synthetics, and metallics. Natural organics such as henna and chamomile have been used for centuries to color hair. Such dyes are placed on the hair and removed when the desired shade has been obtained. They are more difficult to apply, less reliable than manufactured dyes, and less predictable as far as coloring is concerned. Except for an occasional allergic reaction to specific natural ingredients, they are considered harmless.

The use of metal salts to color hair is mentioned in the literature of ancient Rome. Cosmeticians of the times darkened hair by passing it through a lead comb that had been dipped in vinegar. Because the metallic dyes are incompatible with permanent wave solutions and oxidation dyes, they are not widely used by American women. However, American men use them as a subtle method of changing hair coloring. Lead, silver, and copper are most often used, although they are not recommended for moustaches, because of the danger of ingestion or inhalation of the metals, which can be toxic. Lead is also a suspected carcinogen.

The most attention to the possibility of inducing cancer with dyes is on the synthetic dyes. The first synthetic dye to be used on human hair was pyrogallol. It was used for brown shades but was extremely dangerous if ingested or painted over a large area of skin, causing kidney damage and gastrointestinal poisoning. The first of the amino dyes developed and the one most commonly used today in the United States is p-phenylenediamine *(see)*. This dye and the other synthetic oxidation dyes frequently cause dermatitis and other allergic skin reactions, and the laws in most states require that patch testing be done before use. There is evidence that p-phenylenediamine products cause skin cancer in animals, and many European countries will not permit its use. Dyes in use today contain not only the dye itself and the oxididizer but hair conditioners, color modifiers, antioxidants, stabilizers, and other compounds to "treat" hair. The compounds use bases called intermediates *(see)* because their actual dyeing ability comes to the fore only upon oxidation. Modifiers are used to develop the desired shade. Antioxidants protect the compound against unwanted reaction with oxygen, and alkalizers are used because synthetic dyes work best in an alkaline medium. Developers are added to speed up the dyeing process. Permanent hair dye is usually mixed just before application and then left on the hair for a specified amount of time.

In 1972 a middle-aged woman visited her physician. She had made heavy use of two semipermanent hair colorings, and when she later developed acute myeloid leukemia, her doctor decided to test the two colorings to see if there were any correlation between them and her disease. The colorings were 2-nitro-p-phenylenediamine, 4-nitro-o-phenylenediamine, and CI acid black (an azo dye *(see)* with 4-amino-2-nitrophenol). Skin-painting experiments on mice showed that the hair colorings applied at low concentrations caused an early appearance of tumors in two strains of mice. Both colorings were also mutagenic *(see* Ames Test in Introduction, page 7*)*. The doctor and his colleagues concluded that in view of the widespread use of hair colorings, both in the home and by professional hairdressers, it is essential that further studies be done. They said there have been fragmentary reports of a link between the occupation of hairdresser and excess cancer incidence. Three epidemiological studies of bladder cancer noted an excess of hairdressers and barbers with tumors of the urinary tract. Because in each study this excess was based on a very small number of cases, we are still faced with a lack of strong statistical evidence. However, the fact that three studies— separated in place and time—have mentioned this excess strengthens the argument for the existence of a cancer hazard.[356] Adding further evidence, researchers at NCI tested hair-dye chemicals for their ability to cause cancer by feeding them to rats and mice. Preliminary results showed that six hair-coloring ingredients are indeed carcinogenic in animals: 4-methoxy-m-phenylenediamine, 4-MMPD (commonly used in permanent hair color); 2,4-toluene diamine (used in a few permanent hair colors); 4-amino-2-nitrophenol and 2-nitrophenylenediamine (used in many gold and reddish shade high lighters); direct black 38 and direct blue 6 (no longer manufactured). Bruce Ames reported in 1977 that 150 of the semipermanent hair dyes he tested (see Ames Test in Introduction, page 7) were mutagenic. An estimated 70 to 75 percent of the substances that are known carcinogens show up as mutagens in his test. In January 1978 NIOSH reported that a new study of beauticians and cosmetologists shows they have a higher than expected incidence of six kinds of cancer. That study, along with NCI's findings, led NIOSH to recommend that 2,4-diaminoanisole be treated as a human carcinogen. On April 6, 1978, the FDA issued an order that manufacturers place a warning on the label of some permanent hair dyes that reads: "Warning; contains an ingredient that can penetrate your skin and has been determined to cause cancer in laboratory animals." The FDA also proposed that beauty parlors post notices urging customers to check the labels on products used in the salon. As of this writing the FDA has no power to ban the ingredients in hair dyes or even to require manufacturers to demonstrate safety. At most, the FDA can only warn consumers. The 1938 Food, Drug and Cosmetic Act exempted coal-tar dyes from certain provisions of the law. Not everyone agrees that hair dyes are dangerous. Dr. E. Cuyler Hammond, of the American Cancer Society, conducted a 13-year test of 5,000 hairdressers and a matched group of nonhairdressers and did not find any difference in the groups. However, the ACS on February 22, 1978, did issue a statement that said: "The results of studies among beauticians and women who use permanent hair dyes have been mixed. But the regulatory agencies feel that in the absence of hard data, they must be cautious. They feel that because of the wide use by the public, even a small potential risk of cancer caused by little exposure could be associated with significant additional cancer cases. While available information does not prove or disprove that hair dyes cause cancer in humans, the ACS advises caution in the use of the substances under question until more definitive evidence is developed." (A preliminary study by New York University researchers suggests that women who have used hair dyes for 10 or more years face an increased risk of developing breast cancer. Published in the February 1979 issue of the *Journal of the National Cancer Institute*, the use of hair dye by 129 women with breast cancer was compared to 193 matched controls.[357])

In the meantime, if you feel you must dye your hair, consider the following: semipermanent rinses and most blonde tints don't contain 4-MMPD. Processes called streaking or frosting—bleaching strands of hair

—do not touch the scalp. Another process, blonding, bleaches the hair and then adds a toner. Many "golden-blonde" toners are free of the ingredients under suspicion.[358,359] Loving Care and Clairesse do not contain any of the suspected dyes listed, and henna is considered safe because it is a vegetable dye. It is, however, less predictable as far as hair-dye color is concerned.

HAIR DYES. *See* Hair Coloring.

HALOTHANE. An anesthetic, it accelerated tumor spread in rats in the Lobund Laboratory of the University of Notre Dame. The laboratory specializes in the study of the effects of the environment and chemicals on animals raised germ free.[360]

HAMBURGER. Grilled or pan-fried hamburgers may cause cancer. Chopped meat cooked on a metal surface at temperatures higher than 300 degrees Fahrenheit produces mutagens (substances that cause genetic change). The particular mutagens in fried hamburgers have not yet been identified, and they might possibly turn out to be harmless. But 90 percent of all mutagens ever tested cause cancer in laboratory animals. Hamburger mutagens may represent a risk of cancer in people. When hamburgers are done rare or are broiled or cooked by microwave rather than fried, the mutagenic transformation does not take place. The mutagens are not normal constituents of beef tissue but are formed only during heating and evaporation. The longer the cooking, the more mutagenic the hamburger. Further analysis revealed the new mutagen is distinct from two other carcinogens previously identified in cooked meat—benzopyrene, similarly mutagenic and produced by cooking meat over a high heat, and pyrolyzed amino acids from the charred surface of meat cooked directly over a flame.[361,362]

HEMATITE. *Red iron ore, bloodstone, ferric oxide.* Iron oxide with impurities, it is found as a brilliant black to blackish red or brick-red mineral. It has a metallic to dull luster and is the most important ore of iron. Certain varieties are used as paint pigments and for rouge. Its dust is known to cause benign plaques in the lung, but it is also suspected of causing cancer in iron miners. It caused cancer when injected under the skin of rats in 104 milligram doses per kilogram of body weight.[363]

HEPATITIS TYPE-B VIRUS. The relationship between this virus and liver cancer may be as close as the relationship between cigarette smoking and lung cancer, according to Dr. Thomas London of the Philadelphia Institute for Cancer Research. At a meeting of the American Society of Preventative Oncology, he presented the preliminary findings of his research team linking the virus to primary hepatocellular carcinoma. Currently, a human cancer caused by a virus has never been proven, although animal cancers have been verified. How the hepatitis B-virus paves the way for liver cancer is still unknown. Dr. London's studies, done mainly in Africa and Asia, where type-B flourishes, found that better than 90 percent of those who develop liver cancer are type-B hepatitis carriers. Carriers of type-A and other viruses that cause hepatitis or jaundice are not potential victims of liver cancer. There appears to be a progression in liver malfunction toward cancer: from chronic hepatitis to cirrhosis to cancer.[364]

HEPTACHLOR. A cyclodiene member of the chlorinated insecticides that include aldrin, dieldrin, endrin, and endosulfan. Developed in the 15 years following World War II, it was registered in 1952 for use in soil, foliage, and commercial pesticides; for malarial control; and for use against agricultural pests and termites. In tests conducted by the NCI, liver cancer was found in 72 percent of male mice and in 71 percent of the females given high doses, far exceeding the norm. There was no apparent increase of liver cancer in animals given low doses. High-dose females also showed an increased incidence of thyroid tumors. On November 18, 1974, the EPA notified its intent to cancel the regulation of the pesticide heptachlor, except for subsurface ground insertion for agricultural termites and for application to nonfood plants. On August 1, 1976, it banned heptachlor except for use on seed, to control ants on Hawaiian pineapple, and to control the narcissus-bulb fly. Persistent human exposure presumably continued as a result of the existence of the compound in crops, water, and the atmosphere. A zero tolerance level was established for residues on animals, and on vegetable, fruit, and field crops. For four additional vegetables, a tolerance level of 0.1 parts per million was set. Acceptable human intake of 0.005 milligrams per kilogram was established for heptachlor. Average daily intake between 1965 and 1970 was 0.0003 milligrams per kilogram of body weight. In 1970, concentrations of 0.03 ppm were detected in 96 percent of 3,451 hospitalized patients tested. Similar observations of concentrations were made in 1971 and 1972, with some individuals ranging as high as 1.63 ppm. Heptachlor also crosses the placental barrier and has been found in breast milk.[365]

HEREDITY. There is a tendency to inherit a susceptibility for certain kinds of cancer. It may be determined by many things, such as defects in immunity, hormonal patterns, enzyme deficiencies, bone abnormalities, or a tendency to develop benign growths or cysts, as in the colon, breast, or ovaries. A survey of 4,515 Nebraskans showed that when one parent or sibling had cancer, 8.9 percent of the persons checked also had had cancer. In families where two immediate relatives had cancer, the risk to others in the immediate family rose to 16.3 percent and increased to 27.4 percent—more than one in five—for those with three or more close relatives who had had cancer. A number of quite rare hereditary conditions have been definitely shown to enhance cancer risk—one of these is a tendency to form multiple polyps or benign growths in the large bowel. Eventually, all who inherit this condition develop colon cancer. In general, however, immediate relatives of colon-cancer patients face a two to three times greater than expected risk of developing colon cancer themselves. This, of course, could be from dietary habits as well as from heredity.

Retinoblastoma, a rare form of eye cancer, is caused by a genetic abnormality, and the siblings or children of retinoblastoma victims would have a 50 percent chance of getting the disease. The risk of leukemia is increased among persons with mongolism, a disorder in which the cells contain an extra piece of genetic material; as well as among persons with Bloom's syndrome and Fanconi's anemia, inherited conditions in which the gene-bearing chromosomes tend to break. Another usually fatal genetic disorder, xeroderma pigmentosum, which involves an abnormality in the pigment-forming cells of the skin, predisposes its victims to sunlight-induced skin cancer, because their bodies lack the ability to repair the genetic damage to skin cells caused by ultraviolet radiation.

In one type of thyroid cancer, medullary carcinoma, studied by researchers at the Mayo Clinic, in one family, four children and two grandchildren have thus far been victimized by the disease. The Mayo doctors concluded that each member of this family had a 50-50 chance of inheriting the genetic trait that led to this cancer. Early recognition of this genetic factor led to lifesaving surgery for all but one of its victims.

There are "cancer families" in which members develop various forms of the disease. In one family, 8 of 19 members, through 3 generations, developed cancer, including colon cancer, uterine cancer, and lymphosarcoma. Two sisters in the family each developed several different cancers. Dr. Henry Lynch of Creighton University, Omaha, Nebraska, who has done much of the research in the study of "cancer families," said that just as a person's genetic inheritance may confer a particular susceptibility to cancer, it may also result in a relative resistance to this disease. He has also studied families in which cancer is extremely uncommon. Intensive investigation of such families may give clues to enzyme and hormone patterns, supply new insights into the workings of immune systems, and further reveal how heredity and environment interact to cause cancer.[366]

HERPES-2 VIRUS. There has been increasing evidence in the last decade that the herpes-2 virus may be involved in the development of cancer of the cervix. Cold sores and fever blisters are caused by a type of herpes, but the one in question is "herpes genitalis." It is increasingly diagnosed in both men and women, and it is considered a venereal disease. The herpes-2 lesion appears on the genitalia some three to seven days after sexual relations with an infected person. The sores appear to be tiny blisters; these may rupture in a day or two and cause ulcers. The condition usually clears up without treatment within six weeks and leaves no scar. But during the course of the disease there may be pain, burning, fever, and general malaise. A flare-up may occur without reinfection over the next weeks, months, or even years. The second attack is usually of shorter duration and less severe.

In a significant number of cases, women with cancer of the cervix have been found to harbor herpes-2 antibodies. The theory is, therefore, that women who have had either early sex or sex with multiple partners may be more susceptible to herpes-2 infection and consequently to cancer of the cervix. Use of the condom does protect against infection.

HERPES VIRUS DYE-LIGHT TREATMENT. Herpes simplex virus (HSV) infections usually heal, in time, without treatment, but they frequently recur and cause sufficient discomfort and embarrasment to cause many patients to seek some form of therapy. One new treatment method, based on in vitro (cells grown in a culture dish or test tube) investigations, animal studies, and some circumstantial evidence, is photodynamic inactivation of the virus. This is achieved by treating the herpes lesions with a dye, such as neutral red, and then exposing the lesions to light. However, it has been shown that photodynamically inactivated HSV can induce cancerous changes in cells in vitro, suggesting this form of treatment is not without hazard. Furthermore, treatment with the neutral red dye did not demonstrate effectively the frequency of or length of the interval between subsequent recurrences of herpes infections.[367]

HEX. *Hexachlorocyclopentadiene.* A fire retardant and pesticide produced at an estimated rate of 22 million kilograms annually in the United States. Data about its effects on the environment are few. There is no acceptable analytical method to detect hex residues. Because hex vaporizes readily at relatively low temperatures, the National Academy of Sciences recommended a study of atmospheric residues. It also recommended studies of possible products of reaction between hex and other chemicals, how hex is metabolized and its possible carcinogenicity. It is related to Kepone *(see)* and mirex *(see),* both suspected carcinogens.[368]

HEXACHLOROPHENE. *Chlorinated bis-phenol.* Widely used as an antiseptic prior to 1972, it was highly effective against gram-positive bacteria and many pathogenic fungi. The chemical was used as a surgical scrubbing agent, in bathing newborns to prevent staph infections, and in over-the-counter drugs such as mouthwashes, powders, cosmetics, and soaps. It was banned in 1972 by the FDA because it was toxic to the neurological system. It is still used in agricultural chemicals. Hexachlorophene was given in feed to rats for 105 to 106 weeks. According to a summary of the report, included in the *Federal Register,* April 14, 1978, as part of NCI's Carcinogenesis Testing Program, hexachlorophene did not cause tumors in rats under test conditions.

HEXAMETHYLENETETRAMINE. *See* Methenamine.

HEXAMETHYLPHOSPHORAMIDE (HMPA). A solvent used in fiber production, as an ultraviolet inhibitor in polyvinyl chloride, and as a chemical sterilant for insects. Tests performed by the U.S. Department of Agriculture in the 1950s showed no evidence that HMPA causes cancer. Testing in the 1960s by Du Pont de Nemours, interested in using it as a solvent, showed a moderate degree of toxicity. The company, according to staff toxicologist Henry J. Trochimowicz, began long-term testing. These later tests showed that HMPA must be handled with precautions appropriate for a potential carcinogen since relatively low-exposure levels produced malignant nasal tumors in rats. The company then began a series of protective measures in the workplace and devised and refined techniques for measuring HMPA in air and urine. [369]

HEXANE, 1,2:5,6-DIEPOXY. Used as a filling for thermometers instead of mercury and to determine the refractive index of minerals, it may be irritating to the respiratory tract. It causes tumors when inhaled by mice and cancer when applied to mouse skin in 17 milligram doses per kilogram of body weight.[370]

HEXESTROL. See Phenol.

4-HEXYLRESORCINOL. *Resorcinol, 4-hexyl-, caprokol, crystoids, Sucrets.* Used in mouthwashes and sunburn cream, it is a pale yellow heavy liquid that becomes solid upon standing at room temperature. It has a pungent odor and a sharp astringent taste and has been used medicinally as an antiworm medicine and as an antiseptic. It can cause severe gastrointestinal irritation; bowel, liver, and heart damage; and has been reported in concentrated solutions to cause burns of the skin and mucous membranes. Given intravaginally in mice, it caused tumors in 2,480 milligram doses per kilogram of body weight.[371]

HMPA. See Hexamethylphosphoramide.

HIGHWAYS. Persons living near highways may face an increased risk of developing cancer because they are exposed to elevated levels of cancer-causing chemicals produced by automobiles. A population study of a Swiss mountain town from 1958 to 1970 found deaths from cancer to be nine times more frequent among residents living along a well-traveled highway than among those living away from it. This finding suggests a link between cancer incidence and chemical carcinogens associated with highway traffic. Scientists measured the content of polycyclic aromatic hydrocarbons (PAH), a class of compounds, many of which are carcinogens, known to be produced during combustion in car engines. They found PAH levels were significantly higher closer to the highway than in other sections of town or in the surrounding mountains. As another piece of evidence, the scientists analyzed soot samples taken from an automobile exhaust pipe. The chemical pattern of PAH compounds in the soot closely matched the pattern in soils near the highway, providing a powerful argument that car exhaust is responsible for the observed PAH accumulation. The new data demonstrates that auto exhaust and environmental PAH mixtures are far more complex than assumed previously. When carcinogens in air and water are identified, the EPA will try to eliminate them through appropriate regulations, legislation, or court proceedings.[372,373]

HISTAMINE. *Theramine.* Consists of white crystals that are a product of the degradation of histidine. Histamine occurs in animals and humans and is a strong allergen. It is liberated by injury to tissues or whenever a protein is decomposed by putrification. It causes tumors when injected under the skin of rats in 3,000 milligram doses per kilogram of body weight.[374]

HODGKIN'S DISEASE. A cancer of the lymph system. A National Institute of Health-supported epidemiologic study revealed that socioeconomic factors, age, sex, and possibly viruses all may play a significant role in the initiation and progression of the disease. NCI investigators found three major epidemiologic patterns, revealing the importance of socioeconomic and age-susceptibility factors. The first pattern is characterized by high incidence and mortality rates in male children, a low incidence rate in the third decade of life, and a second peak of high incidence in the older age groups. Populations of patients falling into pattern I are generally classified as having a larger proportion of the lymphocyte-depleted or mixed cellularity types (histological subtypes of Hodgkin's disease which are associated with an unfavorable outlook for the patient). This pattern prevails in developing countries wherever industrialization and economic growth are low. Low rates of occurrence of the disease in children and a pronounced initial peak in young adults characterize pattern III. Nodular sclerosis, a hardening of the nodes as a result of inflammation, is the prevalent subtype in this pattern which prevails in wealthy urbanized countries. Pattern II, an intermediate one, appears in rural areas of developed countries, specifically central Europe and the southern part of the United States. In some Eastern countries, there may be a fourth pattern which is characterized by a relatively few number of cases in all age groups.

Hodgkin's disease also seems to vary according to sex. It appears that females are less susceptible than males to the initiation of Hodgkin's disease and more resistant to its lethal effects. Moreover, among children, girls are rarely affected, and the incidence in women is lower and the outlook is better than that for men. Socioeconomic factors also seem to influence the development and progression of Hodgkin's disease. In many communities, plagued with poverty, overcrowding, and poor nutrition susceptibility is high, particularly in children. In the better-developed, wealthier countries, children are usually well nourished and increasingly protected from chronic infectious diseases. In these populations, Hodgkin's disease is uncommon in children, but shows an initial peak in young adults, who have a better outlook for survival than those in less developed countries. The epidemiologic patterns of Hodgkin's disease bear some similarity to those of tuberculosis and mononucleosis. The epidemiologic similarities of Hodgkin's disease to tuberculosis, infectious mononucleosis, and chronic infectious diseases bring attention to the fact that there may be a link between infection and this form of cancer.[375]

HORMONES. They are the secretion of endocrine glands. Hormones are chemical messengers that literally "arouse" us to action. They help us respond to our environment; they influence and are influenced by what we see, hear, feel, eat, and drink, and by external and internal physical events. Under normal circumstances the many minute but powerful secretions work in harmony. When an imbalance occurs, diseases including cancer result. There is now little doubt that hormones are intimately involved in cancer growth, but whether they set the stage for cancer or actually are carcinogens themselves is not clear.

It is certain that hormones are needed for the growth of tissue such as uterine, endometrium, breast, and prostate tissue. The longer the tissue is under hormonal stimulation, the theory goes, the greater its chances for developing cancer. Lending weight to this premise is that it is difficult to induce mammary cancer with a mammary-tumor virus when mice have had their ovaries removed. Similarly, rats who have had their ovaries or pituitary glands removed are protected against the induction of mammary cancer by the carcinogen dimethylbenzanthracene. In rabbits, removing ovaries decreases the effectiveness of the induction of endometrial cancer by the carcinogen methylcholanthrene. In each of these cases the administration of estrogens restored the capacity of the tissues to undergo malignant transformation in response to a cancer-causing agent. Therefore, we can conclude that hormone-responsive tissues require hormonal stimulus to respond to a carcinogen.

If the initial exposure to a cancer-causing agent is a chance phenomenon, then the longer the tissue is stimulated the greater the probability that this event will result in cancer.[376] Besides the animal studies, there are observations that this is also true in humans. It has been demonstrated that cancer of the breast can be prevented by early removal of the ovaries in susceptible women. Men who have cancer of the prostate show marked improvement, but not cure, in 80 percent of the cases when their testes, the source of their male sex hormones, are removed and they are given the female hormone estrogen. As for the female hormone estrogen, in women it has been associated with cancer of the breast and endometrium, and with liver tumors. Men have developed liver tumors after taking androgens, not only for medical reasons but also illegally to build muscle power for sports. While hormones may set the stage for cancer or be carcinogenic, they can also protect against cancer. For example, in Scotland it has been found that lung-cancer patients excrete less of the hormone androsterone than do nonlung-cancer patients. It has also been shown that establishment of blood-borne metastases is the result of a lack of a certain clotting factor in the blood. Androsterone is known to increase that clotting factor. There have also been reports that the female hormone estriol *(see)* protects against breast cancer. When it is found in large amounts in the urine of women, those women do not develop breast cancer.[377] Therefore, the consensus of opinion now seems to be that there are three factors intimately involved with the development of cancer: genetic susceptibility, hormonal status, and cancer-causing agents.[378,379]

HOUSEWORK. Much attention has been paid to the hazards of working in industry but little focused on what may prove to be one of the highest risk occupations—housework. Exposure to the major classes of chemicals takes place in the home. Among these are prescription and over-the-counter drugs; pesticides for household, pet, or garden use; food additives; and cosmetics. In addition, there are the many materials needed or convenient for the operation of the household: adhesives, solvents, soaps, detergents, polishes, and other cleaning supplies; toiletries; air fresheners; hobby supplies; plastic articles and toys; synthetic fabrics; and an almost endless list of other chemicals.[380] Thus, it is not surprising that a study by University of Oregon researchers reported that the risk of dying of cancer for housewives is twice that for working women. Dr. William E. Morton, head of the Health Science Center's Division of Environmental Medicine at Oregon, explained that running a household is the nation's major cottage industry, and yet until now it has been ignored by occupational medicine. He said that the higher cancer death rate among housewives warrants immediate studies to determine whether the effect occurs in other states and, if so, what's behind it. The Oregon researchers could not at first believe their own statistics when they found that the death rate for housewives between 16 to 64 years was 129.8 per 100,000 compared to 82.5 for all other women. They did a second analysis, this time comparing cancer deaths for all women listed on death certificates as housewives, unemployed, or not in the labor force, with those for all employed women. The rates were 102.6 per 100,000 for housewives versus 51.1 per 100,000 for working women. The only cancer-death rate significantly higher than the countywide rate was that for housewives. Dr. Morton found that cancers of the breast, cervix, ovaries, colon, and rectum, uterus, liver, and gallbladder, brain, lungs, and stomach, along with lymphomas, proved to be significantly more common among housewives than among working women. He cautioned against hasty interpretation of the findings, and said they may be confined to just one small metropolitan area, or possibly that poor health kept the women from working during the last year or so of life. However, Dr. Morton did say that he would not be surprised if the suggested risk for housewives turns out to be real. "The home is a complex chemical environment that contains many of the same chemicals that are known hazards in industry." He suspected the risk may be related to the amount of chemicals used.[381]

HYDANTOIN, 5,5-Diphenyl-. *Aleviatin, causoin, danten, dihydantoin.* A white odorless solid that is used as an intermediate *(see)* in the manufacture of pharmaceuticals, textile lubricants, and certain high polymers, including epoxy resins. It causes cancer when injected into the abdomen of rats in doses of 1,370 milligrams per kilogram of body weight and when given orally to rats in doses of 1,500 milligrams per kilogram of body weight.[382] *See also* Dilantin.

HYDRAZINE. A colorless, fuming, hydroscopic liquid derived from sodium hydroxide, chlorine, and ammonia. It is highly toxic when ingested. A strong irritant to the skin and eyes. It is a severe explosive hazard. It is used as a rocket propellant; as an agricultural chemical to prevent potatoes from sprouting; in drugs as an antibacterial; as an antihypertensive; as a polymerization catalyst in spandex fibers; and as an antioxidant in plating material, fuel cells, solder, photo developers, oil-well drilling solutions, and diving equipment. It prevents cells from dividing and has caused cancer when injected into the abdomen in mice in 400 milligram doses per kilogram of body weight. There is an OSHA standard for it.[383]

HYDRAZINE SULFATE. A white crystalline powder that is used in the manufacture of chemicals, in condensation reactions, as a catalyst in making acetate fibers; in the analysis of minerals, slags, and fluxes to determine the arsenic in metals; to separate polonium from tellurium; as a fungicide; as a germicide; and experimentally in the treatment of cancer. It caused cancer when given orally to mice in doses of 1,280 milligrams per kilogram of body weight and when injected in 832 milligram doses per kilogram of body weight.[384]

2-HYDRAZINOETHANOL. *Hydroxyethylhydrazine, ethanol, 2-hydrazino.* Prepared from hydrazine monohydrate and chloroethanol, it is a colorless, slightly viscous liquid used as an intermediate *(see)* in manufacturing processes. It causes cancer in mice when administered orally in 572 milligram doses per kilogram of body weight.[385]

HYDROCARBONS. *See* Polycyclic Hydrocarbons.

HYDROQUINONE. *2,5-Bis (bis(2-chloroethyl) amino) methyl hydroquinone.* Used in bleach and freckle creams and in suntan lotions. A white crystalline phenol that occurs naturally, but it is usually manufactured. It combines with oxygen very rapidly and becomes brown when exposed to air. Death has occurred from ingestion of as little as 5 milligrams, and 2 milligrams have caused nausea, vomiting, and ringing in the ears. It caused tumors when applied to the skin of mice in 800 milligram doses per kilogram of body weight. Hydroquinone mustard causes clouding of the eye lens, and application to the skin may cause an allergic reaction. When injected into the abdomen of mice in 28 milligram doses per kilogram of body weight, it caused cancer.[386,387]

IMIDAZOLE MUSTARD (DTIC). *Imidazole-4-carboxamide; 5-(3,3-dimethyl-1-triazeno).* An inhibitor of metabolites and of histamine *(see),* it is used in the biological control of pests, especially fabric-feeding insects. It was tried as an anticancer drug. It caused lung tumors in mice.[388]

2-IMIDAZOLIDINETHIONE. *See* ETU.

IMMUNITY. Do we all get frequent cancers that our body defeats? Is cancer a breakdown in the immunological system? One clue is in the discovery of a rare immune-deficiency disease that sometimes leads to cancer. For a number of years, Thomas A. Waldmann, M.D., and his colleagues at NCI have studied patients, mostly children with a life-threatening disease called common variable hypogammaglobulinemia (CVH), which is characterized by the patient's inability to make protective antibodies. Ten percent of these patients develop cancer. The scientists grew lymphocytes from 13 patients with CVH in laboratory cultures and found that despite chemical stimulation, they produced from 16 to 37 fewer antibodies than lymphocytes from normal individuals under the same test conditions. After a series of experiments, the investigators discovered that the patients' immune defect was due to an excess of a certain type of T-lymphocytes. These are white blood cells that originate in the bone marrow and migrate through the thymus before becoming active immune agents. These types of cells in CVH patients act as suppressor cells that block antibody production. This may indeed be a clue to why cancer occurs.

Another clue is that the incidence of cancer appearing in patients who have undergone kidney or heart transplants is estimated at 20 to 140 times greater than malignancies found in a comparable age-adjusted population. All of those who have undergone organ transplants from donors other than identical twins also underwent immunosuppressive chemotherapy to offset the normal processes through which their bodies would reject the transplanted organ.

In laboratory animals on which immunosuppressive drugs are tested, malignant as well as nonmalignant tumors arise. These tumors have been traced to viruses that appear to be a necessary intermediate between immunosuppression and cancer in the animal. The immune reaction in these animals appears to interfere with virus elimination and tumor rejection mechanisms, thus the growth of tumors.

What is not known is whether viral infection is a necessary intermediate between immunosuppression and cancer in man, since no cancer viruses in man have yet been isolated with certainty. Immunosuppressed patients are extremely vulnerable to many common nontumor viruses as well as the human wart virus that causes benign skin tumors. It has also been found that drugs used in transplant patients to suppress immunity increase the risk of lymphomas 35 times, the risk of lip and skin cancers 4 times, and the risk of several other cancers 2½ times.

To prevent cancers from occurring in transplant patients, scientists are seeking to stimulate antiviral or antitumor defenses, including interferon production and other systems that would not cause rejections of the transplant.[389,390]

IMURAN. *Azathioprine.* An imidazolyl derivative of mercaptopurine, it is used to fight rejection of transplanted organs in patients. There have been reports of lymphomas developing in patients receiving immunosuppressive therapy after kidney transplants.[391] *See also* Immunity.

INDICAN. *Indol-3-yl-potassium sulfate, urinary indican.* Consists of light brown platelets. It occurs in the urine of mammals and in blood plasma. Can cause cancer when injected under the skin of mice in 5,000 milligram doses per kilogram of body weight.[392]

INDIGO CARMINE. *See* FD & C Blue 2.

INDIGOTINE. *See* FD & C Blue 2.

INDOLE. A white lustrous flaky substance with an unpleasant odor that occurs naturally in jasmine oil and orange flowers. It is also derived from coal tar and from feces. In highly diluted solution the odor is pleasant and is used in perfumes. When injected under the skin of mice in 1,000 milligram doses per kilogram of body weight it causes tumors.[393]

INTERMEDIATE. An organic compound that is a stepping stone between the parent compound and the final product, as in the production of dyes, pharmaceuticals, or other artificial products that develop properties only upon oxidation. For instance, an intermediate is used for hair-dye bases that have dyeing action only when exposed to oxygen.

IONIZING RADIATION. Very short wavelengths that are highly energetic and penetrating rays of the following types:

- Gamma rays, emitted by radioactive elements and isotopes (decay of atomic nucleus).
- X-rays, generated by suddenly stopping fast-moving electrons.
- Subatomic particles, such as electrons, protons, and diatrons when accelerating.

Ionizing radiation can cause mutations in DNA and in cell nuclei; it adversely affects protein and amino-acid mechanisms; impairs or destroys body tissue; and attacks bone marrow, the source of red blood cells. Exposure to ionizing radiation, even for a short period, is highly dangerous and can result in death, either immediately or from cancer many years later. Ionizing radiation can result in leukemia and thyroid cancers as well as other forms of cancer. However, it is also used to cure cancers.[394] *See* X-rays.

IPD. *3,3-Iminobis-1-propanol dimethanesulfonate (ester) hydrochloride.* Synthesized from bis(3 hydroxypropyl) amine and methanesulfonic acid anhydride, it has been found to have an antitumor effect against tumors resistent to nitrogen mustard and has been used for the treatment of myelogenous leukemia. It was tested because it was one of the anticancer drugs administered chronically in the treatment of human cancer. In the study IPD was given by abdominal injection to rats and mice for periods up to

52 weeks. While this study was limited to early deaths and other toxic effects from the drug, the appearance of cancers in the peritoneum near the injection sites in both rats and mice indicated that IPD has a potential for carcinogenic activity in animals under test conditions.[395]

IRON BLACK. *see* Magnetite.

IRON-DEXTRAN COMPLEX. *Imferon.* Used to treat severe cases of iron-deficiency anemia. A risk of carcinogenesis may attend the muscular injection of the iron-carbohydrate complexes. Under experimental conditions such complexes have been found to produce sarcomas when injected in rats, mice, rabbits, and possibly in hamsters in very large doses. The number of tumors produced was relatively small, and such tumors have not been produced in guinea pigs. The long latency period between injection of a potential carcinogen and the appearance of a tumor makes it difficult to measure the risk of this substance in man;[396] however, NIOSH considers it a suspected human carcinogen.[397]

IRON-DEXTRIN COMPLEX. *Ferrigen.* Iron-Carbohydrate complex. *See* Iron-Dextran Complex.

IRON LACTATE. *See* Ferrous Lactate.

IRON-OXIDE, SACCHARATED. *Iron oxide mix; iron sugar; colliron I.V.; ferric oxide, saccharated.* Brown powder used in iron-deficiency anemia. Caused cancer when injected under the skin of mice in doses of 104 milligrams per kilogram of bodyweight.[398] Listed as a positive animal carcinogen by NIOSH.[399]

IRRITATION. Chronic irritation has been associated with the development of cancer. For example, irritation caused by gallstones and bladder stones has been found to be associated with a greater incidence of malignancy in those organs. Infections caused by bacteria, parasites, or other microorganisms may not, in themselves, be dangerous, but the chronic inflammation they cause can lead to a malignancy. If tar is repeatedly placed on the skin, a cancer will develop, but no one is exactly sure why. A chronically infected scar, especially a burn scar, or a chronically infected cervix may set the stage for cancer.

ISONIAZID. *Isonicotinic acid hydrazide, armacide, pyricidin, robisellin, tebecid, zonazide.* An antituberculosis agent derived from gamma-picoline. Severe hepatitis associated with Isoniazid therapy has been reported and may develop months after therapy. It has also caused lung tumors in humans and cancer in mice.[400,401,402]

ISONICOTINIAMIDE, 2-ETHYLTHIO. *Ethionamide.* Minute yellow crystals derived from ethanol and used as an antimicrobacterial in tuberculosis treatment in conjunction with other agents. It causes tumors when given orally to mice in 24 milligram doses per kilogram of body weight.[403]

ISONICOTINIC ACID. A white, practically odorless powder that is slightly soluble in water. Used in the synthesis of isoniazid acid and similar substances *See also* Isoniazid.

ISONICOTINIC ACID HYDRAZIDE. *See* Isoniazid.

ISOPHOSPHAMIDE. Similar to nitrogen mustard *(see)*, it was selected for testing by the NCI because it is a new drug and is one of a series of anticancer agents selected for carcinogenicity screening with rodents. In a carcinogenesis test of this investigational anticancer drug, intraabdominal injections of the compound produced cancers in female mice and rats but not in the males of either species. In rats, uterine leiomyosarcoma was induced by the test compound. A benign mammary tumor, fibroadenoma, also was associated with isophosphamide dosage. Female mice responded to isophosphamide with malignant lymphomas of the blood-building system, which includes the liver, lymph nodes, bone marrow, and spleen.[404]

ISOPROPYL OIL. Used in the production process of isopropanol. It caused cancer of the paranasal sinus, larynx, and lung, and the process has been discontinued.[405]

ISOPROPYL -N-PHENYLCARBAMATE. An antisprouting agent found to cause cancer when given to animals whose skin was subsequently painted with croton oil. It was banned in the United States but nowhere else.[406]

ISOQUINOLINE. *4-((p-Dimethylamino)phenyl) azo; 5-((p(dimethyl-amine)phenyl) azo)-.* Dark red crystals. When in liquid form it has a pungent odor resembling a mixture of anise oil and benzaldehyde. It is used in the manufacture of dyes, in insecticides, and as a rubber accelerator. Found to cause cancer in rats when given orally in doses of from 720 to 3,276 milligrams per kilogram of body weight.[407]

JETS. Since pollutants emitted by jet aircraft are of the same type as those given off by a car, a direct comparison is possible. In one landing and takeoff cycle (LTO), a jet produces as much soot as 2,500 cars produced all day.[408] Total emissions from jet aircraft can be expected to increase in the future because of increasing numbers of flights and the use of more powerful engines. The major pollutants that are emitted by jet aircraft include particulate matter (soot), carbon monoxide, aldehydes, hydrocarbons, and nitrogen oxides. The first of the pollutants, particulate matter, constitutes not only a visual nuisance but is also a potential health problem. The rest, which are not visible, are irritants and in high concentrations can be toxic.

KALE. *See* Antithyroid Compounds.

KAPRON. *See* Nylon.

KEPONE. *Chlordecone.* A chlorinated insecticide. The compound was first introduced in 1958 and has been used as an insecticide against leaf-eating insects, ants, and cockroaches, and as a larvicide against flies. In tests conducted by the NCI, it was found to cause a form of liver cancer. Rats fed high-dose levels of the chemical, and mice at both high- and low-dose levels, exhibited significant increases in liver cancer. In control animals not treated with chlordecone, no liver cancers were found among male or female rats, or among female mice. Clinical effects other than liver cancers also were found among chlordecone-treated animals. These effects included generalized tremors, skin changes, and extensive hyperplasia (abnormal cell growth) of the liver.[409]

In the environment it behaves similarly to mirex and some other organo-chlorine compounds. It degrades slowly, concentrates in biological tissue, and produces both acute and chronic effects more readily in some species than in others. Acute toxic effects observed among workers exposed to relatively high concentrations of it in Virginia included weight loss, neuro-logical impairment, abnormal liver function, skin rash, and reproductive failure. It causes liver tumors in animals and likely would produce them in humans. Therefore, it must be considered a human carcinogen.[410]

Of the estimated 1,600,000 kilograms of Kepone produced in the United States from the 1950s to 1975, as much as 99.2 percent was exported to Latin America, Africa, and Europe. In tropical areas, including Puerto Rico, Kepone has been used extensively to control the banana-root borer. Human exposure to chlordecone can result from consumption of either livestock foraged on Kepone-treated land or fish taken in waters polluted by runoff from the land. Depending on the rate of application, Kepone used on banana plantations could result in chlordecone residues of about 10 parts per million in fish taken from runoff-polluted water. Current FDA permissi-ble levels for Kepone in United States seafood are 0.3 ppm in fish and in oysters and 0.4 ppm in crabs. The EPA canceled the use of Kepone in ant and cockroach traps in 1976 because some pesticides are known to concen-trate in indoor air and dust, and inhalation is a possible hazard. The National Academy of Sciences panel recommended that homes and busi-nesses using the traps be surveyed to determine the extent to which Kepone persists in the air and is a hazard to health.

KERB. *See* Pronamide.

KRAMERIA. *See* Rhatany Extract.

KWELL. *Cyclohexane 1,2,3,4,5,6-hexachloro: lindane (gamma benzene hexachloride one percent) shampoo.* The active ingredient in this shampoo is lindane *(see)*, a parasite killer used in the treatment of head lice and crab lice and their nits. Lindane can penetrate human skin and has a potential for central nervous system toxicity. Animal studies have indicated greater absorption through the skin of the young. Causes liver damage and can cause cancer when given orally to mice in 22 milligram doses per kilogram of body weight.[411,412]

LABORATORIES, SCHOOL. High school and college science labora-tories have been found to contain carcinogenic chemicals. Many state edu-cation and occupational health departments have ordered known carcinogens removed from high school and college classroom shelves. These are substances for which the recommended exposure level is essentially zero.

A survey by Kentucky Labor Department officials found that 90 percent of the 41 four-year colleges and universities in that state had one or more of these cancer-causing chemicals in their labs, as did 5 percent of the high schools. According to a report in the September 1976 *Journal of College Science Teaching*, Arizona, Oregon, Washington, and Utah authorities reported their own scattered instances of finding carcinogens with few or no restrictions placed on them in high school and college chemistry labs. One difficulty in getting these substances off the shelves is that each of the carcinogens is known by a variety of names, so that even the knowledgeable chemistry teacher may need a complete listing to do a thorough search of science-department shelves. Another difficulty is that improperly packaged and disposed of carcinogens may be even more dangerous than they were on the schoolroom shelves. The most frequently found chemical on the Kentucky list was benzidine *(see)*. It has been used in schools primarily as an indicator in quantitative analysis and to stain slides in biology classes. Not long after publicity about the rise of this chemical in the lab appeared, a Chicago chemistry major developed leukemia while in college. Her physician attributed her disease to exposure to benzidine in the laboratory.[413]

LACTOSE. *Milk sugar, saccharum lactin, D-lactose.* Used in infant foods, in bacteriology, for baking and confections, in margarine and butter manufacture, and the manufacture of penillin, yeast, edible protein, and riboflavin. Causes tumors when injected under the skin of mice in 50 milligram doses per kilogram of body weight.[414]

LARYNX CANCER. Some 7,000 people develop this disease each year, and 3,000 people die of it. The symptoms are (1) hoarseness or other persistent voice changes; (2) sensation of lump in the throat; (3) persistent soreness of the neck; (4) difficulty in swallowing. Individuals who use cigarettes and alcohol to excess are more susceptible to cancer of the larynx. The disease is almost never found in nonsmokers and nondrinkers. It is diagnosed by examination of the larynx through the mouth with the aid of a mirror. Cancer of the larynx can be prevented by avoiding cigarette smoking: the risk of developing cancer of the larynx is seven times greater for cigarette smokers than for nonsmokers. Similarly, excess use of alcohol should be curbed. Symptoms of hoarseness should be brought to the attention of a physician if they persist more than two weeks. When detected early, cancer of the larynx may be cured by radiation therapy, surgery, or both. New and improved techniques of treatment will in many cases preserve the normal voice. When there is impairment of speech following treatment, encouraging methods of rehabilitation have been developed.

LASIOCARPINE. A pyrrolizidine alkaloid that is found in the seeds of

Heliotropium lasiocarpum, Heliotropium europaeum, and several other plant species, all members of the family Boraginaceae. It is toxic to the liver of sheep and cattle grazing on *Heliotropium* plants. Acute liver dystrophy in humans caused by *H. lasiocarpum* poisoning was reported in Russia between 1931 and 1945. A test of lasiocarpine was conducted by the NCI to assess the combined effects of a group of known or suspected carcinogens. Lasiocarpine caused liver tumors in both sexes of the rat and leukemia in female animals.[415]

LAUROYL PEROXIDE. *Dilauroyl peroxide.* A white coarse powder that is tasteless, and a faint odor. It is soluble in oils and most organic solvents, is toxic when ingested or inhaled, is a strong irritant to the skin, and is combustible. It is a strong oxidizing material. Used as a bleaching agent and as an intermediate *(see)* and drying agent for fats, oils, and waxes. It is also a polymerization catalyst.[416,417] Causes tumors when inhaled, injected, or painted on mice in doses of from 64 to 38 milligrams per kilogram of body weight.

LEAD. *Acetate, trihydrate, naphthenate, chromate oxide, sugar of lead.* One of the best-known and most-studied of occupational hazards, lead has been recognized as a poison for more than a thousand years. Lead affects the blood-forming tissues in the bone marrow, producing anemia. After many years of lead poisoning, a person may develop kidney complications that can lead to high blood pressure and even to complete kidney failure. Children who eat lead paints show many of the same signs. The damage to their brains can be so great, however, that they may be permanently retarded. Lead may be a weak carcinogen. In one study by Tabershaw/-Cooper Associates, Inc. of Berkeley, California, over 7,000 men who had worked for at least one year in a lead smelter or lead-battery plant and who had been heavily exposed to metals had only slightly higher than expected rates of cancer of the lung, stomach, and large intestine. One problem with lead is that the body stores it for extremely long periods.

Lead acetate or sugar of lead consists of white crystals or flakes with a sweetish taste that absorb carbon dioxide when exposed to air. It is used in the dyeing of textiles; in medicines, waterproofing, varnishes, lead dryers, chrome pigments, gold processes, antifouling paints; as an insecticide and a catalystical level. Rats who had 0.1 to 1 percent of lead acetate in their diet for a year or longer developed kidney tumors. It may be absorbed through the skin and is highly toxic by ingestion, inhalation, or skin absorption.[418]

- Basic lead acetate caused cancer when given orally to mice and rats at 27 milligrams per kilogram of body weight.[419]
- Lead naphthenate consists of a soft yellow resinous semitransparent lead-salt solution. It is used in paint and varnish dryers, wood preserva-

tives, insecticides, and as a catalyst for reactions between unsaturated fatty acids and sulfates in the presence of air. It is toxic when absorbed through the skin and caused tumors when painted on the skin of mice in 48 milligram doses per kilogram of body weight.[420]

- Lead chromate (6+) oxide or basic lead chromate is also called chrome orange or C.I. pigment red. It consists of yellow crystals that are soluble in strong acids and alkalines but insoluble in water. It is derived from the reaction of sodium chromide and lead nitrate. It is toxic when ingested or inhaled and caused tumors when injected under the skin of rats in 150 milligram doses per kilogram of body weight. It is used as a pigment in industrial paints, rubber, plastics, and ceramic coatings. There is an OSHA standard for safe amounts permissible in the air.[421]

- Lead (II) phosphate (3:2) also called lead orthophosphate is a white powder that is insoluble in water. Used as a stabilizer for plastics, it caused cancer when injected into rats in 725 milligram doses per kilogram of body weight.[422]

LEUKEMIA. Leukemia is a generalized disorder of blood-cell production in which abnormal white blood cells accumulate in the blood and bone marrow. These cells seem to appear suddenly in the same bone marrow that previously formed only normal, healthy, mature white cells. Although leukemia rarely produces tumors, it is similar to cancer in several respects and is therefore sometimes called "cancer of the blood." The causes of leukemia are not fully understood. Under special circumstances, ionizing radiation and a few chemicals have been known to induce the disease. Both radiation and some chemicals interfere with the functioning of bone marrow, but how this effect is related to the development of leukemia remains to be determined. Bone-marrow damage resulting from the long-term use of certain drugs has on occasion been associated with the development of leukemia. Leukemia has been reported to occur at higher than average rates among persons exposed to intense radiation. Susceptibility to radiation-induced leukemia varies from one individual to another. This varying susceptibility is one of a number of pieces of evidence indicating that leukemia may have, in part, a genetic basis. This is also suggested by the frequency with which childhood leukemia occurs in identical twins who have the same genetic makeup. It has recently been found that leukemia occurs together with certain congenital defects more often than can be attributed to chance. Viruses that contain RNA and closely resemble the particles known to cause leukemias in many vertebrate animals other than man may also be a cause of leukemia. There is evidence that RNA-containing leukemia viruses (or viral genetic information) are present in a heritable form in all cells of certain species of animals and can be transmitted in a latent form, along with normal genetic information, from parent to offspring. It is possible that residence in certain houses somehow predisposes the occupants to leukemia. Environmental factors may be responsible for some cases of leukemia. These houses tend to have more occupants than other houses, or greater concentrations of elderly people. Several mechanisms (infectious, physical, or chemical) can be envisioned by which occupancy in a given house might predispose its residents to leukemia. Possibly some infectious agent, capable of triggering leukemia under suitable conditions, might be present in dormant form in the structure of the house or in house dust. An unsuspected source of radiation incorporated in the structure of the house or in its surroundings might also contribute to the development of leukemia in the occupants of the house. Or, some leukemogenic chemical might be present in an area of the house. Virologists strongly suspect that cats might be a primary host for the oncogenic virus that appears to have definite possibilities as a producer of leukemia. This virus seems capable of crossing to other species. Such crossing may result in the production of epidemics of contagious malignant disease in man.

There are two kinds of leukemia: (1) chronic—long in duration, and (2) acute—more severe and short in duration. Adults are generally stricken by acute or chronic granulocytic (granular blood cell) leukemia. Acute lymphocytic leukemia (made of lymph cells) usually strikes children, while adults are afflicted by the chronic type. Both children and adults may be victims of acute and chronic monocytic leukemia (monocyte cell). Drugs are used in the treatment of leukemia, and remission is always a possibility —whether it is a temporary or potentially permanent arrest of the leukemic process. Drug side effects are common, and supportive care is necessary. Both drugs and leukemia damage the bone marrow and impair the patient's ability to produce two important blood elements: (1) platelets, tiny disc-shaped particles that prevent hemorrhage, and (2) white blood cells (granulocytes), which help control bacterial and fungal infections. Hemorrhage and infection are the most common causes of death among acute leukemia patients. Transfusions are often necessary to prevent or stop hemorrhaging. Immunotherapy and bone-marrow transplants may also be effective in treatment of leukemia. The long-term survivals recently achieved in some patients with leukemia may include a significant number of cures.

LEUKERAN. *Chlorambucil.* A derivative of nitrogen mustard *(see),* it is used in the treatment of chronic lymphocytic leukemia, malignant lymphomas, and Hodgkin's disease. It is not curative but produces remission. It is easier to handle than nitrogen mustard. It can cause severe bone-marrow depression.

LEUKOPLAKIA. *See* Precancerous Conditions.

LIGHT SKIN. *See* Phaeomelanin.

LINDANE. *1,2,3,4,5,6-Hexachlorocyclohexane HCH.* A pesticide. Also used on the skin of humans as a scabicide and pediculicide (lice destroyer). It is irritating to the skin and can cause liver damage.[423] It has been selected by the EPA for priority attention as a toxic water pollutant and has been selected for testing by the NCI as a suspected carcinogen.[424]

LIVER CANCER. Agents found to cause it are arsenic and vinyl chloride. Workers whose jobs cause them to be susceptible to it are tanners, smelters, vintners, and plastic workers.

LIVER TUMORS. *See* The Pill.

LUNG CANCER. This disease is the leading cancer killer of men and the second leading cancer killer of women in the United States and is one of the swiftest-acting and most lethal forms of malignancies. Eighty percent of its victims die within two years after diagnosis and 50 percent of them within six months. The symptoms of lung cancer are (1) chronic cough, (2) coughing up blood, (3) shortness of breath, (4) recurrent respiratory infections, (5) persistent pain in the chest. The overwhelming majority of cases occur in cigarette smokers over the age of 45. Patients with a past history of tuberculosis also have an increased incidence of lung cancer. People whose occupation brings them in contact with asbestos, chromates, and radioactive materials are more susceptible.

The relationship between occupation and increased incidence of lung cancer raised concern in Texas, where deaths from lung cancer, particularly those living in the heavily industrialized metropolitan area of Houston, rose in the 1970s: fatalities increased by 53 percent, more than double the 25 percent rate of the entire state of Texas for all forms of cancer. The general population of the state increased by about 14 percent during the same period. The exact reasons for the increase are still conjecture, but researchers believe it has to do with petrochemical plants, as well as other industries concentrated in the area.[425]

Cancer of the lung is one form of cancer in which there is a truly effective preventative measure: avoid cigarette smoking. The smoker's risk of getting lung cancer is proportional to the number of years cigarettes have been smoked, the number of cigarettes smoked per day, the age at which cigarette smoking started, and how deeply cigarette smoke is inhaled. Cigarette smoking not only leads to death from lung cancer but also increases the chances of dying from other lung and heart diseases.

Lung-cancer deaths increased by 8 percent annually in white women and almost 10 percent in black women between 1973 and 1976, according to government statistics. The increase was attributed by cancer experts almost entirely to cigarette smoking. They pointed out that females began to indulge heavily in the habit in the mid-1940s and that we are seeing the results now.[426]

In addition to tobacco, the following are considered lung-cancer agents: arsenic, asbestos, bis-chloromethyl ether, chromium, coal tar, dusts, iron oxide, mustard gas, nickel, and petroleum. Workers whose jobs place them at risk for lung cancer include: vintners, miners, asbestos users, textile users, insulation workers, tanners, smelters, glass and pottery workers, retortmen, radiologists, radium workers, and chemical workers.

Occupational exposure to any of the cancer-causing agents mentioned should be avoided or carefully controlled. Adequate safeguards for pure air should be provided if one works in dusty occupations, such as mining, milling, or grinding. Successful treatment of lung cancer depends first on early diagnosis. Some inroads are being made in this area; preliminary results from screening programs have shown that annual chest X-ray exams coupled with three annual deep-cough sputum exams in high-risk individuals can detect cancer very early. However, it is still difficult to diagnose cancer of the lung at a stage when it can be cured. Any lingering lung infection should be suspect and requires prompt medical evaluation.

Patients (more often men) with small-cell anaplastic carcinoma, a malignant proliferation of cells, are receiving a combination of eight drugs. Formerly, they would have been expected to die within 3 months after diagnosis, but they are now living a year or 18 months, and a small number are even remaining disease free for several years. Less progress is being made in extending the lives of patients with the other kinds of lung cancer: squamous cell (scalelike), almost always associated with smoking; adeno-carcinoma (of the glands); and brochiolar (of the branches), a rare form. Recent innovations and advances in computer science, nuclear medicine, and cell biology may also benefit lung-cancer victims in the not-so-distant future. Human small-cell carcinoma cells can now be grown in the laboratory, thus providing a vehicle for the rapid testing of new drugs against this form of cancer.

LUTEOSKYRIN. A fungus from *P. islandicum* Sopp. causes liver tumors in rats and mice. It grows on rice and cereals. Chronic daily ingestion of a few tenths of a miligram by mice for two years was toxic to the liver.[427]

LYMPHOMAS. Cancers of the lymph system.

LYMPH SYSTEM. The circulatory network of vessels, spaces, and nodes carrying lymph, the almost colorless fluid that bathes the body's cells. The system is important in the body's defense against infection.

MAGENTA. *See* Fuchsin.

MAGNETITE. *Black gold, black iron oxide, lodestone, iron ore.* Contains 72 percent iron and is readily recognized by its strong attraction to magnets. It is derived from the action of air, steam, or carbon dioxide on iron and is used as a pigment, as a polishing compound in metallurgy, in medicine, in magnetic inks, in the electronic industry, and as a coating for magnetic tape. It caused tumors when injected into the abdomen of mice in 400 milligram doses per kilogram of body weight.[428]

MALATHION. An organophosphorous insecticide. It was given in feed to rats and mice for 80 weeks. According to a summary of the report, malathion was not carcinogenic in either rats or mice under the test conditions.[429]

MALEIC ANHYDRIDE. *2,5-Furandione; lytron.* Derived from passing a mixture of benzene *(see)* vapor and air over vanadium. Used in polyester resins, in fumaric and tartaric acid manufacture, in pesticides, as a preservative for oils and fats, and for permant-pass resins for textiles. It is a strong irritant to tissue. It caused cancer when injected subcutaneously in doses of 610 milligrams per kilogram of body weight. [430]

MALEIC HYDRAZIDE. Regulates the growth of unwanted "suckers" or about 90 percent of the United States tobacco crop and is also applied to 10 to 15 percent of domestic potatoes and onions to prevent sprouting after harvest. It is highly toxic to humans and has produced central nervous system disturbances and liver damage in experimental animals. It has led to liver and other tumors in some mice. However, other studies, including one done for the NCI and published in 1969, show no carcinogenic effects from it. It has produced genetic damage in plant and animal systems, a fact that often signals a cancer-causing effect.[431]

MALONALDEHYDE. A decomposition product of peroxidized polyunsaturated fatty acids, it has been shown to be a carcinogenic initiator on mouse skin, and it has also been demonstrated to be mutagenic. Eating of peroxidized foods by animals during experiments has been related to heart disease, cancer, and aging. When several types of commercially available food both cooked and uncooked were tested for malonaldehyde, it was determined that beef purchased at the supermarket had the greatest amount of it. Turkey and cooked chicken had high levels, and most cheeses had only a small amount of it. In contrast, many vegetables and fruits had either minute amounts or no malonaldehyde.[432]

MALTOSE. *Malt sugar, maltobiose.* The most common reducing disaccharide, it is composed of two molecules of glucose and is found in starch and glycogen. Its colorless crystals are derived from the enzymatic action of malt extract on starch. It is used as a nutrient, sweetener, culture medium, and stabilizer for polysulfides. It causes tumors in mice when injected under the skin in doses of 500 milligrams per kilogram of body weight.[433]

MAMMOGRAPHY. The use of this special breast X-ray is a comparatively new technology. It is good at finding tiny, presumably curable breast cancers that would otherwise be undetected until they had grown into palpable lumps. The use of mammography for screening apparently healthy women in the NCI program was controversial. Critics of the screening said that the X-rays may cause as many breast tumors as they detect. However, the premise behind the screening was that if cancer were discovered early enough, it could be cured. The technology is being improved and radiological refinements make it possible to get pictures of the breast with lower and lower X-ray dosages. In the meantime the NCI and the American Cancer Society made the following recommendations pertaining to the use of mammography:

- Mammography screening should be available to women over 50.
- For women between the ages of 40 and 49, mammography should be used only for those who have had breast cancer or who have a mother or sister who have had the disease.
- For women between the ages of 35 and 39, mammography should be used only if a woman has previously had cancer in one breast.
- Thermography, the examination of breast tissue by heat rather than X-ray, has not been proved to be valuable and should be dropped from the program, although it should still be studied.
- Mammography should never be used to screen women under 35 years.
- Mammography should be used for women of any age to aid in the diagnosis of a suspected tumor.[434,435]

MANGANESE (ETHYLENEBIS) (DITHIOCARBAMATE). *See Ethylenebisdithiocarbamate.*

MANNITOL. *See Mannomustine.*

MANNITOL MUSTARD. *See Mannomustine.*

MANNOMUSTINE. *Mannitol mustard; mannitol; 1,6-bis(2-chloroethyl)amino-1,6-dideoxy-; dihydrochloride D; degranol; mannitol myleran.* An antineoplastic agent used to treat certain forms of cancer. It can cause nausea, vomiting, and leukopenia. It has caused tumors when given intravenously to rats and cancer when injected in mice in doses of 23 milligrams per kilogram of body weight.[436]

MEGESTROL. *Pregna-4,6-diene-3,20-dione,17-hydroxy-6-methyl-, acetate.* White crystalline solid used as a drug to combat endometrial (uterine) carcinoma and breast cancer. Its effects are palliative. Megestrol has caused birth defects and cancer in women.[437] It has been banned by the FDA for use other than as an antineoplastic.[438]

MELANOMA. An estimated 9,500 new cases of malignant melanoma of the skin occur each year. Of these, approximately 4,500 will be in men and 5,000 in women. An estimated 5,300 people will die of melanoma each year. Incidence rates for malignant melanoma vary widely in geographical areas. The duration and intensity of sun exposure as well as the racial factors that determine the sensitivity of the individual's skin to sunlight appear to be important factors. The observed incidence of melanoma is increasing, perhaps a factor of an aging population longer exposed to the ultraviolet rays.

Moles rarely undergo malignant change. They vary in color from yellow brown to black. A small percentage of "junctional nevi," flat or raised moles, found at the junction of the dermis and epidermis may become malignant. Active junctional nevi contain some changed cells characteristic of early or premalignant lesions. Melanomas apparently develop more frequently from this type of mole. Therefore, an increase in size or pigmentation of a mole should signal an immediate visit to a physician. Excision by a specialist of all malignant lesions is recommended, especially when the mole shows increasing pigmentation, speckling, or a halo of pigment around the base, or when any mole increases in size, bleeds, ulcerates, or crusts. Usually malignant melanomas arise from moles on the lower legs and on mucous membranes. Moles subject to constant irritation or trauma show a relatively high incidence of malignant changes and should be removed.[439,440]

MELPHALAN. A nitrogen mustard that is a strong irritant to the eyes and mucous membranes. Used on rare occasions in medicine to treat malignancies. It is also occasionally used as an insect chemo-sterilant. It caused bone-marrow cancer in patients. *See also* Nitrogen Mustard and Anticancer Drugs.[441]

MERCURY. *Quicksilver.* Until July 5, 1973, it was widely used in cosmetics, including face masks, hair tonics, medicated soaps, bleach and freckle creams. Mercury compounds are heavy silver liquids derived from minerals that occur in the earth's crust. Mercury is potentially dangerous when it enters the body through any of the portals of entry, including the skin. It is still used as a preservative in eye preparations to inhibit the growth of germs. It is now the only use permitted. The ban on mercury was brought about because it was found that its use in bleaching cream and other products over a period of time caused mercury buildup in the body. It caused tumors when injected into the abdomen of mice in doses of 400 milligrams per kilogram of body weight.[442]

MERCURY (ACETATO) PHENYL-. *Norforms, trigosan, tag fungicide.* Used as a herbicide, especially for crabgrass, and as a fungicide. Given intravenously to mice, it caused tumors in 2 milligram doses per kilogram of body weight.[443]

METALS. Shiny chemical elements that conduct electricity and can be found in various shapes. They also form compounds with other elements such as oxygen and sulfur. Metals are of special concern because they occur naturally in the environment. Therefore, we can be exposed to them at work, in the air, and in our food and water. The body is slow in removing many metals, and they may accumulate in tissues and produce long-range effects. A few nonradioactive metal ions have been tested and found capable of inducing neoplasms in animals, generally after parental administration. Subcutaneous, intramuscular, and intrapleural injections of inorganic compounds of beryllium, cadmium, chromium, cobalt, and nickel have led to the formation of sarcomas at the sites of injections in rats and mice. The ingestion of lead acetate by rats at levels of 0.1 and 1 percent of the diet for one year or longer has led to adenomas and adenocarcinomas of the kidney.[444]

METHANE, TRICHLOROFLUORO-. *See* Fluorocarbons.

METHANESULFONIC ACID, ETHYL ESTER AND METHYL ESTER. Prepared from sulfur trioxide and methane, it is used in alkylation and esterification reactions, as a solvent, and as a catalyst in polymerization. It caused tumors when injected into the abdomen of rats and mice and cancer when injected into the abdomens of mice in 36 milligram doses per kilogram of body weight.[445,446] A NIOSH candidate for hazard review for carcinogenesis.

METHANETHIOL, TRICHLORO-. *See* Perchloromethanthiol.

METHAPYRILENE. An antihistamine widely used in over-the-counter sleeping aids was linked to tumors in laboratory animals by an NCI study. Rats fed a compound of the substance and nitrites developed cancer. As the drug has reportedly caused anemia and leukopenia in humans,[447] the FDA has announced plans to ban methapyrilene from sleeping aids pending further study.[448]

METHENAMINE. *Cystogen, formin, hexaform, hexamethylenetetramine.* Consisting of white crystalline powder or colorless crystals derived from ammonia and alcohol, it is moderately toxic. It is a skin irritant and is flammable. It is used as a catalyst in resorcinol-formaldehyde resins and as an ingredient in rubber and textile adhesives. It is a protein modifier and an ingredient of the high explosives. It is also used as a urinary antiseptic. When injected under the skin of rats, it caused tumors.[449]

METHOTREXATE. *Glutamic acid, N-(p-((1,2,4-diamino-6-pteridinyl) methyl)methylamine) benzoyl)-iL; aminopterin.* An antimetabolite used in cancer chemotherapy and to treat bad cases of psoriasis, it has many serious side effects, including liver and kidney damage, diarrhea, ulcerative stomatitis, and hermorrhages. It inhibits folic-acid enzymes and interferes with cell reproduction (cellular proliferation in malignant tissue is greater than in normal tissue). Methotrexate may impair malignant growth without irreversible damage to normal tissue. It is used in the treatment of gestational choriocarcinoma, hydatidiform mold, leukemia, and lymphosarcomas, It causes tumors when painted on the skin of mice or given intramuscularly to rats.[450] As with other anticancer drugs, there is always the possibility that it will later induce cancer in the patient.[451]

METHOXYCHLOR. A synthetic organochlorine insecticide, it is structurally similar to DDT and widely used in agricultural pest control. It is effective against a wide range of insects that attack fruits, vegetables, shade trees, home gardens, forage crops, and livestock. It is used as a spray for barn, grain-storage bins, mushroom houses, dairies, and other agricultural buildings. More than 3 million pounds are used in the United States per year, 2 million of which are used to protect livestock and livestock buildings. It is sprayed on beef and dairy cattle. The remaining one million pounds is used to treat thousands of acres of varied crop land. The major crop use is alfalfa.

Considered an excellent replacement for DDT, risk of exposure is greatest for agricultural workers, farmers, and pest appliers. Relatively ineffective against soil organisms, it is generally applied directly to crops via ground or aerial spraying. As a result, contamination of the atmosphere over a wide area leads to the possibility of inhalation by people residing there. It also has a long residual activity against many species. It was fed to rats and mice for 78 weeks during an NCI test. According to results, methoxychlor was not found to be carcinogenic in rats or mice of either sex under the test conditions.[452]

4-METHOXY-m-PHENYLENEDIAMINE. *See* 2, 4-Diaminoanisole Sulfate and Hair Coloring.

METHYLCHLOROMETHYL ETHER (CMME). *Chlorodimethyl ether, chloromethyl ether, and chloromethyl methyl ether.* A corrosive liquid that smells like hydrogen chloride and formaldehyde, it is usually contaminated with traces of bis(chloromethyl)ether *(see)*, a sister compound and potent carcinogen. The facilities that use CMME make their own and keep it in closed vessels during the production of other products. Millions of pounds are used in the United States each year, chiefly as a chloromethylating agent in the manufacture of resins, the treatment of textiles, and the production of certain drugs. The resins are used to produce high-purity water for electric-plant generators, nuclear-reactor coolants, transistor production, and to treat radioactive wastes. CMME contributes to the production of certain bactericides and is used as a drug to lessen blood cholesterol. It is also used during sugar purification, gelatin production, and as an analytical standard. None of these final products contain CMME according to OSHA. CMME releases vapors that induce coughing and nausea. Skin contact can cause burns, chapping, and dehydration. It is a demonstrated carcinogen. It produces both lung and skin cancers in lab animals. OSHA has strict standards for worker protection involving release, handling, or storage of any substances containing more than one-tenth of one percent of methylcholoromethyl ether.[453]

METHYLENE BIS. A food packaging adhesive, it induced cancer in test animals and was banned by the FDA.

4,4'-METHYLENE-BIS (2-CHLOROANILINE) (MOCA). MOCA is a light yellow or tan solid usually sold in the form of pellets or small clumps and powder. It is characterized as a carcinogen. MOCA is used in 800 to 1,800 workplaces, mainly as a curing agent for polymers containing isocyanates, particularly in the production of polyurethane resins. Some 2 or 3 million pounds of this substance were produced in the United States in 1970. It is also manufactured in Great Britain and Japan, whose total output is believed to be less than 2 million pounds.

It has been demonstrated to induce tumors in rats and mice, although human studies are unavailable. One report involving irritation of the bladder in employees exposed to MOCA has been published. There is little danger from airborne MOCA in general, as tests on fallout plates in work areas have revealed little in the way of airborne particles. Absorption through skin contact of the workers may be a more important route of body entry than inhalation. OSHA has strict standards for workers involved in the manufacture, processing, repackaging, release, handling, or storing of any substance containing more than one percent MOCA. MOCA is often used in a premixed form. Because of this, it produces little dust or vapor hazard.[454]

METHYLENE CHLORIDE. *Dichloromethane.* Prepared by the chlorination of methane, it is a colorless liquid that is used as a solvent for cellulose acetate, in degreasing and cleaning fluids, in aerosol product propellants, and in urethane-foam production. At one time it was also used as an inhalation anesthetic. Methylene chloride belongs to a family of chemicals suspected and, in some cases, known to cause cancer. Vinyl chloride is the prime example. Dow Chemical Company of Midland, Michigan, makes more than 1,000 chemicals, but its production of methylene chloride is among the top 20 in volume. It was removed from aerosol products in December 1978 as part of the fluorocarbon ban for aerosol sprays. Dow denies the chemical is carcinogenic, but chances are that it will be proven so, just as its cousin chemicals are now being found to cause cancer.[455]

N-METHYL-N-FORMYL HYDRAZINE. *See* Mushrooms and Hydrazine.

METHYL METHACRYLATE. *Polymer methacrylate.* A colorless volatile liquid derived from cyanohydrin methanol and dilute sulfuric acid. Used for polymethacrylate resins and the impregnation of concrete. It caused tumors when injected under the skin of rats in doses of 300 milligrams per kilogram of body weight.[456]

2-METHYL-1-NITROANTHRAQUINONE. An intermediate *(see)* in the manufacture of anthraquinone dyes. It is no longer used by the dye industry, but workers exposed to it have had an increase in bladder cancer. It was fed to rats and mice for 78 weeks in NCI tests. It caused cancer of the liver in male rats and was associated with an increased incidence of one benign-tumor type in both male and female rats.[457]

N-METHYL-N-NITROSOUREA. *See* Urea, Methyl Nitroso-.

METHYLTHIOURACIL. *Uracil, 6-methyl-2-thio-, antibason, basecil, methicil, Thimecil.* Crystals with a bitter taste used as an antithyroid substance. It is more active and less toxic than thiouracil, and it is also used for fattening swine and sheep.[458] It caused cancer when given orally to rats in 9,100 milligram doses per kilogram of body weight.[459]

METRONIDAZOLE. *See* Flagyl.

MICROWAVES. Waves that are in the spectrum between ordinary radio waves and the infrared in the electromagnetic spectrum. They are used in radar, and in microwave ovens, burglar alarms, diathermy machines (which treat arthritis, sprains, muscle soreness, and congested sinuses), TV transmitters, automatic garage-door openers, telephone relay systems, and driver-aid call boxes on highways. Environmentalists are beginnning to say, because there are so many microwave-emitting devices, that the country is surrounded by "electronic smog." It has long been known that at high levels, microwave radiation produces enough heat to damage certain tissues. At this high level there is danger of thermal damage to the eyes, testes, gall and urinary bladders, and the digestive tract, because these organs have smaller blood vessels that make them less able to cool themselves after exposure to the heat-produced microwaves. The effects of exposure to low levels of microwaves have long been a subject of controversy. Studies made in Eastern Europe have shown that long-term exposure to low-level microwave radiation might cause headaches, dizziness, fatigue, irritability, loss of judgment, leukemia, cataracts, changes in the blood-brain barrier, heart trouble, cancer, central nervous system disorders, or genetic damage. The prevailing view among Western scientists has been that without significant heat there can be no clinically significant biological effects from microwaves. However, now the view is held that instead of raising temperature the microwave energy may disrupt water molecules bound to protein, thus producing biological changes. If this is the case, people exposed to potentially harmful levels of microwave radiation would have no way of knowing it. In most cases there are no telltale sensory signals. And some studies have indicated that the effects of low-level microwaves could be cumulative, so that radiation levels that might appear safe today could, 20 years from now, produce a host of medical problems. More than ten thousand people work directly with microwave devices, and almost everyone comes in contact with them every day, in schools, hospitals, and in their homes. The United States currently has no standard for environmental exposure, and the occupational limit of 10 milliwatts per square centimeter is 1,000 times higher than the Soviet Union's standard.

In the past, American scientists have not accepted these European reports of harmful effects of low-level, nonionizing radiation, but preliminary tests have found that such exposure may affect the immune system, create anomalies in fetuses, and affect behavioral performance. The General Accounting Office of the United States Congress has concluded that the public may be exposed to dangerous levels of microwave radiation and that the federal government has been negligent in monitoring the problem. Despite the daily exposure of most Americans to microwaves, the government has failed to conduct adequate research on safety-levels systems and set safety standards.[460,461,462,463,464]

Because of these new findings, microwave sources should be effectively shielded by metal screens such as copper mesh or thin steel plates. Any source should be periodically checked with a microwave detector. Since the doors of microwave ovens tend to become loose, ovens should be checked periodically for leakage. The following precautions should be taken in the home: stay at least an arm's length away from a microwave oven while it is in use; switch the oven off before opening the door; keep children from watching through the viewing port of the door while the oven is in use.

MILK (BREAST). *See* Breast Cancer.

MILK SUGAR. *See* Lactose.

MINERAL OIL. It is a mixture of various hydrocarbons. Included in the category of mineral oils is petroleum, shale, lignite, greases, solvents, and cutting oils. Workers are exposed to mineral oil from greasing operations and from fuel-oil mists thrown off by moving machinery parts. An epidemic of skin cancer has occurred in a French area, the Valley of the Arve, Haute Savoie, among workers in metal machinery factories. In 15 years, more than 133 cases of cancer, most of them of the scrotum, have occurred. This is a ratio of 25 per 100,000, more than 36 times the rate for the general population of the area. Cutting oils frequently contain benzopyrene, and the more they are used on machinery, the greater the buildup of these carcinogenic hydrocarbons. Machine oils may cause inflammation of the lungs, and cancer has been found in the scarred lungs of workers exposed to mineral oil.[465,466,467]

MIREX. *1,3,4-Metheno-1H-cylobuto (cd) pentalene.* White odorless crystals derived from benzene *(see)*, it is a pesticide more resistant to degradation in the environment than most other organochlorine compounds—its environmental half-life (time it takes for half the substance to decompose) is 5 to 12 years. Because it is metabolized and excreted slowly, it accumulates in biological organisms and has a high potential to produce chronic effects. This probably accounts for the presence of Kepone residues (Kepone [chlordecone] is a contaminant of mirex and a product of mirex degradation) in mothers' milk in roughly the same areas of the southern United States where mirex was widely used to control the "imported" fire ant. A complicating factor in the assessment of the effects of mirex residues in the environment is that nearly three-fourths of the compound sold in the United States—more than a million kilograms since 1959—has been used as a flame retardant in plastics, sold under the name Dechlorane. The fact that plastics tightly trap or bind the molecules of mirex and inhibit or prohibit their release into the environment may account for the apparent lack of Dechlorane residues in areas other than the southern states. Mirex caused cancer when given orally to mice in 2,222 milligram doses per kilogram of body weight.[468] Because of its potential as a carcinogen and its long-lasting effects, the EPA banned its use on June 30, 1978.[469]

MITOMYCIN C. An antibiotic and antitumor agent produced by streptomyces from soil. It is used in cancer therapy because it cross-links with DNA. It produced sarcomas at the site of administration.[470]

4-MMPD. *See* Hair Coloring.

MNAR. *N⁶ Methylnitroso adenosine.* A chemical made up of a natural component found both in food and in almost every human cell. It frequently causes tumors in both adult mice and in young mice exposed from the time they were fetuses. The findings may have implications for the study of environmentally induced cancer. MNAR is in a class of chemical compounds called nitrosamines *(see)*. These compounds are formed by the interaction of nitrites, commonly found as food preservatives and as amines, which are naturally found in various foods. Nitrosamines can be formed in the human stomach but are also widely found as contaminants of food, air, cigarettes, and various agricultural and industrial chemicals. The process of nitrosation—the combination of nitrites and amines—can be greatly accelerated by the catalytic action of a number of common chemicals found in food and drink. When injected into test animals, nitrosamines have been previously shown to be carcinogenic. But it had been believed that significant quantities of nitrosatable amines are encountered only sporadically by human beings, so that the importance of nitrosamines as a major general public health problem was questionable. In a more recent study, however, it has been shown that an amine constituent (this amine is a component of transfer RNA, a type of nucleic acid found in all cells as well as in food) present in appreciable quantities in most cells can be converted into a carcinogen by interaction with nitrite. The nitrosamine that is readily formed as a result of this interaction is MNAR. The scientists found that MNAR causes tumors in both young and adult mice after either injection or the ingestion of the compound and should be considered a potential human carcinogen because of the widespread occurrence of its component parts.

MNU. *See* urea, Methyl Nitroso-.

MOLES. *See* Melanoma.

MORPHOLINE, 4,4' METHYLENE AND N-NITROSO-. *Bismorphonino methane.* Prepared by dehydrating diethanolamine, it is a mobile hydroscopic liquid used as a cheap solvent for resins, waxes, casein, and dyes. Its fatty acids are used as surface-active agents and emulsifiers. Other compounds of morpholine are used as corrosion inhibitors, antioxidants, plasticizers, viscosity improvers, insecticides, fungicides, herbicides, local anesthetics, and antiseptics. It is irritating to the eyes, skin, and mucous membranes and may cause liver and kidney injury.[471] It caused cancer when injected subcutaneously in rats in 50 milligram doses per kilogram of body weight, and it caused tumors in mice when given orally in doses of 150 milligrams per kilogram of body weight and in hamsters when injected under the skin in doses of 1,060 milligrams per kilogram of body weight.[472]

MOTH BALLS. *See* Naphthalene.

MOTH FLAKES. *See* Naphthalene.

MULTIPLE MYELOMA. Cancer of the bone marrow, characterized by greatly increased numbers of abnormal plasma cells.

MUSHROOMS. A potent cancer-causing agent, N-methyl-N-formyl hydrazine, a derivative of hydrazine *(see)* has been found in a wild mushroom known as the "false morel." Dr. Phillipe Shubik, director of the Eppley Institute for Research in Cancer, Omaha, said that since the false morel *(Gyrometra esculenta)*, eaten by about 100,000 people in the United States, contains this cancer-causing agent, other mushrooms should also be investigated for the presence of similar materials. Dr. Shubik said that the variety of mushroom used most commonly in the United States contains a hydrazine derivative called agaritine. Although it is not known to cause cancer, it is chemically related to other hydrazine derivatives that do. Based on his findings, Dr. Shubik said there is no need for Americans to cut back on their mushroom consumption. However, he suggested that the hydrazine-mushroom-cancer connection should be studied further.[473]

MUSTARD GAS. *Dichlorodiethyl sulfide.* Highly toxic war gas. Causes conjunctivitis and blindness. Can be decontaminated by chloramines or bleaching powder. Its vapor is extremely poisonous and can be absorbed through the skin. It is also used in organic synthesis and in medicine to treat cancer. It causes cancer of the bronchi in workers exposed to it and cancer of the lung, larynx, trachea, and bronchi in cancer patients treated with it.[474]

MYLERAN. *See* Busulphan.

1-NA(ALPHA-NAPHTHYLAMINE). *a-Naphthylamine, fast garnet B., 1-aminonaphthalene, naphthalidam, naphthalidine.* Consists of white to yellow crystals that have an unpleasant odor and are prepared from nitronaphthalene. It turns red when exposed to air. Used in a wide variety of products, including agricultural chemicals (chiefly herbicides), dyestuffs, food colors; it is also a key component in the production of color film. Only one company in the United States is known to produce and sell 1-NA, and this firm distributed almost 7 million pounds in 1972 and imported 60,000 pounds. As an antioxidant, 1-NA is used in the production of paint, plastic, rubber, and petroleum products. It has induced bladder tumors in mice and rats in 25 milligram doses per kilogram of body weight and has strongly been implicated in human bladder cancers as well. There is an OSHA standard for it as a carcinogen to protect workers involved in the manufacture, processing, release, handling or storage of any substances containing more than one percent 1-NA.[475]

2-NA (BETA-NAPHTHYLAMINE). Used in the manufacture of dyes and toning prints. Recognized as the cause of malignant bladder and pancreas tumors. Most susceptible are dyestuff manufacturers and users, rubber workers, and paint manufacturers. It has an incubation period of from 12 to 30 years.[476]

NAPHTHALENE. *Tar camphor. Moth balls, moth flakes.* Consists of white crystalline volatile flakes that have a strong coal-tar odor and are derived from coal tar. Toxic by inhalation. It is used as a moth repellent, fungicide, and emulsion breaker; and in the manufacture of explosives, cutting fluids, lubricants, synthetic resins, synthetic tanning preservative, and solvents. It is also used as a base for a wide variety of dyes. It causes tumors when injected under the skin of rats in 3,500 milligram doses per kilogram of body weight.[477] Dye workers handling naphthalene products have suffered from bladder cancer.[478]

NAPHTHALENEDIOL. *Naphthoresorcinol.* A reagent for sugars, oils, and for gluconic acid in urine, it did not produce cancer when applied to the skin of mice but did when given orally to rats in a dose of 2,600 milligrams per kilogram of body weight.[479] *See also* Naphthalene.

2,7-NAPHTHALENEDISULFONIC ACID, 3,3'-(4,4'-BIPHENY-LYLENE)BIS(AZO)-BIS (5-AMINO-4-HYDROXY)-, TETRASO-DIUMSALT. *Airedale blue, Atlantic blue, C.I. direct blue, diazol blue 2 B.* Used as an intermediate *(see)* for dyes and as a dye, it is produced by the sulfonation of naphthalene *(see).* Causes cancer when injected under the skin of rats in doses of 750 milligrams per kilogram of body weight.[480]

2,7-NAPHTHALENEDISULFONIC ACID, 3,3'-((3,3'DIMETHYL-4,4'-BIPHENYLYLENE)-BIS (5-AMINO-4-HYDROXY)-, TETRA-SODIUM SALT. *Amanil sky blue, C.I. direct blue, Congo blue.* Caused cancer when given orally to rats in 440 milligram doses per kilogram of body weight and when injected under the skin of rats in 1,088 milligram doses per kilogram of body weight.[481] *See also* Naphthalene.

1,3-NAPHTHALENEDISULFONIC ACID, 6,6'-((3,3'-DIMETHYL (1,1- BIPHENYL) -4,4' -DIYL) BIS (AZO)) -BIS(4- AMINO -5- HY-DROXY)-, TETRASODIUM SALT. *C.I. direct blue 53, Evans blue dye, diazol pure blue, Geigy blue 536.* Determined by a NIOSH review to be an animal carcinogen.[482]

2,7-NAPHTHALENEDISULFONIC ACID, 3,3'-((3,3'-DIMETHYL-4,4'-BIPHENYLYLENE)-BIS(AZO))BIS(5-AMINO-4-HYDROXY-, TET-RASODIUM SALT. *Amanil sky blue, benzamine blue, benzo blue 3B, C.I. direct blue 14, Congo blue, tripan blue, etc.* Determined by a NIOSH review to be a positive animal carcinogen.[483]

1,3-NAPHTHALENEDISULFONIC ACID, 7-HYDROXY-8-((4-SUL-FO-1-NAPHTHYL)AZO)- TETRASODIUM SALT. *Acid brilliant scarlet 3R, acid ponceau 4R, acid red 18, brilliant scarlet 3R, coccine, cochineal, red 4R, C.I. food red 7, Victoria scarlet red, etc.* Made by sulfonating naphthalene *(see),* it causes cancer in rats when given orally in doses of 2,600 milligrams per kilogram of body weight.[484]

2,7 -NAPHTHALENEDISULFONIC ACID, 3 HYDROXY- 4-((4-SUL-FO-1-NAPHTHYL)AZO)-, TRISODIUM SALT. *Acid Amaranth, food red 2, naphthalene (see), and sulfonic acids.* Causes cancer when fed to rats in 1,080 milligram doses per kilogram of body weight.[485] *See also* **FD & C Red No. 2.**

2,7-NAPHTHALENEDISULFONIC ACID, 3-HYDROXY-4-((2,4,5-TRIMETHYLPHENYL)AZO)-, DISODIUM SALT. *Sodium ponceau 3, extended D and C red No. 15, FD & C red No. 1.* Caused cancer when fed to rats in 730 milligram doses per kilogram of body weight.[486] FD & C red No. 1 has been determined to be a positive animal carcinogen and is being studied by NIOSH for hazard review as a cancer-causing agent.[487]

2,7-NAPHTHALENEDISULFONIC ACID, 3-HYDROXY-4-(2,4,5-XYLYLAZO)-, DISODIUM SALT. *Acid leather red, acid scarlet, calcolake scarlet 2R, C.I. acid red 26, C.I. food red 5, D & C red no. 5, etc.* Determined by NIOSH to be a positive animal carcinogen, it is now undergoing a NIOSH hazard review.[488]

2-NAPHTHALENESULFONIC ACID, 6-HYDROXY-5-((p-SULFOPHENYL)AZO)-, DISODIUM SALT. *Acid yellow, AF yellow no. 5, C.I. food yellow 3, food yellow 3, orange yellow, sun yellow, FD & C yellow lake no. 6.* Caused tumors when injected under the skin of rats in 2,750 milligram doses per kilogram of body weight.[489] *See* **FD & C Yellow No. 6.**

1-NAPHTHALENESULFONIC ACID, 4-HYDROXY-3-((6-SULFO-2,4-XYLYL) AZO)- DISODIUM SALT. *See* **FD & C Red no. 4.**

NAPHTHALIDAM. *See* **1-NA.**

NAPHTHENIC ACID, ZINC SALT. Derived from petroleum and made up of a derivative group of the compound naphthalene *(see)*. When lead, cobalt, and manganese are part of these acids, health hazards can arise from either the acid or the metal or both. These acids are irritating to the skin and mucous membranes.[490] EPA pesticide candidate for additional carcinogenic studies as of February, 1976.[491]

2-NAPHTHOL, 1-((2,5-DIMETHOXYPHENYL)AZO)-. *See* **Citrus Red No. 2.**

2-NAPHTHOL, 1-((4-(o-TOLYLAZO)-o-TOLYL)AZO)-. *Candle scarlet B, C.I. solvent red 24, dispersol red PP, fast oil red B, fat ponceau R, brilliant red B, scarlet red, waxoline red O.* Caused cancer when injected under the skin of rats at 512 milligrams per kilogram of body weight.[492] A NIOSH candidate for a hazard review since it has been determined to be a positive carcinogen for animals.[493]

2-NAPHTHOL, 1-(2,4-XYLAZO)-. *A.F. red no. 5, Ceres orange RR, oil orange KB, Somalia orange 2R, Sudan red.* Causes tumors when injected into the abdomen of mice at 80 milligrams per kilogram of body weight.[494] Since NIOSH considers it a positive animal carcinogen, it is now a candidate for hazard review.[495]

1,4-NAPHTHOQUINONE. Prepared by chromic acid oxidation of 1,4 aminonaphthol, it has yellow needles and is used in dyes. *(See* Naphthalene.*)* Causes tumors when painted on the skin of mice at 2,000 milligrams per kilogram of body weight.[496]

1-NAPHTHYLAMINE. *See* 1 NA.

2-NAPHTHYLAMINE. *See* 2-NA.

2-NAPHTHYLAMINE. *2-Aminonaphthalene.* Prepared by heating B-naphthol with ammonium sulfite. Its white to reddish crystals are used in the manufacture of dyes. It caused cancer in a wide variety of animals, including the rat, mouse, monkey, dog, and hamster.[497] Naphthalene derivatives have caused urinary bladder tumors in dye workers.[498] There is an OSHA standard for it as a carcinogen.

2-NAPHTHYLAMINE, N-ETHYL-1-((p-(PHENYLAZO) PHENYL) AZO)-. *Ceres red 7 B, C.I. solvent red 10, lacquer red 13 B, oil violet, Sudan red 7 B.* Causes tumors when fed orally to rats in 17 milligram doses per kilogram of body weight.[499] *See also* 2-NA.

2-NAPHTHYLAMINE, 3-METHYL-. Caused cancer when injected in rats and mice. *See also* 2-Naphthylamine.

2-NAPHTHYLAMINE, 3-METHYL-, HYDROCHLORIDE. Causes tumors when given orally to rats in doses of 390 milligrams per kilogram of body weight.[500] *See also* 2-NA.

2-NAPHTHYLAMINE, 1-(o-TOLYLAZO)-. *A.F. yellow no. 3, C.I. food yellow 11, C.I. solvent yellow 6, oil yellow. See also* 2-NA.

NASAL CAVITY, SINUSES. Agents considered most carcinogenic to the sinuses are chromium, isopropyl oil, nickel, wood and leather dusts. High-risk occupations for this form of cancer are glass, pottery, and linoleum workers; battery makers; nickel smelters; mixers; roasters; electrolysis workers; wood, leather, and shoe workers.

NCI. National Cancer Institute.

NICKEL AND NICKEL COMPOUNDS. Occurring in the earth's crust, it is a lustrous white hard metal that is used as a catalyst for the hydrogenation of fat. Nickel may cause skin rashes in sensitive individuals. Ingestion of large amounts of the soluble salts may cause nausea, vomiting, and diarrhea. Nickel causes cancer in rats, rabbits, hamsters, and guinea pigs both by injection and by inhalation, and in amounts as little as 15 milligrams per kilogram of body weight.

Gaseous nickel carbonyl, used in many organic solvents, is the most dangerous of the nickel compounds. It is highly volatile; it is also soluble in fats, thus it is presumably able to penetrate cellular membranes. Metastasizing pulmonary tumors have been experimentally induced in rats by inhalation of nickel carbonyl. In men, nickel dust, nickel sulfide, nickel carbonate, nickel oxide, nickel carbonyl, and nickelocene have reportedly caused cancer in the nasal cavities, larynx, and lungs after exposure of 3 to 25 years.

Nickel sulfide, also called heazlewoodite, causes cancer when injected into rats and mice. Nickel acetate causes cancer when injected intramuscularly in rats.[501,502,503]

NICKEL (2+) OXIDE. *Nickelous oxide, nickel oxide, green nickel oxide.*

A green powder that becomes yellow in acids. Used in nickel salts, porcelain painting, and in fuel-cell electrodes. Causes cancer when injected into mice and rats at from 100 to 200 milligram doses per kilogram of body weight.[504] There is an OSHA standard for it.

NICOTINE, 1'-NITROSO-1-DEMETHYL. *Nitrosonornicotine.* An alkaloid derived from tobacco. A thick, watery-white oil, it turns brown on exposure to air that is the product of distilling tobacco with milk of lime. Highly toxic when ingested, inhaled, or absorbed through the skin. Causes tumors when injected into the abdomen of mice in 3,300 milligram doses per kilogram of body weight.[505]

NIOSH. National Institute of Occupational Safety and Health. *See* Introduction, page 12.

NITRATE. *Potassium and sodium.* Potassium nitrate, also known as saltpeter and nitre, is used in gunpowder and fireworks and as a color fixative in cured meats. Sodium nitrate, also called Chile saltpeter, is also used as a color fixative in cured meats. Both nitrates are used in matches and improve the burning properties of tobacco. They combine with natural stomach saliva and food substances (secondary amines) to create nitrosamines *(see),* powerful cancer-causing agents. Nitrosamines have also been found in fish treated with nitrates. Nitrates have caused deaths from methemoglobinemia (it cuts off oxygen from the brain). Because nitrates are difficult to control in processing, they are being used less often. However, they are still employed in long-curing processes, such as country hams, as well as dried, cured, and fermented sausages. In the early seventies, baby-food manufacturers voluntarily removed nitrates from their products. The U.S. Department of Agriculture, which has jurisdiction over processed meats, and the FDA, which has jurisdiction over processed poultry, have asked manufacturers to show that the use of nitrates is safe. If the manufacturers cannot prove their safety, the USDA and FDA will then decide, on the basis of available information, whether nitrates should be banned.

Nitrates change into nitrites on exposure to air. Our major intake of nitrates in foodstuffs comes primarily from vegetables or water supplies that are high in nitrate content, or from nitrates used as additives in the meat-curing process. Nitrates are natural constituents of plants. They occur in very small amounts in fruits but are high in certain vegetables—spinach, beets, radishes, eggplant, celery, lettuce, collards, and turnip greens—as high as more than 3,000 parts per million. The two most important factors responsible for large accumulations of nitrates in vegetables are the high levels of fertilization with nitrate fertilizers and the tendency of the species to accumulate nitrate.[506] *(See* Nitrosamines.*)* Environmental nitrate pollution should be reduced, and products containing nitrates as preservatives and coloring should be avoided.

NITRITE. *Potassium and sodium.* Potassium nitrite is used as a color fixative in the $125 billion a year cured meats business. Sodium nitrite has the peculiar ability to react chemically with the myoglobin molecule and impart red-bloodedness to processed meats, to convey tanginess to the palate, and to resist the growth of *Clostridium botulinum* spores. It is used as a color fixative in cured meats, bacon, bologna, frankfurters, deviled ham, meat spread, potted meats, spiced ham, Vienna sausages, smoked-cured tuna fish products, and in smoked-cured shad and salmon. Nitrite combines with natural stomach and food chemicals (secondary amines) to create nitrosamines *(see)*, a powerful cancer-causing agent. The U.S. Department of Agriculture, which has jurisdiction over processed meats, and the FDA, which has jurisdiction over processed poultry, asked manufacturers to show that the use of nitrites was safe and that nitrosamines were not formed in the products, as preliminary tests showed in bacon. If the manufacturers cannot, then the USDA and the FDA will decide, on the basis of available information, whether nitrites should be banned. Processors claimed that there was no chemical substitute for nitrite. They said alternate processing methods could be used, but the products would not look or taste the same. (Baby-food manufacturers voluntarily removed nitrites from their products in the early seventies.) The FDA has found that adding vitamin C (ascorbic acid) to processed meats prevents or at least retards the formation of nitrosamines. In May 1978 the USDA announced plans to require bacon manufacturers to reduce their use of nitrite from 150 to 120 parts per million and to use preservatives that retard nitrosamine formation. Processors would be required to keep nitrosamine levels to 10 ppm under the interim plan.

But in August 1978 a new concern about nitrite was raised. The USDA and the FDA issued a joint announcement that the substance had been directly linked to cancer by a Massachusetts Institute of Technology study. MIT's Dr. Paul M. Newberne reported that in his experiments rats receiving nitrites in their diet developed significantly more cancers of the lymphatic system than did rats receiving no nitrites. The FDA said this effect differs from the effect of nitrites combining with secondary amines to create nitrosamines, because this latter effect causes tumors in different organs but not in the lymphatic system. Furthermore, the MIT researcher said, nitrite appears to promote tumors rather than initiate them as nitrosamines do. The FDA-USDA statement said the agencies were now evaluating the risk-to-benefit ratio of using nitrites. If nitrites are removed, would botulism result? (Nitrites are the most effective preservative against the deadly botulism spores.) At the time of the report, the USDA allowed 120 ppm, but the agency proposed a reduction to 40 ppm by May 1979. Monsanto, the only manufacturer in the United States of sorbic acid and potassium sorbate, maintained that the lower amount of nitrites could be used immediately if 0.26 percent potassium sorbate were added. The company claimed bacon treated this way tasted and looked the same as bacon with the higher amounts of nitrites. Some scientists claim that sorbic acid alone could replace nitrites in all processed meats.

If you must eat nitrite-laced meats, include a food or drink high in vitamin C at the *same time*—for example, orange juice, grapefruit juice, cranberry juice, and lettuce. The vitamin C prevents the transformation of nitrates and nitrites to nitrosamines *(see)*.

5-NITROACENAPHTHENE. Used in Japan as a dye intermediate *(see)* but produced in the United States solely for use in research, it was given in feed to rats and mice for 78 weeks. It proved carcinogenic to the liver in female mice. The chemical was also carcinogenic in rats, causing clitoral and breast cancers in females and lung and ear-canal cancers in rats of both sexes. The test did not provide evidence for carcinogenicity of the compound in male mice.[507]

5-NITRO-o-ANISIDINE. An intermediate *(see)* in the manufacture of dyes, it was given in feed to rats and mice for 78 weeks. It caused cancers of the skin and skin glands in male and female rats, clitoral gland cancers in female rats, and liver cancers in female mice.[508]

4-NITROBIPHENYL (4-NBP). *4-Nitrodiphenyl, p-nitrobiphenyl, p-nitrodiphenyl.* Usually sold in the form of needlelike crystals, it is presently used only in laboratories in cancer research and as an analytic standard. It causes bladder cancer in humans and dogs. OSHA has strict standards for the protection of workers, including laboratory workers, involved in the manufacture, processing, release, handling, or storage of any substance containing more than one-tenth of one percent of 4-nitrobiphenyl.[509]

NITROFEN. An agricultural pesticide used as a selective contact herbicide for pre- and postemergent control of annual grasses and broad-leaf weeds on a variety of food crops. Agricultural workers and manufacturers are exposed through skin absorption and by inhalation. The general public is exposed through ingestion due to possible persistent residual quantities of nitrofen on food crops. Adverse effects on agricultural workers following excessive exposure over prolonged periods included a reduction of hemoglobin and white blood cell counts, inhibition of cholinesterase (an enzyme in the heart muscle), and abnormalities in red-blood and serum-enzyme levels. The chemical was given to rats and mice for 78 weeks. It proved to be a liver carcinogen in mice of both sexes and in female rats.[510]

NITROFURAZONE. *Furacin, 2-furaldehyde, 5-nitro-semicarbazone, alcomycin, babrocid, furacillin.* Prepared from 2-formyl-5-nitrofuran and semicarbazide, it consists of pale yellow needles. It is used in topical antibacterial formulations for the skin, ear, nose, and eyes. It is also used for burn patients. It produces liver, kidney, and breast tumors in rats at high doses. No tumors were reported in dogs or monkeys, although the animals died from toxic effects of the drug.[511] The drug works by inhibiting the enzymes necessary for carbohydrate metabolism in bacteria. It was formerly used as an antibacterial and growth promoter in chickens, turkeys, and swine but was banned by the FDA when it was shown to cause cancer in animals.[512]

NITROGEN MUSTARD. A class of compounds with a fishy smell and an ability to bring tears to the eyes. They are named from their similarity in structure to mustard gas. The sulfur of mustard gas is replaced by an amino nitrogen. Cancer chemotherapy by alkylating agents was discovered while scientists were conducting secret research during World War II. The full story was not published until 1963. The remarkable sensitivity of normal lymphoid tissue to the cytotoxic action of the nitrogen mustards led to a test on one mouse with a transplanted lymphoma. The encouraging results of that test led to more extensive investigations, and eventually related compounds were developed for clinical use to treat malignancies. Among them busulfan (Myleran), cyclophosphamide (Cytoxan), Leukeran, and 1-phenylalanine mustard (Melphalan) *(see* all*)*. Nitrogen mustard caused cancer when injected or given intravenously to mice in very small doses. Unfortunately, many of the cytotoxic drugs have been found to cause cancer years after being used to combat cancer.[513,514]

NITROGUANIDINE. *Guanine,1-ethyl-3-nitro-3-nitroso.* Long, flat, flexible, lustrous needles derived from guanidine nitrate and used in high explosives, especially flashless propellant powder. It is also used as a chemical intermediate *(see)*. It causes cancer when given orally to mice and hamsters, when injected into rats and mice, and when painted on the skin of mice.[515]

2-NITROPHENYLENEDIAMINE. *See* Hair Coloring.

2-NITRO-p-PHENYLENEDIAMINE. A hair-dye ingredient, it was given in feed to rats and mice for 78 weeks. It caused liver cancer in female mice under NCI test conditions. There was no convincing evidence for carcinogenicity of the compound in male mice or in male or female rats.[516]

3-NITROPROPIONIC ACID. A naturally occurring nitro chemical found in plants, nuts, and fungi, it was given by stomach tube to rats and mice for periods of between 104 and 110 weeks. According to the NCI report, 3-nitropropionic acid was not carcinogenic in female or male mice under the test conditions. In male rats there was an increased occurrence of liver and pancreas tumors, primarily benign, but no conclusive evidence that the chemical was carcinogenic.[517]

NITROSAMINES. In 1970, Dr. William Lijinski and Dr. Samuel Epstein reported in the British journal *Nature* that nitrosamines are environmental cancer-causing agents and that they could be produced by the interaction of sodium nitrite *(see* Nitrite*)* and secondary amines (normal breakdown products of proteins). Secondary amines, especially dimethylamine and morpholine, are virtually everywhere: in common foods such as ham, frankfurters, milk, coffee, tea, beer, and fish, with the largest amount in fish (hundreds of parts per million); in human saliva; in human stomachs; in pesticides; in drugs; in the air. They are also used in industrial processes.

Besides being produced by the above reaction, nitrosamines are also formed by the interaction of nitrogen dioxide and nitrous oxide, both of which are principal products of oil, coal, and gas combustion, including motor-vehicle exhaust. Such nitrosamines in the environment did not receive much public attention until 1975 when Ralph Nader's Public Interest Research Group asked Thermo Electron Corporation, a Waltham, Massachusetts, instrument manufacturer, to take atmospheric nitrosamine measurements. In one locale, a missile-fuel plant in Baltimore, Maryland, which used nitrosamines in the manufacture of fuel for Air Force Minutemen missiles, levels of minute amounts were found in the air. Local residents were alarmed and the government shut the plant down.

Nongovernment calculations show that a person ingests 0.5 micrograms of dimethylnitrosoamines (DMN) if he eats four slices of cooked bacon with nitrite levels permitted by the old standard. He inhales 0.8 micrograms after smoking a pack of cigarettes. However, if he breathes air containing 1 microgram per cubic meter DMN for 24 hours, he will inhale 10 to 14 micrograms of DMN. One important factor missing in the picture is how nitrosamines behave in the human respiratory system. An EPA epidemiologist says that while nitrosamines have been shown to form in the digestive system, a counterpart has not been noted for the respiratory tract. If nitrosamines do, indeed, form there, then the population may be even more at risk for cancer than previously supposed. Cancer researchers have tested nitrosamines on dogs, monkeys, parrakeets, rats, mice, hamsters, guinea pigs, and rainbow trout—each group has contracted cancer. Moreover, each has developed a variety of cancer types suggesting that nitrosamines do not limit their harmful effects to one organ. As far back as 1954, researchers reported nitrosamines to be among the most efficient cancer inducers known—a single dose can cause a malignancy in some animals.[518]

Nitrosamines have been discovered in urban air, soil, water, and sewage treatment wastes, in places ranging from New York City to Alaska. Unlike other pollutants that have a limited number of sources, nitrosamines are generated from chemicals found almost everywhere. Nitrosamines may be one of the major causes of cancer today. Animal studies have shown that in low doses they encourage other weak cancer-causing agents to increase their malignant potential. There is *no direct* evidence linking nitrosamines to human cancer. Many scientists feel this is because nitrosamines are so prevalent that it is difficult to show a cause and effect. Since every animal group tested produced cancers when exposed to nitrosamines, it is safe to assume that humans are also at risk.[519] *See also* Nitrites for foods that prevent nitrosamine formation.

N-NITROSODIMETHYLAMINE (DMN). *Dimethylamine, nitrous dimethylamide, N,N,-dimethylnitrosoamine, dimethylnitramine, etc.* A poisonous yellow liquid, it has been used as an industrial solvent in the manufacture of rocket fuel. Although it has been patented for use as an antioxidant, as a softener for copolymers, and as an additive for lubricants, it is not known to be used for these purposes now. The one known producer stopped making it before an OSHA emergency temporary standard came into effect. It has been demonstrated to be carcinogenic in many laboratory animals, including rats, mice, rabbits, and several species of fish. Therefore, it is assumed to be carcinogenic for humans as well. OSHA standards for it as a carcinogen protect workers involved in the manufacture, processing, release, handling, or storage of any substance containing more than one percent of N-nitrosodimethylamine.[520]

N-NITROSODIPHENYLAMINE (DBN). *Nitrous diphenylamide, diphenylnitroso-amine.* Yellow to brown or orange powder or flakes used in the manufacture of rubber and as a pesticide. It causes cancer when given orally to rats in doses of 3,900 milligrams per kilogram of body weight, when given subcutaneously to rats in 10 milligrams per kilogram of body weight, when given orally to mice in doses of 3,650 milligrams per kilogram, when given orally to guinea pigs in 46 milligram doses per kilogram, when given orally to hamsters in 7,500 milligram doses per kilogram, when injected under the skin of hamsters in 7,500 milligram doses per kilogram. It is currently being tested by the NCI for carcinogenicity.[521]

NITROSOETHYLUREA. *See* Urea, Ethyl Nitroso and Urea, Methyl Nitroso.

NITROSOMETHYL UREA. *See* Urea, Methyl Nitroso.

NMU. *See* Urea, Methyl Nitroso.

NONANE, 1,2,:8,9-DIEPOXY. A colorless liquid, soluble in alcohol, it is flammable, irritating, and narcotic in high concentrations. Used in organic synthesis and biodegradable detergents. Causes tumors when inhaled by mice in 3,800 milligram doses per kilogram of body weight.[522]

17-alpha-19-NORPREGNA-1,3,5 (10)-trien-20-YN-17-01,3-Methoxy-. *See* Estradiol.

NUCLEAR RADIATION. The incident at the Three Mile Island nuclear reactor plant near Harrisburg, Pennsylvania, in the spring of 1979, alarmed the world. Something that could not be seen, heard, or felt might escape from a concrete container and cause cancer in people who lived near it, within a radius of several miles. If there had been a large release of nuclear radiation at Three Mile Island, it might have spread fallout over a considerable distance, but not as far as an above-ground nuclear-bomb test would have done. Although nuclear-weapons tests were supposedly conducted far from human habitation, the detonation of such devices scatters radioactive materials in all directions, but mostly upwards. The materials that get into the stratosphere are dispersed across the earth and eventually wind up in foodstuffs practically everywhere. Material hurled directly into the lower atmosphere, however, as a nuclear-reactor accident might do, comes to earth fairly quickly and is not spread as far. When fallout is present in the lower atmosphere, it is ingested and inhaled. It gets into water supplies and is deposited directly on food plants and on the soil. It is eaten by meat-eating and milk-producing animals. Thus practically everything eaten or inhaled in the area is contaminated to some extent. How far the radioactive fallout spreads when it is in the lower atmosphere depends a great deal on weather conditions. Rain brings it down to earth, and wind spreads the contamination.

It is a fact that nuclear radiation and fallout can cause cancer. The people of Hiroshima and Nagasaki, Japan, who survived exposure to atomic bombs have been carefully studied during the ensuing years by the Atomic Bomb Casualty Commission. The result has been solid information that a single exposure at high doses produces leukemia in humans. It also increases the incidence of cancer of the lung, breast, and thyroid.[523] A University of Utah study reported in 1979 that nuclear-bomb tests in Nevada in the 1950s have caused increased leukemia deaths in neighboring Utah. Dr. Joseph L. Lyon, co-director of the Utah Cancer Registry, showed that the cancer death rate among children in southern Utah has been 2½ times that of children born before or after the tests. Dr. Lyon said that 15 to 20 youngsters died who would not have died without the tests. The deaths began to rise in 1959 and peaked in 1967 and declined as the testing was moved underground, he reported.[524]

It was also reported that nearly 4,300 sheep grazing downwind from Nevada nuclear tests died in the spring of 1953 after absorbing up to 1,000 times the maximum amount of radioactive iodine allowed for human beings. More than 230 claims have been filed with the Department of Energy (the successor to the Atomic Energy Commission) by cancer victims and their families, in Utah, Arizona, and Nevada. They charge the tests have caused cancer and deaths.[525]

NYLON. *Silon, furon, amilan, caprolon, enkalon, mirlon, perlon.* Clear or white opaque plastic. The name *nylon* was dedicated to public domain, Oct. 27, 1938, at the Herald Tribune Forum where the product itself was introduced. It has many uses in fabric, finishings, sutures, and tow ropes among them. It causes tumors when injected under the skin of rats in doses of 123 milligrams per kilogram of body weight.[526]

NYTOL. *See* Methapyriline.

OCCUPATIONS. According to a current study conducted by John Hickey, James Kearney, and their associates at Research Triangle Institute for NIOSH, the following industries are at highest risk for exposure to carcinogens (in descending order of hazard):

- Industrial and scientific instruments (solder, asbestos, thallium).
- Fabricated metal products (nickel, lead, solvents, chromic acid, asbestos).
- Electrical equipment and supplies (lead, mercury, solvents, chlorohydrocarbons, solders).
- Machinery, except electrical (cutting oils, quench oils, lube oils).
- Transportation equipment (constituents of polymers or plastics, including formaldehyde, phenol, isocyanates, amines).
- Petroleum and products (benzene, naphthalene, polycyclic aromatics).
- Leather products (chrome salts, other organics used in tanning).
- Pipeline transportation (petroleum derivatives, metals used in welding).

The chemical industry ranked twelfth. Investigators combined potency exposure and annual production to conclude that the ten most hazardous industrial chemicals are, in order, asbestos, formaldehyde, benzene, lead, kerosene, nickel, chromium, coal tar-pitch volatiles, carbon tetrachloride, and sulfuric acid. The Research Triangle results differ from previous studies because those previous studies generally considered only the volume of the carcinogens and not the amount of exposure. Previous studies ranked the chemical industry very high, for example, because it manufactures hazardous materials in lots of tons or more. But the large quantities of materials may be actually manufactured by a small number of people, so the volume of carcinogens may grossly overestimate the potential hazard. In contrast, John Hickey of Research Triangle said that the manufacture of scientific and industrial instruments requires relatively small amounts of carcinogenic materials. But these materials are used in the hand fabrication of devices, so the total exposure—and thus the total risk—is very high. The fabrication of metal and electrical products both rank high for the same reasons. Hickey said that the single most severe problem in many industries is the presence of carcinogenic dusts *(see)* in the workplace. New methods of control of dusts must be developed. Another severe problem is the venting of areas where carcinogens are made. In many cases the venting system now in place does little good and, in some instances, it even blows carcinogens back in the faces of workers. Research Triangle Institute's report is basically a library study, and the investigators neither visited nor tested potential carcinogens.[527]

OIL OF CALAMUS. *See* Calamus.

OLEIC ACID. *Cis-9-octadecenoic acid, red oil.* Obtained from various animal and vegetable fats and oils. It is colorless but on exposure to air turns yellow to brown. It has a rancid odor. It is used as a defoaming agent; as a synthetic butter, cheese, and spice flavoring; as a lubricant binder in various foods; and as a component in the manufacture of food additives. It has low oral toxicity and is mildly irritating to the skin. It caused tumors when injected under the skin of rabbits in 3,120 milligram doses per kilogram of body weight and when painted on the skin of mice in 62 milligram doses per kilogram of body weight.[528,529]

OLIVINE. *Iron magnesium silicate.* A mineral consisting of a silicate of magnesium and iron that is used in making refractories. It caused tumors when injected into mice in 400 milligram doses per kilogram of body weight.[530]

ORAL CONTRACEPTIVES. Pills currently available consist of estrogen and/or progesterone. The regulatory agencies have taken little action about the induction of liver tumors in women by some of these agents. Concerned scientists feel that some oral contraceptives may either be direct-acting carcinogens or that they prepare the body for action by other carcinogens. The possibility of removing oral contraceptives from the market is not politically feasible at this time, even if it is desirable from the viewpoint of cancer prevention. In justifying their withdrawal, given the present evidence, it would be necessary to weigh the threatened population increase against the tumor burden that might be induced. *See also* The Pill, Estrogens, Progesterone, and Hormones.

ORLON. *See* Acrylonitrile.

OSHA. *Occupational Safety and Health Administration.* This organization has been able to enact human-exposure standards for only 20 of the estimated 2,000 chemical carcinogens. As a result, the agency proposed to categorize all toxic chemicals into one of four groups until separate standards can be generated for each. Temporary standards would be set for entries in the top two categories. The OSHA proposal would class chemicals by health risk. Those that caused cancer in humans, in two mammalian test species, or in repeated tests of one species would enter category I. Chemicals reported to be carcinogenic but that lacked firm corroborative evidence would make up category II. Two optional groups, III and IV, would contain chemicals requiring further data development and chemicals that are suspected carcinogens but are not found in American workplaces.

According to internal administration documents, the federal government is failing to protect the safety and health of its own employees, and as a result, the costs of worker sickness and injury are skyrocketing. OSHA has been criticized for not policing United States agencies, and for cracking down only on businesses, especially small businesses. The Supreme Court has ruled that OSHA inspectors can no longer conduct surprise health and safety checks at workplaces without a warrant. It is still hoped that effective inspections can still be carried out.[531,532]

OSTEITIS DEFORMANS. *See* Precancerous Conditions.

OSTEOGENIC SARCOMA. One of the most common and serious of malignant bone tumors, it usually occurs in young people.

2-OXETANONE. *See* B-Propiolactone.

OXYMETHOLONE. *Anadrol, adroyd, anapolon.* A potent anabolic and androgenic drug, it enhances the production of red blood cells. It is used in the treatment of anemias caused by deficient red-cell production. It is illegally taken by athletes who wish to enhance their muscle strength. It has caused liver cancer and leukemia.[533]

OZONE. Although the concentration of ozone in the stratosphere is only a few parts per million, it plays an important role in the life cycle on earth by absorbing nearly all the remaining shortwave solar ultraviolet (UV) radiation, as well as most of the longer rays. Thus the ozone layer shields the earth from most of the harmful UV radiation. A depletion of the ozone would allow increasing amounts of harmful radiation to reach the earth's surface, adversely affecting plant, animal, and human life, as well as causing changes in the climate. Recently, considerable attention was paid to the effect of human-related activities on the ozone equilibrium. It had been theorized that the release of various chemical compounds into the environment such as halogens, nitrogen fertilizers, and emissions from subsonic and supersonic aircraft have and will continue to deplete the ozone field. Current estimates of the amount of stratospheric ozone destroyed by release of gases—used as refrigerants and as propellants in some aerosol sprays—appears to be roughly twice what the committee, the National Research Council Assembly of Mathematical and Physical Sciences' Committee on the Impacts of Stratospheric Changes, reported in 1976, although they are within the upper limit of uncertainty allowed by the committee in April 1978. Inhalation of ozone gas produced tumors in mice and there is an OSHA standard for it.[534]

PAB. *See* p-Aminobiphenyl.
PABS. *See* Sulfanilamide.
PARAFFIN. *Alkane.* A class of alphatic hydrocarbons. The physical form of these hydrocarbons varies with increasing molecular weight, from gases (methane) to waxy solids. They occur principally in Pennsylvania and midcontinent petroleum. They are used in the manufacture of ointments, paraffin paper, and candles; for fixing drawings; waterproofing wood, cork-paper, and leather; in the manufacture of varnishes; in lubricants; to cover food products; in floor polishes; cosmetics; electrical insulators; and for extraction of perfumes from flowers. Paraffins have caused tumors when implanted in mice in doses of 600 milligrams per kilogram of body weight.[535]
PARATHION. An organophosphorus pesticide, it was given in feed to rats and mice for 80 weeks. It was carcinogenic to the adrenal glands of male and female rats, but the evidence was not statistically conclusive. The compound was not carcinogenic in either sex of mice under the test conditions.[536]
PATULIN. *Peniciden, clavacin, claviformin.* A substance derived from

the metabolism of a number of fungi and molds. It is also found in rotten apples, which can be incorporated along with good apples in the processing of apple cider and apple juice. It was found in 37 percent of supermarket samples of apple juice and cider. The highest amount found was 440 parts per billion, the average was 70 ppb. Patulin injected into rats has caused tumors. These tumors were subcutaneous—they formed at the point of injection. Although preliminary feeding tests have yet to produce tumors, patulin is a suspected human cancer-causing agent because of its chemistry.[537]

PCB (POLYCHLORINATED BIPHENYLS). These are highly toxic and persistent chemicals primarily used as insulating fluids in heavy-duty electrical equipment in power plants, industries, and large buildings across the country. Small capacitators containing PCBs are found in many home appliances—air-conditioners, microwave ovens, fluorescent lights, and in some television sets. PCBs have also been used for other industrial purposes —plasticizers in paints, adhesives, and caulking compounds, and as hydraulic and heat-transfer fluids, some of which are still in service. They are also used for "carbonless" duplicating paper. Evidence from studies of occupational exposures to PCBs and accidental poisonings indicate that it is toxic to the nerves, causes cancer, and has adverse skin and liver effects. PCBs have also been associated with birth defects, cancer, and immunological defects in laboratory animals and genetic defects in microorganisms.

PCBs bioaccumulate in fish and wildlife, posing a threat to the human food chain. High PCB levels in the Great Lakes and the Hudson River threatened commercial and sport fishing. PCBs are so widely distributed throughout the world that they have been found in air samples taken 2,000 miles off the Atlantic Coast and in ice samples extracted from the Antarctic ice sheet. Because of the persistence of these chemicals, this environmental burden is not expected to diminish in the near future.[538] Of the roughly 1.25 billion pounds of PCBs that have been purchased by industries in the United States since their introduction in 1929, there are about 750 million pounds still in use, another 300 million pounds are in landfills and dumps, most of them uncontrolled, and 150 million pounds are simply loose in the environment. The Environmental Defense Fund has asked that the FDA invoke a zero tolerance of PCBs in the food supply. The tolerance is now set at from 5 to 2 parts per million.[539]

PCP (PENTACHLOROPHENOL). A widely used compound, it is effective in killing weeds and eradicating slimy molds. It is used in many herbicides and fungicides and as a wood preservative. About 200 million pounds are produced in the world every year. It is known to cause mutations in laboratory animals and is suspected of being a carcinogen. A high incidence has been detected in human urine and seminal fluid, and in many foodstuffs, including some soft drinks and candy bars. In one study of 60 students, all had low amounts of this toxic and persistent chemical in their urine. Fifty percent also showed traces of polychlorophenoxy acids, widely used chemicals in herbicides (were also used as defoliants in Vietnam). The fact that levels as high as 70 parts per billion were detected in seminal fluid has significant implications for birth defects and genital carcinoma. A spot survey of food and paper products bought in local supermarkets suggested the food chain is a major source of human contamination. Residues of PCP averaging 10 ppm in bread, cereal, noodles, rice, sugar, wheat, powdered milk, and soft drinks were found. It was also found in the city's drinking water and in high-quality bond paper. It was found in candy, where scientists theorized that the chemical moved into the confection either from the wrapping paper or from the contaminated sugar.[540]

PDB. *See* Benzene.

PENCILS. *See* Diarylanilide Yellow.

PENICILLIC ACID. An antibiotic substance produced by fungi. It has caused cancer when injected under the skin of rats in 61 milligram doses per kilogram of body weight and under the skin of mice in 608 milligram doses per kilogram of body weight.[541]

PENICILLIN G. *Compocillin G, liquacillin, benzylpenicillinic acid.* Obtained by the extraction of sodium benzylpenicillum with ether or chloroform, it is used as an antimicrobial. Allergic reactions may occur. It caused cancer when injected under the skin of rats in 1,300 milligram doses per kilogram of body weight.[542]

PENIS CANCER. *See* Circumcision.

PENTYLAMINE, N-METHYL-N-NITROSO-. *Methylamylnitrosamine, nitrosopentylamine.* It is used in the manufacture of dyestuffs, as a solvent, and in pharmaceuticals. It caused cancer when given to rats in 330 milligram doses per kilogram of body weight.[543]

PERCHLOROMETHANETHIOL. Occurs in "sour" gas of West Texas, in coal tar, and in petroleum distillates. Also found in urine after the ingestion of asparagus. It is produced in the intestinal tract by action of bacteria. It has the odor of rotten cabbage and is used as an intermediate *(see)* in the manufacture of jet fuels, pesticides, fungicides, plastics, synthesis, and methionine. It may cause nausea and in high concentrations is a narcotic. It caused cancer in rats when inhaled in 15 milligram doses per kilogram of body weight. There is an OSHA standard for it.[544]

PEROXYACETIC ACID. *Sodium salt.* Colorless liquid with a strong odor, it is used in bleaching textile, paper, oils, and waxes and is also used as a polymerization catalyst, bactericide, and fungicide, especially in food products. It is a synthetic glycerol. Inhalation caused tumors in mice in 311 milligram doses per kilogram of body weight.[545]

PEROXYBENZOIC ACID, t-BUTYL ESTER. *Perbenzoic acid.* It is prepared from benzene. Peroxybenzoic acid has an acrid odor and is very volatile. It is used to convert ethylene compounds into oxides. It caused tumors when inhaled by mice in 241 milligram doses per kilogram of body weight.[546]

PEROXYBENZOIC ACID, p-NITRO-. *See* Peroxybenzoic acid, t-Butyl Ester.

PERSONALITY. The human mind and body are tied together in an extraordinarily complex fashion. A number of investigators have suggested that certain psychological personality factors may be precursors of cancer and of recovery from cancer. In one study begun in 1946 by Caroline Bedell Thomas of Johns Hopkins Medical School, psychological tests were given initially to medical students and then followed up each year with questionnaires about health. This has led to a startling and unexpected finding. Those who had developed cancer—48 by 1977—had strong personality similarities to those who committed suicide. They were generally "low-gear" people, given to holding in their emotions, whose relationships with their parents had been much more cold and remote than those of individuals who developed other kinds of diseases.

In a study performed at the NCI it was found that patients who relapsed after treatment for malignant melanoma (skin cancer) were those who tended to minimize (or repress) their illness. A similar study of women with breast cancer had the same results. Those who expressed a high degree of anger toward not only their disease but their doctors lived longer than those who were compliant and cooperative.[547]

In animals, stress has been identified as a precursor of cancer: anxiety and fear caused by shipping and handling are stressors for mice. A strain of mice carrying a cancer virus developed cancer 92 percent of the time when they were exposed to moderate, chronic, or intermittent stress, while similar mice protected from such stress developed cancer only 7 percent of the time. It has been suggested that the physiological effects of stress lead to an impairment of the body's defense system and thus to a presumed increase in susceptibility to cancer. The loneliness, alienation, and isolation that have been found among cancer patients in "personality" investigations might have weakened their immune systems and led to increased susceptibility to cancer.[548] *See also* Emotions.

PERTHANE. *P,P'-Ethyl-DDD.* This organochlorine insecticide was fed to rats and mice for 105 weeks. According to the NCI, test results suggested a carcinogenic effect of the compound in female mice livers, but the incidence of liver tumors was not statistically significant compared with control animals. The compound was not found carcinogenic under the test conditions in male mice or in rats of either sex.[549]

PESTICIDES. There are several classifications of pesticides: insecticides, rodenticides, fungicides, herbicides, and fumigants. Pesticides help to control weed and insect pests. Reduction of damages from pests increases storage life of food and can increase the nutritional quality of the product. Pesticides have been used to control specific insects that are vectors of diseases. United States insect-borne diseases controlled by pesticides include malaria, plague, equine encephalitis, spotted fever, and endemic typhus. Most pesticides are poisonous and can be hazardous to the user, the environment, and the food consumer. Pesticides that reach the consumer generally do so by the oral route. Thus, stomach and bowel cancers are of particular interest to agronomic and agricultural scientists.

Pesticides may promote or induce cancer. One type of pesticide, hydrocarbons (DDT, for example), is not acutely toxic to human beings unless exposure is excessive, as in ingestion or massive body contact, when they cause nervous excitation, convulsion, coma, and then death. Another group of insecticides, the organophosphate esters, has similar toxic effects but differs in degree of toxicity. These insecticides all are readily absorbed through the skin and may also be inhaled or ingested. Acute symptoms following massive exposure include vomiting, dizziness, tremors, and convulsions. Such exposure can be fatal. Other insecticides cause skin and lung irritation: dithiocarbonates, a group of chemicals commonly used as fungicides, are highly irritating to the skin, eyes, and respiratory tract. Chronic effects of long-term exposure are not known precisely, but allergic reactions and effects on the hormones have been observed. There is also concern that these chemicals may cause cancer or damage the genetic material in the body.

Tests for pesticides frequently establish the ability of the compounds to promote not induce cancer. A further complication is that of multiple carcinogens, one adding to another. The sale and use of some 2,000 pesticide products containing 23 potentially hazardous ingredients has been restricted by the EPA to farmers and commercial users who have been certified and shown competent to use the product safely. What happens to the rest of us when exposed to pesticides in the air and on our food and in the animals and fish we eat is yet to be determined.[550,551,552,553,554]

PETROLEUM. *Coal tar, crude oil, mineral oil, rock oil, Seneca oil.* A highly complex mixture of paraffinic, naphthenic, and aromatic hydrocarbons containing a low percentage of sulfur and trace amounts of nitrogen and oxygen compounds. It is believed to have originated from both plant and animal sources millions of years ago. In the United States the chemical basis of petroleum varies with locale. In general, Pennsylvania crudes are aliphatic (wax based). Western crudes are aromatic (asphalt based) and midcontinent crudes are mixed bases. The most important petroleum fractions obtained by cracking or distillation are various hydrocarbon gases: butane, ethane, propane, naphtha of several grades, gasoline, kerosene fuel oils, gas oil, lubricating oils, paraffin wax, and asphalt. From the hydrocarbon gases, ethylene, butylene, or propylene are obtained. These are important industrial intermediates *(see)* as they are the source of alcohols, ethylene glycols, and monomers for a wide range of phenol, toluene, and xylene products, as well as hundreds of other products, including proteins for animal feed. (About 5 percent of petroleum consumed in the United States is used as feed stocks by the chemical industry.)

Petroleum is flammable and is moderately toxic by ingestion. It can cause local skin irritations. It caused tumors when painted on the skin of mice in 40 milligram doses per kilogram of body weight.[555] Many petroleum derivatives are known or suspected carcinogens. Approximately 65,000 petroleum and petrochemical workers are being observed for the development of ailments, from simple colds to cancer and other life-threatening diseases, and 10,000 retirees are being followed for mortality causes. It will be several years before the researchers can make any generalizations regarding petroleum exposure and disease because the subjects in a prospective epidemiological study, such as this one, must be followed for a substantial period of time in order to have statistically valid findings. Some preliminary studies have suggested a possible relationship between geographic proximity to petrochemical plants and increased incidence of cancer. A study by the NCI found that between 1950 and 1969 there was a significantly higher death rate from respiratory-tract cancers among people living in areas where the petroleum industry was heavily concentrated than in those where it was not. There was also a significant increase in skin, testis, stomach, and rectal cancers in these petroleum-industry regions. However, other possibly significant factors, such as smoking history, personal and family history, and other sources of industrial and environmental exposure, were not measured. Another study of 20,000 petroleum refinery workers suggested that mortality from all causes and total cancer mortality were less than expected when compared with those of the general public. But, deaths from certain cancers of the lymphatic system were slightly higher, although not to the level of statistical significance.[556]

PETROLEUM RESIDUES. *See* Petroleum.

PETROLEUM WAXES. *See* Petroleum.

PHAEOMELANIN. This is a red brown or blond pigment produced in human hair and skin. It is easily shattered by ultraviolet light and oxygen, and this destruction (demonstrated for the first time in 1977) may be the key to skin cancer. When sunlight hits phaeomelanin, it is broken into 17 molecular fragments, forming a powerful "superoxide ion" known to cause biological damage. Red and blond phaeomelanins have very different photochemical properties than the black or dark brown eumelanins. Ultraviolet light destroys phaeomelanin. This would explain the poor tolerance to ultraviolet light and the greater susceptibility to skin cancer found in redheads and blonds. Phaeomelanin is unaffected by ultraviolet light in the absence of oxygen, but simultaneous exposure to light and oxygen probably produces quick destruction of pigment.[557]

160

PHENACETIN. *Acetophenetidin.* Consists of white crystals that result from the interaction of p-phenetidin and glacial acetic acid. It is moderately toxic by ingestion. Phenacetin is used as an analgesic medicine. According to studies in West Germany, there is strong indirect evidence of a relationship between chronic phenacetin abuse and malignant tumors of the urinary tract. Since 1969, there have been 5 cases of malignant tumors of the kidney among 115 cases of chronic nephritis due to abuse of phenacetin-containing drugs. In five patients, three men and two women, the total amount ingested had been between 1.4 and 7.3 kilograms over a period of 14 to 22 years. In two patients, the cancer developed after abuse had stopped. The average latency time from the beginning of the abuse to the manifestation of the tumor was 21 years.[558] Three animal tests conducted to confirm clinical observations, however, proved negative.[559]

PHENANTHRENEQUINONE. *Phenanthrene 9.* Orange red crystals that turn a dark-green color when exposed to air. It is used in organic synthesis and dyes. It caused tumors when painted on the skin of mice in 2,000 milligram doses per kilogram and is suspected of being a human carcinogen.[560]

PHENAZINE. *Azophenylene.* A tricyclic compound consisting of yellow crystals, it is used in organic synthesis, in the manufacture of dyes, and as a larvicide. It is obtained by passing aniline vapor through a red-hot tube. It caused tumors when implanted in mice in doses of 7 milligrams per kilogram of body weight.[561]

PHENESTERINE. A chemotherapeutic agent once used to combat cancer. It caused lung tumors in mice.[562]

PHENFORMIN. A synthetic oral hypoglycemic agent used to control maturity-onset diabetes. There was no evidence under NCI tests that the drug caused cancer. However, test procedures were not up to standard, and the early deaths of male mice before the time when cancer might develop made carcinogenicity testing equivocal. An analysis of the data did indicate the theoretical possibility of tumor induction, although no tumors were detected during the test.[563]

PHENOBARBITAL. See Barbiturates.

PHENOL. *Carbolic acid, phenic acid, phenylic alcohol.* A class of aromatic compounds derived from benzene and a constituent of coal tar. One danger of handling the phenols is that they are so easily absorbed through the skin. Among the phenols are cresols, xylenols, resorcinol, naphthols. It also occurs in urine and has the characteristic odor present in coal tar and wood. It is a general disinfectant and anesthetic for the skin. Ingestion of even small amounts may cause nausea, vomiting, circulatory collapse, paralysis, convulsions, coma, and greenish urine, as well as tissue damage of the mouth and gastrointestinal tract. Death after ingestion results from respiratory failure. Fatalities have been reported from ingestion of as little as 1.5 milligrams.

Fatal poisoning can also occur through skin absorption. Although there have been many poisonings from phenolic solutions, phenol continues to be used in commercial products. A concentration of one percent applied for several hours to prevent itching from insect bites and sunburn caused gangrene, a result of spasm of small blood vessels under the skin. A concentration of 2 percent caused gangrene, burning, and numbness.[564] Phenol is used in shaving creams and hand lotions. It is also used as a solvent for refining lubricating oils, in germicidal paints, pharmaceuticals, dyes, and slimicides. It caused cancer when painted on the skin of mice in 4,000 milligram doses per kilogram of body weight.[565] There is an OSHA standard for skin (5 parts per million).

PHENOL, PENTACHLORO-. See Pentachlorophenol.

PHENYLALANINE MUSTARD. See Melphalan.

PHENYLAZO-2-NAPHTHYLAMINE. Yellow dyes made from aniline (see).

PHENYLENEDIAMINE, m, o, AND p. Most permanent home and beauty-parlor hair dyes contain this chemical or a related one such as 4-nitro-o-phenylenediamine. Colorings that contain it are called oxidation dye, amino dye, para dye, or peroxide dye. PPD was first introduced in 1890 for dyeing furs and feathers. It comes in about 30 shades and is used as an intermediate (see) in coal-tar dyes. The color penetrates the hair shaft and dyes it permanently. May produce eczema, bronchial asthma, gastritis, skin rash, and death. Can cross-react with many other chemicals, including azo dyes (see) used for temporary hair colorings. Can also produce photosensitivity. Europeans will not allow PPD in their products but use safer p-toluenediamine instead. Before using permanent hair dyes, beauticians and individual users are supposed to test a patch of skin to determine if there is an adverse reaction. PPD has been known to cause cancer in animals for many years.[566] See also Hair Coloring.

m-PHENYLENEDIAMINE, 4-(1-NAPHTHYLAZO). C.I. solvent brown I. It caused cancer when given orally to rats in 34 milligram doses per kilogram of body weight.[567,568] See also Phenylenediamine.

m-PHENYLENEDIAMINE, 4-(PHENYLAZO)-, HYDROCHLORIDE. Brilliant oil orange Y base, chrysoidine G. It caused cancer when given orally to mice in 31 milligram doses per kilogram of body weight.[569] See also Phenylenediamine.

p-PHENYLENEDIAMINE. See Hair Coloring.

PHENYLTOIN. See Dilantin.

PHOSPHINE OXIDE,TRIS (1-AZIRIDINYL)-. See Triethylenephosphoramide.

PHOSPHINE OXIDE,TRIS (1-(2-METHYL) AZIRIDINYL)-. See Triethylenephosphoramide.

PHOSPHINE SULFIDE,TRIS (1-AZIRIDINYL)-. See Triethylenethiophosphoramide.

PHOSPHORIC ACID, TRI-2-PROPENYL ESTER. *See* Triallyl Phosphate.

PHOTODIELDRIN. Dieldrin-free photodieldrin, a breakdown product of the pesticides aldrin and dieldrin, was given to rats and mice for periods ranging from 59 to 80 weeks. It is more toxic than dieldrin to rats and mice but less toxic to dogs, chickens, and pheasants. It is not produced commercially. It was selected for study because it is a photochemical conversion product of dieldrin. Under test conditions of the NCI it was not carcinogenic in rats or mice.[570]

PICLORAM. Systemic herbicide regulated by the EPA. Employed only for nonfood use to control broad-leaf weeds and woody plants. There is a persistent environmental problem of long-term low-level human exposure. Picloram was given to mice and rats for 80 weeks. According to an NCI report, under these test conditions the incidence of neoplastic nodules of the liver was suggestive of the ability of the compound to cause benign liver tumors in rats. In mice, picloram was not found to cause tumors.[571]

THE PILL. An estimated 8 to 10 million American women take "the pill," and 25 million others have taken it in the past. An association between use of oral contraceptives and liver tumors has been confirmed. The American College of Surgeons' Commission of Cancer reports on a five-year study of liver tumors, both malignant and benign, in almost 500 hospitals across the nation. Some 543 liver tumors were discovered. A history of oral contraceptive use was found in nearly half of the liver-tumor victims. Also, tumor symptoms were more severe among users.

In another study reported to the American College of Obstetricians and Gynecologists in Anaheim, California, in 1978, it was stated that women 27 or older who have been on the pill for four years or more run at least 200 times the normal risk of liver tumors. And women under 26 years who have used oral contraceptives for four years or more are 19 times as likely as nonusers to develop the tumors. While liver tumors do not occur very often, they are less rare among young women than had previously been believed. Many patients have vague and nonspecific complaints, and doctors have been unaware of this particular diagnostic possibility.[572] A few cancers of the liver have been reported in women using oral contraceptives, but it has not yet been determined whether the drug caused them. Sequential oral contraceptives (no longer marketed in the United States) have been implicated as a cause of uterine cancer. These pills involved taking estrogen alone for a number of days and then with progestogen *(see)* for several days. Oral contraceptives on the market today contain either an estrogen-progestogen combination or progestogen alone. The combination pills are in greater demand.

Pill choosers have been found to have a higher rate of uterine cervical dysplasia, a precursor of cervical cancer, *before* they decided to take oral contraceptives as a means of birth control. A National Institute of Child

Health and Human Development study determined that the suspected higher incidence of cervical cancer in oral-contraceptive users may, therefore, be due to preexisting body and behavioral differences in the women themselves and not in the contraceptives. Women choosing the pill differed from those choosing the IUD in that they had higher income and a lower body weight. Dysplasia was found in 8.3 percent of the pill choosers compared to 4.8 percent of those who chose all other methods. This suggests to researchers that prior differences, not fully understood, in susceptibility to cervical cancer may explain the correlation between the use of the pill and cervical cancer.

As for other correlations between the pill and cancer, the FDA notes that estrogen has been found to cause cancer in laboratory animals and that this suggests that because oral contraceptives contain estrogen, they may also cause cancer in humans. Animal studies have shown that long-term continuous administration of either natural or synthetic estrogens in certain species increases the frequency of cancers of the breast, uterus, cervix, vagina, ovary, liver, and pituitary gland. Synthetic progestogens, none currently contained in oral contraceptives, have also been noted to increase the incidence of mammary nodules, benign and malignant, in dogs. The FDA states that studies to date in women taking currently marketed oral contraceptives have not confirmed that oral contraceptives cause cancer in humans. The agency advises women who have had cancer of the breast or sex organs, or unexplained vaginal bleeding, not to use the pill. It has definitely been determined that there is an association between estrogens taken during and after the menopause and cancer. There is also some evidence now that estrogens in oral contraceptives taken by younger women may also cause cancer of the endometrium (uterus) in females under 40 years. In 30 cases of adenocarcinoma of the endometrium submitted by physicians to a registry, nearly all the cancers occurred in younger women who had used a sequential oral contraceptive. These products are no longer marketed. No statistical association is yet evident suggesting an increased risk of endometrial cancer in users of the current oral contraceptives, but individual cases have been reported.

Several studies have also been reported as finding an increased risk of breast cancer in women taking oral contraceptives or estrogens. In one, a significant risk was suggested for a subgroup of oral contraceptive users with documented benign breast disease after two to four years on the pill. One other study indicated an increasing risk of breast cancer in women taking postmenopausal estrogens—this risk rose with duration of follow-up. A reduced occurrence of benign breast tumors in users of oral contraceptives has been well documented. In a prospective study of women with cervical abnormalities, there was an increase in severity and of conversion to cancer in situ (incipient, symptomless form) in oral contraceptive users compared to nonusers. This became statistically significant after three to four years on the pill. Nonreversal of dysplasia within the first six months on oral contraceptives is suggested as predictive of progression to cancer. A 10-year Kaiser-Permanente study of 17,942 patients in Walnut Creek, California, determined that women who use birth-control pills for more than 4 years face almost twice the risk of developing malignant melanoma. The studies, based on 90,000 women years of oral contraceptive use, were among the largest and longest duration inquiries to date. The report was published in the *British Journal of Cancer,* December 1977.

Therefore, women who have a strong family history of breast cancer or who have breast nodules, fibrocystic disease, recurrent mastitis (inflammation of the breast), abnormal mammographies *(see),* or cervical dysplasia should not take the pill. If they insist on taking it, they should be monitored with particular care. There is a question whether healthy women should be taking a powerful medication such as the pill over a long period. If you wish to avoid the possibility of daily ingesting a cancer-causing agent, choose another method of contraception. *See also* Estrogens, Progesterone, Hormones, Estradiol, and Estrone.[573,574,575]

PIPERONYL SULFOXIDE. An insecticide enhancer, it was given in feed to rats and mice for 104 and 105 weeks. It caused liver cancer in male mice under the test conditions. The compound was not carcinogenic to rats or to female mice.[576]

PIVALOLACTONE. An intermediate *(see)* in the production of polymers *(see),* it was given orally by stomach tube to rats and mice for 103 weeks. It caused cancer of the stomach in male and female rats but under test conditions it was not carcinogenic in mice.[577]

PLASTIC FOOD WRAP AND PACKAGING. A petroleum derivative. It is not biodegradable. Some create toxic smoke when burned. In 1975 the FDA approved a plastic acrylonitrile Coke bottle. But in 1977 rats fed large doses of acrylonitrile lost weight and developed abnormalities, such as lesions of the central nervous system. Another study showed migration of the chemical into the contents after the Coke bottle was kept at a temperature of 120 degrees for six months. The FDA proposed a ban on the product. An FDA official noted that acrylonitrile is not the only troublesome chemical. Some types of polyvinyl chloride (PVC) packages are also suspected carcinogens. PVC liquor bottles were prohibited in 1973, although PVC is used in other packages. Other commonly used plastics in the $15 billion a year food-packaging industry include polyethylene *(see),* polypropylene, and polyesters.

PLUMBANE, TETRAETHYL-. *See* Tetraethyl Lead.

POLONIUM. A naturally occurring radioactive element. This element may be a long-sought link between cigarette smoking and lung cancer in man. Polonium, which emits alpha radiation, is present in small amounts in tobacco as a natural contaminant. For a man smoking two packs of cigarettes a day, polonium deposited from smoke in the bronchial linings may deliver a radiation dose at least seven times, and perhaps much more, than the normal background-radiation exposure of nonsmokers. Polonium may constitute a significant initiator of neoplasia (abnormal growth) in the bronchial tissue of a cigarette smoker. Though it has long been known that ionizing radiation can produce cancer in man, this report suggested that radioisotopes in cigarettes are involved in the production of lung cancer. Polonium is vaporized at the burning temperature of the cigarette and is carried into the lungs by attaching itself to the smoke particles. Most of the polonium is eventually taken up by scavenger cells (phagocytes) and carried over the bronchial lining of the throat.

Genealogically, polonium is the daughter of an isotope of lead (Pb^{210}) and a granddaughter of radium (Ra^{226}). The element is present in all green plants: it is absorbed through the roots, and also to a lesser extent, it is absorbed by the leaves through "natural fallout" in the atmosphere. The element is in no way related to atom-bomb fallout. The radioactive half-life (time it takes for half the amount of a substance to be eliminated) of polonium is 138 days, which assures ample time for the translocation of the particles to the bronchi to take place. The minimum dose delivered by these particles for an individual smoking two packs a day for 25 years would be about seven times the normal background exposure. This estimate does not take account of the radiation dose arising from Pb^{210} (lead) absorption in smoke, either from beta particles emitted by Pb^{210} and Bi^{210} (bismuth) or from the polonium daughter which would arise in the lungs from lead absorption. In addition, this calculation neglects the slowing effect of smoke on ciliary action. For these reasons it is believed that this estimate is probably conservative, and the dose could be 100 rem or more for this process. It is likely that the element is concentrated in specific regions of the bronchi and that in the case of an individual smoking two packs a day over a 25-year period, local doses from this concentration process may range from several hundred rem to over a thousand rem. Particles that penetrate the upper air passages come in contact with the mucus-covered surface of the bronchi where they tend to adhere and to remain in contact with the bronchial mucosa for varying periods of time, depending on the type and nature of the particles.

Polonium, though only one of several naturally occurring alpha emitters present in the tobacco leaf, is particularly important because it is volatile (vaporizes) at the burning temperature of the cigarette. Earlier measurements of radioactive potassium (K^{40}) and of radium isotopes present in tobacco were made by British researchers. However, the isotopes studied by them were found not to be volatile at the burning temperature of the cigarette and thus could not deliver a significant radiation dose. From the standpoint of polonium concentration in the smoke, they found there was little difference between filter and nonfilter cigarettes.[578]

POLYCHLORINATED BIPHENYLS. *See* PCBs and Aroclor.

POLYCYCLIC HYDROCARBONS. These are members of a broad class of chemicals produced by incomplete combustion of organic matter. Cigarette smoke, vehicle exhaust, forest fires, and even charcoal-broiled meat have been shown to contain substantial quantities of these potent carcinogens. The original discovery of their cancer-causing potential was made in the late 1700s when Sir Percivall Pott made his correlation between cancer and chimney sweeping in England. Benzopyrene *(see)* was isolated from coal tar in 1933 and determined to be a carcinogen. It is now believed that diol epoxides, which are formed during the metabolism of polycyclic hydrocarbons as a result of the action of certain enzymes, are responsible for the cancer-causing potential of these chemicals. Evidence is now strong, for instance, that the smoke-related carcinogen benzopyrene is activated in the body to a diol epoxide, which in turn has considerably stronger activity in the Ames Test *(see* Introduction, page 7*)* than does the parent compound.[579]

POLYDIMETHYLSILOXANE RUBBER. *See* Silastic.

POLYETHYLENE. *Alathon, alkathene, lupolen.* A polymer *(see)* of ethylene, it is a product of petroleum gas or the dehydration of alcohol. One of a group of lightweight thermoplastics that have a good resistance to chemicals, low moisture absorption, and good insulating properties. Used in hand lotions and hair dressings, wire and cable coatings and insulations, rubber and plastics, paper and container coatings, liquid polishes and textile finishes. It caused tumors when implanted in rats in 2,120 milligram doses per kilogram of body weight and when injected under the skin of mice in 330 milligram doses per kilogram of body weight.[580]

POLYETHYLENE GLYCOL (PEG). *Carbowax, lutrol.* Any of several condensation polymers *(see)* of ethylene glycol. It is clear, colorless, odorless, and its form can range from viscous liquid to waxy solid. It is used as a chemical intermediate *(see)* in plasticizers, softeners, humectants, and lubricants, and as a base for cosmetics, particularly hand lotions, hair dressings, and various lotions. It is also used in metal and rubber processing. A permissible additive to food and animal feed, it has no known skin toxicity, but implants in mice of 420 milligram doses per kilogram of body weight have caused cancer.[581]

POLYETHYLENE GLYCOL MONOSTEARATE. *MYRJ 45, polyoxyethylene (8) stearate.* A series of derivatives of fat-forming acids. A waxy material ranging from water dispersible to water soluble. It is used as an emulsifier and dispersing agent in food and pharmaceuticals—a flavor disperser in ice creams and an emulsifier in bakery products. It was fed to rats as one-quarter of their diet and resulted in the formation of bladder stones and subsequent tumors.[582] It is added to bread to make it feel fresh.

POLYETHYLENE TEREPHTHALATE film. *Mylar.* A polyester film available in seven types. It is used for electrical and industrial packaging purposes. It caused tumors when injected under the skin of rats in 50 milligram doses per kilogram of body weight.[583]

POLYMER. A substance or product formed by combining many small molecules (monomers). The result is essentially recurring long-chain structural units that have tensile strength, elasticity, and hardness. Examples of polymers (literally; "having many parts") are plastics, fibers, rubber, and human tissues.

POLYNUCLEAR COMPOUNDS. A widespread group of aromatic compounds synthesized mainly in the combustion of organic materials. They have four or more closed rings, usually of the benzoid type, and are present in all kinds of soot and smoke. They occur in tobacco smoke, in smoked fish and meat, in coal and coal-tar pitch, and in the atmosphere of all urban areas, as well as in increasing quantities in rural areas, mainly as a result of the discharge of the exhaust gases from gasoline and diesel engines. We are exposed to complex mixtures of these substances, and exposure occurs under a variety of circumstances and through different routes. One of the most publicized and well-studied of these carcinogenic substances is benzopyrene *(see).* Exposure to mixtures of polynuclear compounds has been reported to be associated with human cancer, particularly with epitheliomas (tumors) of the scrotum and other skin cancers in chimney sweeps, wax pressmen, and cotton-mule spinners, as well as with skin cancer in workers exposed to various mineral oils and lung cancer in gas workers.[584]

POLYP. A small stemlike growth that may occur in the mucous membranes of various parts of the body, such as the intestines or the nose. *See also* Precancerous Conditions.

POLYURETHANE FOAM AND PLASTIC. A thermoplastic polymer *(see).* In foam it can be used in both flexible and rigid forms. Density varies from 2 to 50 pounds per cubic foot. The flexible foam is used in furniture, mattresses, laminates, insulations, floor leveling, seat cushions, and to absorb crude-oil spills on seawater. The rigid form is used for furniture, packaging and packing, marine floatation, auto components, cigarette filters, light structures such as boat hulls, and soundproofing insulation. Plastic polyurethane is used for products that are resistant to weather, abrasion, and organic solvents. It tends to harden and become brittle at low temperatures. It is used as a sealant and caulking agent; in adhesive films; and in auto linings, bumpers, and fenders. It caused tumors when implanted in rats in 325 milligram doses per kilogram of body weight.[585]

POLYVINYL ALCOHOL (PVA). *Polyviol, vinol, rhodoviol.* A synthetic resin prepared from polyvinyl acetates by replacement of the acetate groups with hydroxyl groups. Dry, unplasticized PVA powder is white to cream colored and softens at about 200 degrees Fahrenheit. It is used in the plastics industry in modeling compounds, surface coatings, and films resistant to gasoline. It is also used in textile sizes and finishes; in the manufacture of artificial sponges; in pharmaceuticals; in lipsticks, setting lotions, and various creams. It caused cancer when injected under the skin of rats in 2,500 milligram doses per kilogram of body weight.[586]

POLYVINYL CHLORIDE (PVC). *Chloroethylene polymer.* Derived from vinyl chloride *(see),* it consists of a white powder or colorless granules that are resistant to weather, moisture, acids, fats, petroleum products, and fungus. It has many uses in modern life, including plumbing, piping, conduits, siding, gutters, window and door frames, raincoats, toys, gaskets, garden hoses, electrical insulation, shoes, magnetic tape, film, sheeting, containers for toiletries, cosmetics, and household chemicals, fibers for athletic supports, lining for reservoirs, adhesive and bonding agents, tennis-court playing surfaces, flooring and phonograph records. However, its use as a plastic wrap for food, including meats, and for human blood has alarmed some scientists. Human and animal blood can extract potentially harmful chemicals from the plastic. The chemicals are added to polyvinyl chloride to make it flexible, and they migrate from the plastic into the blood and into the meat in amounts directly proportional to the length of time of storage. The result can be contamination of the blood causing lung shock, a condition in which the patient's blood circulation to the lungs is impeded.[587] PVC has also caused tumors when injected under the skin of rats in doses of 100 milligrams per kilogram of body weight.[588]

POLYVINYL PYRROLIDINONE, POLY(1-VINYL-2-PYRROLIDI-NONE), POLYMERS 1-6. A faintly yellow solid plastic resin resembling albumin. It is used to give a softer set in shampoos, hair sprays, and lacquers and as a carrier in emollient creams, liquid lip rouge, and face rouge. It is also used as a clarifier in vinegar and a plasma expander in medicine. Ingestion may produce gas, fecal impaction, and damage to lungs and kidneys. It may linger in the system several months to a year. It has been combined with procaine and administered subcutaneously as an alleged cure for many ailments. In a New Jersey hospital, two patients seen for treatment of tumors of the arm had a history of procaine-PVP injections. In one case, PVP material was found in the liver. Repeated injections of PVP in rabbits produced a foam-cell storage phenomenon in the spleen, lymph nodes, bone marrow, adrenal gland, liver, lungs, and thymus.[589,590]

POTASSIUM ARSENITE. *See* Arsenic Compounds.

PRECANCEROUS CONDITIONS. There are a number of benign diseases which have been associated with the development of cancer:

- *Leukoplakia.* Clinically, a precancerous condition characterized by thickened white patches of epithelium on the mucous membranes, especially of the mouth and bladder. The step from leukoplakia to malignancy has been postulated to be related to many factors, including local irritation, vitamin deficiency, and poor oral hygiene; but there is no conclusive evidence about any of these. It is known that when multiple patches of leukoplakia are found in the oral cavity, multiple malignant tumors may follow. Leukoplakia of the urinary bladder can precede or accompany bladder cancer. Leukoplakia also occurs in the mucous membranes of many other organs, including the pharynx, esophagus, cervix, conjunctiva, and penis, but the association between these areas and malignancy is not as strong as with the bladder and mouth.

- *Carcinoma in situ.* Sometimes called intraepithelial cancer, it is a benign, asymptomatic neoplastic condition, characterized by microscopic appearances of individual cells suggesting cancer, but without the spread to adjacent structures, or metastases to distant lymph nodes or organs. It is most common in the uterine cervix but is often seen in the oral cavity and elsewhere. Carcinoma in situ of the cervix has probably been studied more than any other benign neoplasm, but there is still disagreement about the nature of events that may lead to invasive cervical carcinoma.

- *Osteitis deformans.* Paget's disease of the bone seems to be related to several forms of bone cancer. Although osteosarcomas predominate, other types of bone cancers have also been found in association with it. When cancer develops in an area affected by osteitis deformans, it is usually where the disease is most advanced and has been present for many years. Such tumors are highly malignant and survival is usually short.

- *Benign polyps.* These are extremely common, in fact, very few of us escape them. They may occur almost anywhere in the skin, digestive tract, reproductive organs, respiratory tract, or elsewhere. Study of the possible malignant transformation of benign polyps is complicated by the fact that in its early stages cancer often looks like a benign polyp. Microscopic examination is required to tell the difference.

- Benign polyps of the nose and uterine cervix are generally agreed to have no relation to cancer of these same organs. Polyps of the endometrium (uterine lining) are often associated with carcinoma, which may be entirely confined to the polyp. It is difficult to tell at an early stage whether the polyp is cancer free. Polyps of the stomach are rare, and it is not known whether they forecast cancer. However, stomach carcinoma is more common among patients with multiple gastric polyps than among those with single polyps. Pernicious anemia has been reported to precede an increased incidence of both gastric polyps and carcinoma.

- It is commonly agreed that villous papillomas—a type of bladder or mammary tumor—are premalignant. Polyps found in familial polyposis, a condition characterized by dark spots on the lips and multiple intestinal polyps and thought to be hereditary, indicate a susceptibility to malignant disease in the lower digestive tract. So too does ulcerative colitis. However, the significance of benign adenomatous polyps found in the colon or rectum of more than 20 percent of the adult population is not conclusively known despite extensive study.[591]

PRENATAL. The most infamous example of prenatal exposure inducing cancer in the offspring is DES *(see)*, the synthetic estrogen. There are other suspected cancer-causing agents that may also cross the placental barrier. Among them are immunosuppressants, which may cause reticulum-cell sarcomas in children; vinyl chloride *(see)*, which may cause angiosarcomas of the liver; benzene; Chloramphenicol; or alkylating agents *(see all)*, which may cause leukemia; oral contraceptives *(see)*, which may cause benign liver tumors; and androgenic anabolic hormones *(see)*, which may cause malignant liver tumors. Malignancies have developed in children whose mothers were given hydantoin *(see)* for epilepsy during pregnancy.[592]

PRINTING-TRADE WORKERS. Susceptible to cancer of the lung and bronchus.[593]

PROCARBAZINE HYDROCHLORIDE. *Natulan.* An experimental anticancer drug, it causes cancer when given orally to rats and mice and when injected in mice.

PROFLAVINE. *3,6-Diaminoacridine.* A synthetic acridine dye that earlier in this century was found to have bacteriostatic and bacteriocidal properties when applied to the skin. During World War II it was widely used as a wound antiseptic. With the advent of more specific and less-toxic antibiotics, its clinical use declined until it was reintroduced with ultraviolet light for the treatment of psoriasis and herpes-2 virus infections *(see)*. Repeated applications of the compound alone, to the skin or in subcutaneous implant, showed neither promoting nor carcinogenic action, although present tests may suggest it is carcinogenic in female mice. They had an unusually high incidence of liver cancer in the control male mice and an unusually high incidence in all female mice, including controls. Furthermore, the positive control compound was tested in the same room as proflavine and may have contributed to the findings.[594]

PROGESTERONE, PREGN-4-ENE-3,20-DIONE. *Luteal hormone, progesterol, progestin, progesterone, prolidon, synovex.* An off-white or white colorless crystalline powder that is stable in air. A female hormone that when injected inhibits gonadotropin production, which in turn prevents follicular maturation and ovulation. Available data indicates that this does not occur when the usually recommended oral dosage is given in a single daily dose. Beagle dogs treated with medroxyprogesterone acetate developed mammary nodules, some of which were malignant (although nodule occurrence appeared in control animals, they were intermittent in nature, whereas nodules in drug-treated animals were larger, more numerous, and persistent, and there were some breast malignancies with metastases). The significance of progestogens to humans has not yet been established.[595] *See also* The Pill, Hormones, and Oral Contraceptives.

PROLACTIN. *Luteotropin, lactogenic hormone (LTH).* One of the hormones secreted by the anterior lobe of the pituitary gland. It aids the growth of the mammary gland and initiates milk secretion. It also influences the activity of the uterus, increasing the secretion of progesterone. It is used as a medicine. Its increased production by the drug chlorpromazine has been associated with an increase in growth of breast cancers. Reserpine *(see)* also increases the flow of prolactin, which may account for the correlation between women taking reserpine (an anti-high-blood-pressure and tranquilizing drug) and the incidence of breast cancer noted among them. Some researchers have also proposed that high levels of fat in the diet induce increased production of prolactin, hence the association between dietary fat and breast cancer noted by the epidemiologists.[596]

PRONAMIDE. *Kerb.* This pesticide, used mainly on lettuce, alfalfa, and, to a lesser extent, on berries, turf, commercial nursery plantings, and sugar-beet seed, caused cancer in mice. The EPA on January 15, 1979, proposed that the continued use of pronamide be allowed, but with additional precautions to reduce potential risks to humans. EPA Assistant Administrator Steven Jellinek said: "In general, EPA concluded that for all uses the economic benefits of pronamide outweigh its risks. Most pronamide is used on lettuce in California and Arizona, which produce most of this country's lettuce. Without pronamide, the estimated loss to lettuce and alfalfa growers would be approximately $17.3 million annually. Pronamide is used primarily as a herbicide to control weeds, which compete with lettuce and alfalfa. Other herbicides available for weed control of these crops are not always as effective, and for lettuce these uses would result in additional labor costs for growers who would have to control the weeds by hand or mechanically."

Pronamide has been in use since 1969. The EPA said that by requiring pronamide applicators to be trained and by reducing the amount of pronamide residue on the lettuce, potential risks would be reduced.[597]

PROPANE,1,3,-EPOXY-2,2-DIMETHYL-. *See* Epichlorhydrin.

1-PROPANOL, 3, 3, -IMINODI-, DIMETHANESULFONATE (ester), HYDROCHLORIDE. A chemotherapy agent used to treat cancer. It caused lung tumors in mice.[598]

PROPANOLIDE. *See* b-Propiolactone.

b-PROPIOLACTONE (BPL). *2-Oxetanone, betaprone.* Prepared by the condensation of ketene in formaldehyde liquid. A versatile intermediate *(see)* in organic synthesis used to sterilize vaccines, grafts, and plasma. It caused cancer in rats, mice, guinea pigs, and hamsters. There is an OSHA standard for it as a carcinogen.[599]

PROPIONIC ACID, 3-NITRO-. *See* 3-Nitropropionic Acid.

PROPYLTHIOURACIL, 6- PROPYL -2- THIOURACIL. *Propacil, prothyran.* A thyroid depressant, it causes changes in the white blood cells. It also causes skin rashes and drug fever. It is prepared from the condensation of ethyl b-oxocaproate with thiourea. It caused cancer when given orally to rats and hamsters, and tumors when given orally to mice and guinea pigs, in doses from 37 to 1,137 milligrams per kilogram of body weight.[600]

PROSTATE CANCER. There are 38,000 new cases of cancer of the prostate each year, and approximately 18,000 men die of this disease each year. The symptoms are (1) difficulty in urination; (2) pain or persistent-pressure discomfort deep in the pelvis; (3) frequent urinary tract or prostate infections; (4) blood in the urine. Cancer of the prostate is a disease of males of middle age and older. There is no question that there are changing cancer death rates by age and race in the United States. Prostate cancer remains a serious problem among blacks. Attempts to identify other high-risk groups, possible sexual or transmissable factors, and socioeconomic factors involved have been instituted and preliminary reports given. These areas must be watched closely since there may be a particular group of individuals who, with further identification, could benefit from improved methods of screening and preventing prostate cancer. It should be noted that even this limited amount of information has not been previously available. Careful case control studies of blacks in Washington, D.C., compared with those in Africa have suggested that factors other than original racial origin, such as environmental factors, may be affecting prostate-cancer growth rates. This is a significant epidemiological advance.

The prostate can be examined by a physician during a rectal examination. This examination will uncover anything suspicious that might indicate cancer of the prostate. The occurrence of cancer of the prostate cannot be controlled since the causes are not known. However, the death rate can be greatly lowered if men, especially those over 50, are familiar with the above symptoms of the disease. Cancer of the prostate is the second most common cancer among men in the United States and is the most common cancer among black males. When nonwhite rates were examined by age and birth cohort, it was found that peak rates occurred at every age in the cohort of 1896 to 1900, and declined thereafter. The etiology, or cause, of prostate cancer remains essentially unknown.[601,602]

PROTEIN. The effect of dietary protein on tumorigenesis in laboratory animals is diverse. Depending upon the type of malignant tumor, a wide spectrum of response to low, high, or adequate protein intakes were studied. Thus, while chronic marginal protein undernutrition predisposed rats to an early occurrence, as well as a high rate, of cancer of the adrenal gland and the lymphoid organs, high protein intake increased their susceptibility to urinary papillomas. For other types of tumors, principally those occurring in the pituitary, thyroid, and pancreas, the highest rate of morbidity (disease) was obtained when rats were fed a diet adequate in protein content. In another study with rats, increasing protein in the diet fivefold (from 9 to 45 percent) had no significant influence on the incidence of three different types of tumors—spontaneous mammary carcinoma, benzopyrene-induced skin tumors, and sarcoma. It was observed that feeding a high-protein diet to rats resulted in an earlier appearance of mammary adenocarcinoma, whereas malignant hepatic (liver) tumor induced by azo dyes tended to be inhibited by increasing the amount of dietary casein (a protein obtained from milk). It is postulated that protein probably increases the resistance of the liver to hydrocarbons. An attempt has been made to explain the widely varying effects of protein on different tumors, analyzing the impact of protein nurtriture on the endocrine system and the immune system. These two systems represent opposite forces with respect to their role in oncogenic processes. It is postulated that the net effect of protein nurtriture on the endocrinological and immunological systems determines the type and prevalence of tumors.[603]

PSORIASIS. A chronic disease of the skin of unknown causes but thought to be related to arthritis. It persists for years with periods of remission and recurrence and is characterized by reddish skin and dry silvery scales that drop off. *See also* Anthralin and Methotrexate.

PURINE, 6-((1-METHYL-4-NITROIMIDAZOL-5-YL)THIO)-. *See* Imuran.

PVC. *See* Polyvinyl Chloride.

PYRAZINEAMIDE. This antituberculosis drug was fed to rats and mice for 78 weeks. It was not carcinogenic in rats or in male mice. In female mice early deaths and the small size of the control group precluded a conclusion on the carcinogenicity of the compound.[604]

PYRAZINECARBOXAMIDE. *See* Pyrazineamide.

PYRENE. A hydrocarbon that occurs in coal tar. It is used in biochemical research as a carcinogen. It caused cancer when applied to the skin of mice in 10 milligram doses per kilogram of body weight.[605]

PYRENE, INDENO(1,2,3-cd)-. *2,3-Phenylenepyrene.* Determined a positive carcinogen in animals by a NIOSH review, it is a candidate for a NIOSH hazard review. EPA has also selected it for top-priority attention as a toxic water pollutant.[606]

3,6-PYRIDAZINEDIONE,1,2-DIHYDRO-. *See* Maleic Hydrazide.

PYRIDINE. A slightly yellow or colorless liquid that has a nauseating odor, a burning taste, and is slightly alkaline on reaction. It is soluble in water, alcohol, ether, benzene, and fatty oils, and is toxic when ingested or inhaled. It has a tolerance of 5 parts per million in air, and it is flammable.

It is used as a solvent in the synthesis of vitamins and drugs, as a solvent in waterproofing and rubber chemicals, as a denaturant for alcohol and antifreeze mixtures, and as a dyeing assistant in textiles and fungicides.

PYRIMETHAMINE. *Daraprim.* A chemotherapeutic agent, it is used to prevent malaria and to treat toxoplasmosis (an infection that can cause extensive or fatal damage to the eyes or the central nervous system). In humans it has produced megaloblastic anemia and leukopenia,[607] and in mice it has caused lung tumors.[608]

PYRROLIZIDINE ALKALOIDS. Derived from green plants—*Senecio, Crotalaria, Heliotropium,* and other genera—they were among the first natural products to be claimed to be carcinogenic. Acute and chronic poisoning of farm livestock by pyrrolizidine alkaloids has been well known for a long time. In man, acute poisoning has been observed only as a result of either the occasional contamination of cereals or the use of native herbal medicines or "bush teas." Small doses in the laboratory produce progressive lesions in the liver and in the lungs: they keep the cells from dividing and cause liver cancer in up to 25 percent of the rats fed a diet containing 0.5 percent dried *Senecio longilolus.* A high incidence of liver tumors in Africa may incriminate pyrrolizidine alkaloids.[609]

QUICKSILVER. *See* Mercury.

QUINALDIC ACID, 4,8-DIHYDROXY- and 8-HYDROXY-. *Xanthurenic acid.* Used for the determination of copper, zinc, and uranium with which it forms insoluble salts. Causes tumors when implanted in mice in 160 milligram doses per kilogram of body weight.[610]

QUINALDINE, 5-((p-(DIMETHYLAMINO) PHENYL) AZO)- and 4-NITRO-, 1-OXIDE. A colorless oily liquid that becomes reddish brown on exposure to air, and is highly irritating to mucous membranes. It is used in the manufacture of dyes, pharmaceuticals, fine organic chemicals, and acid-base indicators. Causes tumors when injected under the skin of mice in doses of 120 milligrams per kilogram of body weight. When injected into rats, it causes cancer in doses of 540 milligrams per kilogram of body weight.[611,612]

QUINAZOLINE. It consists of leaflets from petroleum ether. Has the odor of quinoline and a slightly bitter taste. Caused tumors when painted on the skin of mice.[613]

QUINOLINE, 4-((4-Bis (2-CHLOROETHYL) AMINO)-1-METHYL-BUTYL) AMINO -7- CHLORO-DIHYDROCHLORIDE and 3-BRO-MO-4-NITRO-, 1-OXIDE. A basic nitrogen compound occurring in coal tar, and obtained from it, but more frequently obtained by synthesis from aniline. Used in medicine to preserve anatomic specimens and in the manufacture of copper quinolate. It caused cancer when injected into the abdomen of mice in 8 milligram doses per kilogram of body weight, and it caused tumors when injected under the skin in 120 milligram doses per kilogram of body weight.[614]

8-QUINOLINOL. *Bioquin, oxin, oxychinolin, 8-oxyquinoline, tumex.* Derived from o-aminophenol with o-nitrophenol, it is a white crystalline powder used as a fungistate (inhibits the growth of fungi without destroying them) and as an internal disinfectant. Causes cancer when given orally to rats in a dose of 29 milligrams per kilogram of body weight and tumors when injected into mice in 80 milligram doses per kilogram of body weight.[615]

p-QUINONE DIOXIME. A rubber vulcanization accelerator, it was fed to rats and mice for 104 weeks. It proved carcinogenic in female rats, causing bladder cancer. The compound did not cause cancer in male rats or in mice of either sex under NCI test conditions. Compounds found to be carcinogenic in these animal tests are generally considered to be capable of causing cancer in humans. The tests do not provide information, however, that could be used to predict the frequency at which cancers might be produced in human population under actual conditions of exposure.[616]

QUINOXALINE,5-((p-(DIMETHYLAMINO) PHENYL) AZO)-. *See* Phenylenediamine.

RADIATION. Radiation is generally divided into two categories: ionizing and nonionizing radiation. Ionizing radiation corresponds to X-rays; alpha, beta, and gamma rays; and neutrons. The energy of these rays is so great that when they interact with the atoms that make up all matter, they actually break up the atoms, remove electrons from them, and cause them to develop an electric charge. A charged particle is called an ion. When ionizing radiation, such as X-rays or the radiation from radioactive material, interacts with the body, it interacts with the atoms of the body and damages them. Ionizing radiation is widely used in industry, medical and dental X-rays, and nuclear-power reactors. Nonionizing radiations do not possess enough energy to ionize atoms but can cause burns, and damage the eyes, skin, or other organs of the body. Ultraviolet radiation is the portion of the sunlight that causes sunburn. The symptoms of overexposure to ultraviolet radiation are the same as severe sunburn: reddening of the skin, blistering, and pain. Also, an increased chance of skin cancer is present. There is no legal limit for exposure to ultraviolet radiation. Ionizing radiation is the most serious because it injures cells of the body and can lead to many illnesses, including cancer and genetic damage. It can be immediately fatal in large doses.

People cannot feel radiation, so they may be unaware of being exposed. One theory is that radiation need strike the sensitive part of the cell only once to create a chance that it will become cancerous. Another theory proposes that the sensitive part of the cell must be "hit" several times for

176

it to cause a possibility of cancer. Whichever theory is correct, radiation is certainly a threat. Several scientists who have studied radiation have recently stated that there is no safe level of radiation, and that any dose, no matter how small, can cause leukemia and other forms of cancer. There is no safe level of exposure, and no dose of radiation can be so low that the risk of it causing a malignancy is zero. There is also the belief that at least 30 percent of all X-rays are unnecessary and only subject a patient to unnecessary risks. The prenatal infant and the child are more sensitive to radiation than the adult. Leukemia and other forms of cancer are significantly higher in children whose mothers were X-rayed during pregnancy. This ionizing radiation has the ability to cause congenital anomalies.

Cancer can be induced in any tissue where cancer occurs naturally. The observation that antenatal diagnostic radiography causes a small but definite increase in childhood cancer is good evidence of this. Radiation-associated thyroid carcinomas were reported in patients who had been irradiated during childhood for thymic enlargement, recurrent tonsillitis, acne, and impetigo (a skin disease). In Newfoundland it was discovered that radiation-induced lung cancer was prevalent in workers in the fluorspar mines. Radiologists evidenced an increased incidence of leukemia before proper techniques and caution were used. A study conducted by the *Boston Globe* found an increased evidence of cancers, including leukemia, among workers exposed to low levels of radiation at the Portsmouth Naval Shipyard in Maine: deaths from cancer were reportedly twice the national average, deaths from cancer of the lymph glands were 125 percent higher than the national rate, and deaths from leukemia were 450 percent higher than the national rate.

Radiation alone may not always cause tumor development, but when combined with viral, biochemical, or other factors, the potential for tumor induction often is enhanced. This was found in an investigation where rats were fed subtumorigenic amounts of ethionine, a substance known to cause liver cancer, and then treated with radiation. The group receiving ethionine had a greater number of mammary tumors than did the control rats. Escape of radioactive gas from some luminous watches poses a potential hazard. The women who painted the luminous watch dials between 1916 and 1929 used to point their brushes with mouth moisture and as a result swallowed untold quantities of radium and mesothorium. These women showed a great prevalence toward leukemia and osteogenic sarcoma.

That radiation can cause cancer in humans was dramatically demonstrated by the increased incidence of leukemia in Japanese who received high exposures of atomic radiation in 1945. There has been a rise in the incidence of leukemia and a few statistically significant increases in other somatic cancers in the survivors of Hiroshima and Nagasaki. Fallout from nuclear weapons tests can affect the public health by producing somatic and genetic damage. Fallout affects the air, water, and food, and contaminates the human body. Though nuclear tests are conducted at great distances from human habitations, the detonation of a nuclear device scatters the radioactive materials in all directions, but mostly upward.

The radioactive material that gets into the stratosphere is dispersed very widely and eventually shows up in foodstuffs all over the world, except for those elements that have decayed by the time they descend into the lower atmosphere. Material which is hurled directly into the lower atmosphere comes to earth fairly soon and is not dispersed as widely as the stratospheric fallout. When fallout is present in the lower atmosphere, it is ingested by inhalation. Fallout also settles into water supplies and is deposited directly on food plants and on soil. Thus, practically everything ingested, either by inhalation or by way of food and drink, is contaminated to some extent. Radioactive fallout enters plants directly by deposition on the surface and indirectly by way of the roots that draw nutriments from the soil. It enters meat supplies by way of the food and drink our meat-producing animals ingest; it enters milk and milk products in the same way. It is usually rain that brings it down to the ground. Such variable factors as wind and rain determine to a considerable extent the time and the place at which radioactive debris enters our foods. For now, nuclear plants should be put farther away from where they can do damage, and unnecessary X-ray treatments should be avoided, particularly by pregnant women.[617,618,619,620,621,622,623,624,625,626,627,628,629,630]

Greater progress has been made in monitoring and controlling occupational hazards due to ionizing radiation and radioactive chemicals than is the case with carcinogenic chemicals. At the present time, estimates of the proportion of workers exposed to ionizing radiation vary between 2 and 8 percent. Three main groups of workers have been studied and shown to incur a high incidence of occupational cancers: (1) radiologists (develop skin cancer, leukemia, precancerous changes, and malignancies); (2) workers in industries producing luminous goods that have radium deposition in the body (develop bone cancer); (3) uranium and other miners (develop lung cancer).

Of these three groups, the first two are now subject to control measures, and the appearance of cancer in each group has a low probability. The incidence of lung cancer in uranium miners is still an important problem, and there is also evidence of lung cancer in other miners including those working with hematite, fluorspar, and other ores. This is attributed to the high concentration of radon (a radioactive gas formed by the disintegration of radium or uranium), combined with the presence of mineral dust and other irritants. Epidemiological studies of groups with a high risk of occupational cancer from radiation are taking place in different countries, and the combined data are being collected by the World Health Organization, the United Nations Scientific Committee on the Effects of Atomic Radiation, and the International Commission of Radiation Protection in order to evaluate the risk. Several areas require attention: (1) early diagnosis and dosimetry (measurement) of radioactive contamination are important contributors to the prevention of radiation-induced cancer and include the use of whole-body counters to determine dose and the development of biological and clinical indications of irritation; (2) methods to prevent the retention of and to facilitate the elimination of radioactive substances from the human body using different kinds of pharmaceutical agents could be important; (3) preselection of people for the radiation industries is recommended, and a list of contraindications to radiation work should be prepared. (Such contraindications should include young people, women of childbearing age, and, in general, persons suffering from skin and blood diseases and nonmalignant tumors); (4) medical supervision of workers is of great importance and should include examinations before, during, and after employment. (The ability to select high-risk groups would enable such examinations to be intensified in those who are most in need of them. A long-term postemployment examination is of special importance for an evaluation of the possible appearance of occupational cancer due to the carcinogenic effects of radiation); (5) investigation of the combined effects of different chemical and physical agents is recommended, bearing in mind the existing epidemiological data on the synergistic effects in the following examples: the combined effect of mineral dust, fumes, and radiation in uranium and other miners; the combined effect of smoking and radiation in miners; and the possible combined effects of radiation and other factors, for example, X-rays from frequent radiological examinations in workers with asbestos or in those with lung diseases such as silicosis or other pneumoconiosis.[631]

RADIOACTIVE DUSTS. Radioactive particles can be borne by dust, creating a serious hazard for workers who breathe the dust. This hazard particularly affects underground miners. Radon is a radioactive gas produced by the natural decay of uranium and radium, but its presence is by no means limited to uranium and radium deposits. It can exist in a variety of metal and nonmetal mines. The Mining Enforcement and Safety Administration reports that in the United States measurable amounts of radon have been found in mines producing clay, iron, fluorspar, tungsten, copper, and zinc. Radon escapes from rock into open areas of the mine. When the miner inhales it, his whole body is in effect exposed to radiation. The hazard is limited because most radon is exhaled within its half-life (the time required for half the amount of a substance to be eliminated) of 3.8 days. Far more dangerous are the decay products of radon—radionuclides with an average half-life of 30 minutes. Unlike radon, which is exhaled, these decay products quickly attach themselves to solid surfaces like dust particles.

When miners inhale these dust particles, the radiation attacks those areas in the nose, throat, and lungs where the dust particles are deposited. The dose of radiation a uranium miner's lungs receive from these dust particles is 20 times greater than from inhaled radon. The lung cancer rate among miners is more than four times the expected rate.[632]

RADIOLUMINESCENT PAINT. The Nuclear Regulatory Commission's Office of Standards Development issued a report on radiation doses resulting from exposure to watches and clocks containing tritium and promethium paint. Tritium and promethium are used to provide luminosity on the hands and dials of timepieces. The maximum individual whole-body dose for persons involved in the distribution, use, repair, and disposal of watches or clocks containing tritium paint is 0.9 millirem per year under normal conditions. (A millirem is one thousandth of a dosage of any ionizing radiation that will cause the same amount of human tissue damage as one roentgen of X-ray.) The maximum individual whole-body dose during any accident was 59 millirems from ingestion of an amount equal to about half the tritium—2 millicuries—in one watch. (A millicurie is one thousandth of a grain of radium.) A maximum accidental dose of 230 millirems to the gastrointestinal tract was estimated to be equal to the ingestion of about half the average amount of promethium–45 microcuries—in one timepiece. The report stated, however, that the likelihood of such exposures is very low.

The use of tritium and promethium in such products was authorized in 1961 and 1967, respectively, by the former Atomic Energy Commission, the NRC's predecessor. Although the NRC staff continues to believe the products provide an acceptable degree of safety and that the risk is extremely small, the staff has undertaken a separate study to evaluate the environmental effects of all consumer products containing radioactive material. As part of its continuing regulatory review, the staff will evaluate the environmental effects of the manufacture, use, and disposal of these products.[633]

RADIUM. This brilliant white solid luminescent substance is found in Colorado, Africa, and France. Radiation-protection standards for all radioactive isotopes in body tissues are based on experience with radium. The present radium standard has been predicated on the relatively small sample of radium-poisoning cases first identified in 1931 by Dr. H. S. Martland. From this sampling he cited 18 radium deaths and mentioned 30 patients alive at the time. In 1956 a Boston- and Chicago-area study identified 50 cases, some of which were the same mentioned by Martland.

It is estimated that in the New Jersey-New York-Philadelphia area, more than a thousand persons were exposed to radium and a few other radioactive isotopes. Most of the radium cases were found among former watch-dial painters. However, occupational exposure to radium also occurred among physicists and chemists, and clerical, maintenance, and office staffs in places using radium. Some persons acquired body burdens (refers to presence of radium in body) during medical treatment or diagnosis with radioactive material, including Radithor and Thorotrast. Others used nostrums that contained radium or radon (a gas produced by the decay of radium or uranium) for inhaling, drinking, or bathing. Some were contaminated as a result of radiation accidents or through the use of radioluminescent paints. A well-studied group of radium victims included 30 psychotic patients at Elgin State Hospital, Illinois, who received radium from 1930–1932.

The radium-dial painters case, however, was the most infamous. The workers were exposed from World War I until about 1925. Out of 800 women there were about 50 who overexposed themselves to radium by dipping their brushes in mesothorium and then touching the brushes to their lips. At the time Dr. Martland issued the first warning that the workers were being poisoned, 18 had already died. Five others, whom the doctors said were hopelessly ill, sued the company and were known in the press as "The Five Who Are Doomed to Die." Dr. Martland reported that deaths from radium occurred between 1916 and 1925, from four to six years after exposure, and were due to jaw necrosis and aplastic anemia. From 1924 to 1928 two deaths were due to bone cancer. From 1928 to 1931 additional bone cancers developed and other symptomatic and asymptomatic bone lesions were noted.

In 1952 Boston researchers reported 30 cases due to radium poisoning. Among them were 8 malignancies: 3 osteogenic sarcomas, one giant cell tumor of the bone, one fibrosarcoma of the knee joint, and 3 epidermoid carcinomas of the paranasal sinuses. The present maximum permissible body burden, based on the radium cases, is 0.1 micrograms of radium. In the Massachusetts study the malignancies all arose in patients with body burdens greater than one microgram. There were few symptoms referable to radium poisoning with levels of 0.5 to 1microgram and no cases with a level lower than 0.5 micrograms.[634]

RADIUM BROMIDE. *See* Radium.

RADIUM CHLORIDE. *See* Radium.

RADIUM SULFATE. *See* Radium.

RAPESEED OIL. Brownish yellow oil from a turnip-like annual herb of European origin. Widely grown as a forage crop for sheep in the United States, it has a distinctly unpleasant odor. It is used chiefly as a lubricant and in rubber substitutes, but is also used in soft soaps and in some margarines. Can cause acnelike skin eruptions. When rats were fed a diet high in rapeseed oil over a lifetime, they showed significantly greater degenerative changes in the liver and a higher incidence of kidney damage than animals fed other vegetable oils. In Canada it has been decreed prudent not to use rapeseed oil. *See also* Antithyroid Compounds for thyroid tumor effects.

RAUWOLFIA SERPENTINA. *See* Reserpine.

RESERPINE. *Rauwolfia serpentina, Serpasil.* A crystalline alkaloid extracted from the shrubs of the genus *Rauwolfia,* it is used in the treatment of high-blood-pressure emergencies, in which it is necessary to reduce blood pressure rapidly, and in psychiatric conditions to control symptoms of severe agitation. At one time it was used by an estimated 4 million Americans under a variety of drug trade names. However, in 1974 the British medical journal, *The Lancet,* reported three medical studies suggesting that the risk of breast cancer for women over 50 years old was three to four times higher if they were taking reserpine and related drugs used for hypertension and psychosis. The studies were made separately in Boston, Massachusetts; Bristol, England; and Helsinki, Finland. The studies grew out of what was called an "entirely unsuspected finding" of a drug-surveillance program carried out by Boston University Medical Center in 24 Boston-area hospitals in 1972. After the initial discovery in Boston, the findings were pursued further by a cancer-study unit at Oxford University and by a team at the University Hospital, Helsinki. *The Lancet* said the conclusion of all three studies was that the higher risk of breast cancer among reserpine-takers was related both to dosage and the duration of treatment with *Rauwolfia* derivatives. The reports indicated that women of premenopausal age taking the drug were less likely to develop breast cancer. The Boston survey also implicated *Rauwolfia* as a risk factor in several other rarer forms of cancer: cancer of the brain, uterus, ovary, pancreas, skin, and kidney. But no increased risk was detected for cancer of the lung or bowel. The Boston study compared the case histories of 1,350 women; the English study, 2,138 women; and the Finnish study, 876 women. The current *Physicians' Desk Reference,* widely used by physicians for prescribing information, does not mention cancer as a potential side effect of the medication. However, it does mention breast engorgement and pseudolactation, conditions known to be associated with prolactin *(see)*, the hormone correlated with breast cancer, in some cases. The drug is now recommended for use only in "emergency-type" situations.[635,636]

RESORCINOL. *See* 4-Hexylresorcinol and Phenol.

RHATHANY EXTRACT. *Krameria.* A synthetic flavoring derived from the dried roots of either of two American shrubs, *Krameria triandra* and *K. argentea.* Used in the raspberry, bitters, fruit, and rum flavorings for beverages, ice cream, ices, candy, chewing gum, and liquor. Also used as an astringent. It has a low toxicity when taken orally, but large doses may produce gastric distress. Caused cancer when injected subcutaneously in rats.[637]

RHODAMINE B. Consists of green crystals or reddish violet powder that is very soluble in water. Used as a dye, especially for paper, and as a reagent for antimony, bismuth, cobalt, gold, manganese, mercury, and thallium. It caused cancer when injected under the skin of rats.[638]

RICINOLEIC ACID. A mix of fatty oils found in the seeds of castor beans. Castor oil contains 80 to 85 percent ricinoleic acid. This oily liquid is used in soaps, added to Turkey red oil, and in contraceptive jellies. It is believed to be the active laxative in castor oil. It is also used as an emollient. It caused tumors when given subcutaneously to rabbits in 3,120 milligram doses per kilogram of body weight.[639]

ROUGHAGE. *Dietary fiber.* Doctors have been exploring its usefulness in preventing coronary and diverticular disease, colon cancer, and gallstones. Colon cancer is one of the diseases of Western civilization. Diverticular disease, heart disease, gallstones, polyps, hiatus hernia, and colon cancer all share the same geographical distribution factors: where these diseases occur there is increased fat, protein, sugar, and other refined carbohydrates in the diet. Along with this there is a tremendous decrease in the amount of fiber in the diet. In rural Africa, where people have a high-fiber diet, colon cancer is virtually unknown. In Western countries it is the commonest malignancy after lung cancer.

With high-fiber diets there is a shortened fecal-transit time. With low-fiber diets there are increased numbers of anaerobic bacteria in the stools. These bacteria degrade bile salts and the results are toxic. These toxic products are seen as carcinogenic when combined with slow fecal-transit times, and small feces are thus held in the bowel for a prolonged period and in a more concentrated form than they would be if the stools were large and bulky. Thus, when the diet lacks fiber, the colonic mucosa is exposed to a higher concentration of toxic agents for a longer period of time.

The causes of colon cancer are multiple, but high-fiber diets may be an important way to help prevent this disease. In addition, the use of dietary roughage as a specific treatment has been definitely proven in the relief of constipation and in the management of diverticular disease.[640] *See also* Fiber and Diet.

RUBBER-MILL WORKERS. Subject to cancer of the bladder.[641]

SACCHARIN. An artificial sweetener in use since 1879, it is 300 times as sweet as natural sugar but leaves a bitter aftertaste. It was used along with cyclamates *(see)* in the experiments that led to the banning of the latter in 1969. The FDA proposed restricting saccharin to 15 milligrams per day for each kilogram of body weight or about one gram a day for a 150-pound person. Then, on March 9, 1977, the FDA announced that the use of saccharin in foods and beverages would be banned because the artificial sweetener had been found to cause malignant bladder tumors in laboratory animals. The ban was based on the findings of a study sponsored by the Canadian government that found that 7 out of 38 animals developed tumors, 3 of them malignant. In addition, 100 offspring were fed saccharin, and 14 of them developed bladder tumors. In contrast, 100 control rats were not fed saccharin and only 2 developed tumors. At the time of the FDA's announcement, 5 million pounds of saccharin were being consumed per year, 74 percent of it in diet soda, 14 percent in dietetic food, and 12 percent as a "tabletop" replacement. There was an immediate outcry, led vociferously by the Calorie Council, an organization made up of commercial producers and users of saccharin. The FDA, urged by Congress, then delayed the ban.

Saccharin has also exhibited mutagenic activity (genetic change) in the early-warning Ames Test for carcinogens (see Introduction, page 7). When administered orally to mice, mutagenic activity was demonstrated in the urines of these animals as well as in tissue tests. Highly purified saccharin was not mutagenic in tissue tests, but the urines of mice to which this material had been administered exhibited mutagenic effects on another strain. Two other sweeteners, neohesperidin dihydrochalcone and xylitol, had no detectable mutagenic activity.[642] Congress's Office of Technology Assessment, in view of the evidence to date, strongly endorsed the scientific basis of the FDA's proposed ban. "This review of animal studies leads to the conclusion that saccharin is a carcinogen for animals," the OTA panel said. Clouding the risk assessment, however, is that up to 20 parts per million of unknown chemical impurities contaminated those doses fed rats in the Canadian study that led to the FDA move. (Panel members noted, though, that the impurities level was much lower than in commercially available saccharin.) The impurities themselves proved mutagenic in the Ames Test.

The federal government is now conducting a nationwide study of bladder cancer victims to see if saccharin alone or with other factors causes this kind of cancer in humans as it does in rats. The NCI and the FDA said their study will look at the cases of 3,000 bladder-cancer patients to try and determine which factors contribute to the disease. The life-styles of the patients will be contrasted to 6,000 persons without cancer to see what roles such factors as drinking water, cigarettes, occupational exposures to chemicals, and the artificial sweetener may play in the disease. In the meantime, some scientists feel that it might be beneficial if regular users of saccharin would occasionally discontinue its use for several days and thus allow tissue clearance. Reports of NIH chemicals indicate that saccharin accumulates in the bladder with prolonged administration of normal doses; however, the data also indicate that saccharin was rapidly cleared from the bladder tissue when it was withdrawn from the diet.[643]

On November 6, 1978, the Committee of the Institute of Medicine and National Research Council reported that it had reached the conclusion that saccharin is a "potential carcinogen in humans." The extremely low potency of saccharin as a carcinogen was emphasized by the committee. However, they expressed special concern that children under 10 years of age were consuming diet sodas and other saccharin-containing products in increasing amounts. Exposure in children, the committee noted, may have special significance because of the long time required for some cancers to develop. There were some "worrisome data" regarding consumption by women of child-bearing age, children, and teen-agers. The concern about fetal exposure grew out of earlier findings of increased bladder cancers in male rats fed high-saccharin diets or born to mothers who were on high-saccharin diets during pregnancy. The committee concluded that it is most likely that saccharin, acting by itself, is the carcinogenic agent, rather than any impurities that may be associated with its manufacture.

The FDA was expected to recommend a ban on the artificial sweetener in 1979, but before the ban could take effect, the artifical sweetener would remain on the market for at least another year. In the meantime, proponents of saccharin were expected to launch a campaign to save the sweetener.

SACCHARUM LACTIN. *See* Lactose.

SANAMYCIN. *See* Actinomycin C.

SARCOSINE. *N-Methylglycocoll, N-methylaminoacetic acid.* Deliquescent crystals with a sweet taste. It is very soluble in water, slightly soluble in alcohol, combustible, and has a low toxicity. Used in the synthesis of foaming antienzyme compounds for toothpastes, cosmetics, pharmaceuticals.

SCHISTOSOMA. A parasite found in the waters of the Nile Valley. It has been associated with bladder cancer found among the natives of this area.

SELENIUM. Selenium sulfide used in dandruff treatment and dandruff shampoo was determined a carcinogen in 1979.

SELENIUM DERIVATIVES. Compounds containing this element at low levels in the diet appear to act as essential nutrients for several mammalian and avian species. At high levels in the diet these derivatives are toxic to the liver and have been reported to induce tumors in rats. Inorganic selenium compounds occur naturally in many soils, and the element is incorporated into plant protein, partly as seleno-methionine and seleno-cystine. In some areas the forage contains high amounts of organic selenium compounds and is toxic to livestock. In some experiments, liver tumors were induced in rats fed diets of 5 to 10 parts per million of selenium for well over a year. Another report has claimed that 3 ppm of sodium selenite in drinking water for two years increased the incidence of benign and malignant tumors in rats. For a variety of reasons scientists say that none of these findings is conclusive evidence for or against liver cancer being induced by selenium derivatives and that further work, especially with long-term studies in several rats strains, should be done.[644]

SEMICARBAZIDE. *Aminourea, hydrazinecarboxamide.* Consists of snow-white crystals that are derived from hydrazine sulfate and potassium cyanate and are soluble in water. It is used as a reagent for aldehydes and ketones and to isolate hormones and certain fractions from essential oils.

Caused tumors when given orally to mice in 42 milligram doses per kilogram of body weight. The NCI has been testing it since 1976.[645]

SENECA OIL. *See* Petroleum.

SERPASIL. *See* Reserpine.

SERPENTINE. Yellow rods or leaflets derived from the roots of *Rauwolfia serpentina*. *See also* Reserpine.

SEVIN. *See* Carbamic Acid.

SEX. *See* Herpes-2 Virus.

SHOE INDUSTRY. Those workers in the press and finishing rooms develop a higher than normal incidence of nasal cancer.[646]

SILASTIC. A trademark for polydimethylsiloxane rubber, a composition comparable in physical character to milled and compounded rubber prior to vulcanization. Shows excellent resistance to compression, weathering, and thermal conductivity. Water absorption is low. Used in diaphragms, gaskets and seals, hose, coated fabrics, wire and cable, and insulating components for electronic parts. It caused cancer when implanted in rats in 1,500 milligram doses per kilogram of body weight.[647]

SILICA. A possible link between the second most abundant element on earth, silicon—12 percent of all rocks—and the commonest type of ovarian cancer, cystoma, has become the focus of work at the University of California, San Diego Medical School. Dr. Kurt Benirschke, professor of preproductive medicine, and his research associates think there is reason to believe that the introduction of silica into the internal organs of the body may be related to the development of cystoma—a type of ovarian cancer that is undetectable until it is malignant. Silica, in the form of talcum, has previously been found to cause damaging adhesions to develop in the abdomen around the ovaries and in the genital tract when deposited by the surgeon's gloves during an operation. The same "glove-caused" type of adhesions are sometimes found in the ovaries of women with cystoma. Aside from surgery, the introduction of silica can occur through douching or inserting a talc substance into the vagina from a powdered condom. In one case, a woman was found to have a silica deposit in her abdomen from douching with a common soap powder that uses silicate as a filler. Preliminary tests researching the silica-cystoma link have shown the growth rate of tissue cultures treated with silica to be markedly lower than that of an untreated group. In many cases, the silica was found to actually destroy the cells.[648]

SILICIC ACID. The jellylike precipitate obtained when sodium-silicate solution is acidified: the proportion of water varies with the conditions of preparation and decreases gradually during drying and ignition, until relatively pure silica remains. During drying the jelly is converted to a white amorphous powder, or lumps. It is used as laboratory reagent and reinforcing agent in rubber.

SILICON. *See* Nylon.

SILICONE RUBBER. Derived from silica, which comprises 12 percent of all rocks, it is water repellent, adherent, and stable over a wide range of temperatures. It is used in cosmetics and to waterproof and lubricate products. It caused tumors when implanted in rats in 125 milligram doses per kilogram of body weight.[649]

SILVEX. *See* Dioxin.

6-12 INSECT REPELLENT. *1,3-Hexanediol, 2-ethyl-, ethyl hexanediol, carbide 6-12.* Slightly oily liquid used as an insect repellent. Moderately irritating to mucous membranes but not to skin.[650] It is currently being studied by the NCI and the EPA for carcinogenesis.[651]

SKIN CANCER. There are 120,000 new cases of skin cancer each year, and approximately 5,000 deaths are attributed to skin cancer yearly. The symptoms are (1) any persistent firm swelling of the skin; (2) any nonhealing ulcer or sore; (3) any enlarging or darkening moles. People more susceptible to skin cancer are (1) those with extremely fair skin; (2) those who are highly exposed to sunlight; (3) those with a previous history of skin cancer or malignant moles; (4) those with scars from burns or who have skin changes as a result of radiation therapy; (5) those who have moles that are located on soles of their feet or in areas that are irritated by tight clothing or by the use of a razor (these moles are more likely to become malignant); (6) those who have parts of their bodies exposed to dirt, irritation, or extreme weather conditions that cause inflammation, cracking, and soreness.

Any suspicious lesion should be examined by a physician and removed. All skin lesions that are removed should be examined in the laboratory to determine if they are malignant or not. Protective clothing, such as sun hats and light covering over exposed portions of the body, should be worn by individuals who are exposed to the sun for long periods of time, especially if they have fair skin. Doctors can recommend special lotions and ointments that filter out harmful rays of the sun. Excessive sunbathing increases the risk of skin cancer. Chronic contact with arsenic and coal-tar derivatives should also be avoided since these agents play a role in the development of skin cancer. Workers at risk for skin cancer include insecticide makers and sprayers, oil refiners, vintners, smelters, and farmers. Arsenic *(see)* has also been associated with skin cancer.[652,653]

SMOKING. Over the past 25 years a strong association between smoking of cigarettes and lung cancer has been reported by many investigators. No one now seriously disputes that lung-cancer deaths occur much more frequently among cigarette smokers than nonsmokers. Research studies indicate that tobacco smoking, and particularly cigarette smoking, is associated with a shortened life expectancy. About 300,000 Americans die prematurely each year from diseases related to smoking. Cigarette smoking is a major cause of lung cancer, emphysema, heart disease, and chronic bronchitis. Tobacco smoking is also strongly associated with cancers of the larynx, mouth, esophagus, and urinary bladder. Smoking is associated with an increased risk of stroke and other circulatory diseases. In most diseases related to smoking the health hazards are directly proportional to the number of cigarettes smoked per day, the earlier the age at which smoking starts, and the number of years smoking has continued. Fortunately, those who quit smoking begin to decrease the risk to their health as soon as they quit. The risk of heart attack and stroke is measurably decreased within one year.

Smoke, a product of burning, contains hundreds of chemical substances, including nicotine, tars, and carbon monoxide. Nicotine indirectly causes the blood vessels to constrict, which in turn forces the heart to pump faster and faster, increasing the stress on the cardiovascular system. Tars in smoke take the form of tiny particles that settle onto the membranes of the breathing passages and the delicate lung tissues. Tars contain chemicals that have produced cancer in experimental animals. Carbon monoxide reduces the oxygen-carrying ability of the blood by driving the oxygen from the red blood cells. As much as 10 percent of the oxygen that would normally be carried by the red cells is driven out by the carbon monoxide.

The risk of death from lung cancer is 10 times greater for the average male smoker than for the nonsmoker. Fewer than 10 percent of those who develop lung cancer live more than five years. Cigarette smoking is a major factor associated with the two principal diseases that constitute chronic obstructive pulmonary disease—chronic bronchitis and pulmonary emphysema. These diseases are cripplers and can also kill. Cigarette smoking is causally related to higher death rates from heart attack, stroke, and other circulatory diseases. Smoking makes the heart beat faster, raises the blood pressure, and narrows the blood vessels of the skin. Nicotine makes the heart contract more strongly and more often. Some of the same mechanisms that increase the risk of heart attack also increase the danger of stroke among cigarette smokers. And women as well as men are affected. Women who are heavy smokers are 5 times as likely to die from lung cancer as nonsmoking women. Females who smoke have more illness each year and are more likely to suffer from heart disease, bronchitis, and emphysema. Women who smoke during pregnancy increase the risk of having stillborn infants or babies who die soon after birth.

Tobacco smoke is the most serious interior air pollutant. A nonsmoker in the company of a smoker breathes in smoke not only from the burning end of the cigarette but from the exhaled smoke as well. At least 40 carcinogenic and 9 co-carcinogenic substances have been detected in tobacco smoke, and this is not a definitive number. At least two-thirds of the toxic substances in tobacco smoke—including carcinogens—are not taken in by the smoker but are emitted into the surrounding area where the passive smoker (nonsmoker) is forced to inhale them. Almost without exception the carcinogens in tobacco smoke reach the lungs, whereas the coarse soot particles of industrial air pollution are mostly retained in the nose. Unlike most toxins, carcinogens accumulate steadily until critical threshold values are reached. There are at least half a dozen studies that prove that the children of smokers suffer more frequently from respiratory disorders than the children of nonsmokers. It has been proven conclusively that patients with severe circulatory disorders could find their health significantly compromised by the cumulative effects of toxic substances in passive smoking.

The nonsmokers who inhale the smoke from pipes and cigars are exposed to greater quantities of irritants than in exhaled cigarette smoke. Cigars and pipes have a longer burning period than cigarettes and also produce a greater volume of smoke. Since smoke from pipes and cigars generally is not inhaled, the smoke contains greater quantities of irritants that add to the discomfort of adjacent people. Most cigarette smokers filter out some of the irritants when they inhale. Pipe and cigar smoke is especially irritating to the eyes, nose, throat, and breathing passages. There are higher levels of some damaging compounds in pipes and cigars—such as phenol and benzo(a)pyrene—compared to cigarettes. Although the exact effects of cigar and pipe smoke on nonsmokers have not yet been determined, such smoke probably is even more harmful than cigarette smoke. In a half-hour, smoke from 9 cigars polluted the air as much as smoke from 42 cigarettes. Both cigar and cigarette pollution raise the level of carbon monoxide above the safety limits set for workers in industry. Yet, because of the known health hazards of cigarettes, more and more people are switching to pipes and cigars. Because most pipe and cigar smokers do not inhale, hot smoke filled with harmful particles and noxious gases does not bombard their lung tissue and seep into their bloodstream. As a result, their chances of developing coronary heart disease or severe lung diseases—such as chronic bronchitis, emphysema, and lung cancer—are less than those of cigarette smokers. When people who smoke pipes and cigars do inhale, their chances of developing serious heart and lung diseases are even higher than cigarette smokers. These chances increase in direct proportion to how deeply they inhale and how often. There is a special danger for cigarette smokers who switch to pipes and cigars. Some studies show that smokers who switch have established patterns of inhaling and often inhale unintentionally. The amount inhaled is proportional to the time the lit pipe or cigar is held in the mouth. Even tobacco smoke that is not inhaled, however, still affects the sites it touches. Hot smoke lingers inside the mouth and can travel into the throat and windpipe, even into the upper breathing passages. Smoke—which may be dissolved in the saliva and absorbed by the mucous membranes of the mouth—can be swallowed and enter the digestive tract. Inhaling is not necessary to expose all these sites to the harmful effects of hot smoke. Because of such exposure, the incidence of cancer of the mouth, throat, larynx (voice box), and stomach are as high, and even higher, for cigar and pipe smokers as for cigarette smokers. And pipe smoking seems to be a direct cause of cancer of the lip. Some experiments with mice indicate there is a higher degree of cancer-causing agents in cigar and pipe tars than in cigarette tars. Malignant skin tumors grow more rapidly and in larger numbers in animals whose skin has been painted with cigar tars than cigarette tars. In general, smokers who limit themselves to just pipes and cigars live longer than cigarette smokers—but they do not live as long as nonsmokers. There is some evidence that cigarette smokers who cut down on cigarettes and substitute cigars and pipes do decrease somewhat their chances of premature death. But at the same time people who smoke cigars and pipes have higher premature death rates for certain specific cancers such as cancer of the lip, mouth, throat, larynx, and stomach. Choosing what you will smoke, in effect, determines which diseases you develop. Choosing not to smoke is the alternative. Smokers of little cigars face all the hazards of cigar and pipe smokers and, if they inhale, all the damaging effects suffered by cigarette smokers as well. Most brands of little cigars have even higher levels of tar and nicotine than cigarettes. And, little cigars are manufactured, packaged, sold, and often smoked like cigarettes.

People also switch from nonfilter cigarettes to filter cigarettes. It has been proven, statistically, that the smoking of filter cigarettes appears to reduce the risk of lung cancer when compared with the smoking of nonfilter cigarettes; but overall, nonfilter cigarettes appear to be safer than filter cigarettes for both men and women. Nonfilter-cigarette smokers appear to live two to three years longer than those smoking filter cigarettes. Filter-cigarette smokers have fewer cases of lung cancer than nonfilter-cigarette smokers, but the overall risk factors of filter-cigarette smokers are greater than the risk factors of nonfilter-cigarette smokers. While filter-cigarette smokers may have fewer cases of lung cancer than nonfilter-cigarette smokers, they do have more cases of cardiovascular diseases than nonfilter-cigarette smokers. The higher death rates of filter-cigarette smokers may be explained in terms of higher concentrations of carbon monoxide in their smoke. Carbon monoxide in cigarette smoke appears to be the major contributing factor to the increased death rates for cardiovascular diseases. Carbon monoxide is more prevalent in filter-cigarette smoke than in that of nonfilter cigarettes.

In August 1978, Dr. Gio Batta Gori, deputy director of cancer prevention at the NCI, raised a furor when he was quoted as saying some cigarettes now have so little tar, nicotine, and other harmful elements that they can be called "less hazardous" and can even be smoked in "tolerable" numbers without "appreciable" ill effects on the average smoker. Cancer experts immediately refuted the idea that any cigarette could be safe, and Dr. Gori quickly stated that the only safe cigarette is an unlit one. However, he gave the following list of brands that were "less hazardous" than others. The following is a list of them, along with the number that can be smoked each day without "appreciable harm":

Carlton Menthol	23	L & M Long Lights (100s)	6
Now Menthol	18	Lark II	6
Stride	17	Tareyton Lights	6
Carlton	16	Kent Golden Lights	5
L & M Flavor Lights (King)	8	Real Menthol	5
Lucky 100	8	Benson & Hedges Lights	4
True	8	Newport Lights Menthol	4
True Menthol	8	King Sano	3
Decade	7	King Sano Menthol	3
Pall Mall Extra Mild	7	Merit	3
Decade Menthol	6	Merit Menthol	3
Iceberg (100s)	6	Real	3
Kent Golden Lights Menthol	6	Tempo	3

But no matter how you rationalize, cigarette smoking is bad for you. As researchers work to further elucidate the correlation between cancer and smoking, do the following:

- If you are not a smoker, do not start. If you are a smoker, stop.
- If you must smoke, smoke a pipe or a cigar rather than cigarettes.
- If you must smoke cigarettes, smoke as few as possible (certainly under a pack a day), inhale as little as possible, and discard each cigarette as soon as possible.
- Choose one of the cigarettes known to be less harmful.
- If you are a cigarette smoker and 40 years or older, try to get into one of the large programs that test sputum and take X-rays periodically to detect cancer early.

SNEEZING GAS. *See* Arsine, Diphenylchloro-.
SODIUM CARBOXYMETHYL CELLULOSE. *See* Carboxymethyl cellulose.
SODIUM CYCLAMATE. *See* Cyclamates.
SODIUM SUCARYL. *See* Cyclamates.
SOLDER. A metal or metallic alloy used when melted to join metallic surfaces and usually applied, by means of a soldering iron or a blowpipe,

with a flux such as rosin, borax, or zinc chloride. It usually contains lead *(see)*. Now considered to contribute to cancer in those who work in industrial and scientific instrument plants and in electrical equipment and supplies plants.[654]

SOMINEX. *See* Methapyrilene.

SORBIC ACID. *Acetic acid, hexadienic acid, hexadienoic acid, sorbistat.* It consists of a white free-flowing powder that is obtained from the berries of the mountain ash and is also made from chemicals in the factory. It is used in cosmetics as a preservative and humectant. A mold and yeast inhibitor, it is also used in foods, especially cheeses, and beverages. Used as a replacement for glycerin in emulsions, ointments, embalming fluids, mouthwashes, toothpastes, various cosmetics. A binder for toilet powders and creams, it produces a velvetlike feel when rubbed on the skin. In large amounts, it is sticky. When injected subcutaneously in 2,600 milligram doses per kilogram of body weight, it caused cancer.[655]

STEEL-FINISHING PLANTS. Cancer hazards are usually linked to coke plants and particularly to coke-oven areas. There is, however, a high incidence of bladder, respiratory, and kidney cancer in other workers in the steel industry. Lung-cancer cases were numerous among workers in steel-finishing operations. These findings suggest that cancer-causing agents may be more widespread in steel manufacturing than had previously been thought, although the study does not link the cancers with specific substances.[656] *See also* Coke.

STELAZINE. *See* Chlorpromazine.

STERIGMATOCYSTIN. A close relative of the aflatoxins *(see)*, it is formed by several *Aspergillus* species. It is less toxic than the aflatoxins, but it does produce liver tumors. [657]

STEROIDS. *See* The Pill and Hormones.

STILBENE. *4-Aminostilbene, 4-stilbenamine.* It is derived from benzoin and used in the manufacture of dyes and optical bleaches. Caused cancer when injected subcutaneously in rats in 31 milligram doses per kilogram of body weight, when given orally to rats in 625 milligram doses per kilogram of body weight, and when injected into the abdomen of rats in 300 milligram doses per kilogram of body weight. It caused tumors when given orally to mice in doses of 18 milligrams per kilogram of body weight.[658]

4,4'-STILBENEDIOL,alpha,alpha-DIETHYL-. *See* DES.

STILBESTROL. *See* DES.

STOMACH CANCER. Each year there are 20,000 new cases of stomach cancer and 17,000 people die of this disease. The symptoms are (1) persistent discomfort and pain in the upper central abdomen; (2) indigestion which is persistent; (3) vomiting of blood. Ulcers and ulcer symptoms may be mistaken for stomach cancer and vice versa. People with no acid in the stomach, patients with pernicious anemia, and those with gastritis and gastric polyps are more susceptible to stomach cancer. The disease can be diagnosed by X-ray of the stomach (a GI series). The physician may find tenderness in examining the central portion of the abdomen. The finding of blood in the stool may also be a clue to the presence of stomach cancer. The occurrence of cancer of the stomach cannot be controlled since the causes are not known. However, the death rate can be greatly lowered if people, especially those over 45, are familiar with the symptoms of this disease. *See also* Diet, Bran, Roughage, and Food.

STRESS. *See* Emotions.

STROBANE. *Terpene polychorinates, dichloricide aerosol, dichloride mothproofer.* Yellow waxy solid with a pleasant pine odor. It is used as an insecticide against army worms, boll weevils, cotton aphids, fleahoppers, and Southern green stink bugs. A mixture of chlorinated terpene isomers prepared from camphene and pinenes, it may be mildly irritating to the skin. Large doses cause central nervous system stimulation. It is not recommended for use in dairy barns or milking animals. It can be absorbed through the skin, and liver injury has been reported.[659] Caused cancer when given orally to mice in 1,272 milligram doses per kilogram of body weight.[660]

STRONTIUM. A substance that if deposited in the bones leads to an increased possibility of bone cancer and leukemia. Radioactive strontium that is eaten in milk products replaces the calcium in the bones and stays in the body, emitting radiation to the bones and surrounding tissues. During the years when the world's nuclear powers were testing atomic bombs in the atmosphere, there was a great deal of public concern about the spread of strontium throughout the world. Although atomic tests have stopped, workers exposed to strontium are still affected by it, but the concern has diminished. When a radioactive particle passes through a cell, it interacts with the atoms and molecules that make up the cell and breaks them up. It may destroy the cell permanently or else cause it to stop functioning properly. How radiation causes this damage is not well understood, but the results of exposure are widely documented. One effect of exposure to radiation is an increased incidence of cancer. The government has set a legal limit of 5 rems (roentgen equivalent man) per year for radiation exposure, but a worker who is exposed to this much radiation has a 50 percent greater chance of developing cancer than an unexposed person.[661]

STYRENE. Derived from ethylene and benzene in the presence of aluminum chloride, it is moderately toxic by ingestion and inhalation. Used in polystyrene plastics, resins, and protective coatings. It caused tumors when given to rats in 19 milligram doses per kilogram of body weight and cancer when injected subcutaneously in mice in 94 milligram doses per kilogram of body weight.[662] It has been found in both drinking water and waste-water treatment plants. Recent EPA studies have revealed that toluene, styrene, and xylene are present in drinking-water supplies of about 20 American cities. A similar observation has been made in certain Canadian water supplies. Researchers have found these compounds not only in potable water but also in human blood. It is very difficult to establish whether direct cause and effect exist, but it is clear that possible connections between water-treatment practices and health effects should be studied more extensively. A recent study indicated that there is a 44 percent higher incidence of gastrointestinal- and urinary-tract cancer in population groups drinking chlorinated water than in matched cohort groups drinking nonchlorinated water. While halogenated hydrocarbons (those with benzene or chlorine added) generally have been assumed to be responsible for increased health risks, it is clear that long-term effects of low-level exposure to aromatic hydrocarbons such as benzene in drinking water should also be assessed.[663]

SUCCINIC ANHYDRIDE. *Succinyl oxide, butanedioic anhydride.* Usually made from succinic acid and acetic anhydride, it consists of colorless light needles that are moderately toxic and irritating. It is used as a hardener of resins and in the manufacture of chemical and pharmaceutical esters. Caused cancer when injected under the skin of rats in 2,600 milligram doses per kilogram of body weight.[664]

SUGARS. A series of early reports from Japan, and later Italian studies, indicated that very frequent subcutaneous injections of concentrated solutions of glucose, galactose, fructose, and some di- and polysaccharides in the rat for a two-year period produced low incidences of sarcomas in the site of the injection. While these effects could not be repeated by some other researchers, the impression has been left in the literature that concentrated solutions of various sugars indeed have this property. In a recent well-controlled study with purified mono- and disaccharides, the positive results obtained earlier could not be verified except for a borderline result with sorbose (a sugar). It has been suggested that the positive results may have been due to carcinogenic impurities, possibly related to the charcoal frequently employed in the decolorization of sugar preparations.[665]

SUGAR SUBSTITUTES. *See* Cyclamates, Saccharin, and Xylitol.

SULFANILAMIDE. *Antistrept, astrocid, bacteramid, septinal, sulfanil, therapol.* Used for vaginal infections, it can cause a depression of white blood cells. Its crystals are prepared from the action of ammonia on acetylsulfanilyl chloride. It was formerly used as an antibiotic and still used to treat certain infections in animals. May produce goiters (enlarged thyroids). Rats appear especially susceptible to the goitrogenic effect of sulfonamides (sulfenilamide is a crystalline sulfonamide), and long-term administration has produced thyroid malignancies in the species.[666]

SULFANILAMIDE, N(sup 1)-2-THIAZOLYL-. *Azoseptale, norsulfasol, thiazamide, thiozamide. See* Sulfanilamide.

SULFATHIAZOLE. *See* Sulfanilamide.

SULFIDE,Bis (2-CHLOROETHYL). *See* Mustard Gas.

SULFONAMIDE,4-(ETHYLSULFONYL)-NAPHTHALENE-(HPA) (ENS). *See* Sulfanilamide.

SULFURIC ACID. *Oil of vitriol, green vitriol, iron vitri*[ol] concentrated, it gives off sulfur-trioxide gas and sulfuric strongly irritating to the respiratory tract. In solution, it is skin and teeth. Lung scarring and emphysema may follow It is used in the manufacture of iron compounds, other sulfat ing baths, fertilizers; as food and feed supplements; in pestici ink, etching, and engraving; as dye for leather; and as a cat tumors when injected under the skin of mice in 1,600 milligr kilogram of body weight.[667]

SULFURIC ACID, DIETHYL ESTER. *See* Diethyl Sulfa[te]

SULFURIC ACID, DIMETHYL ESTER. *See* Dimethyl Sul

SULFURIC ACID, ZINC SALT. *See* Zinc Sulfate.

SULFUR MUSTARD GAS. *See* Sulfide, Bis (2-Chloroethyl).

SULFUROUS ACID, 2-(p-t-Butylphenoxy)-1-METHYLETHYL- CHLOROETHYL ESTER. *See* Aramite.

SUN. The effect of sunlight on a person's skin varies with the amount of ultraviolet light that an individual can take. The amount a person can take depends largely on the thickness of his skin and, to a lesser extent, on pigmentation. Photosensitivity is a problem for many who attempt to tan from the sun. Phototoxicity is an exaggeration of the sunburn reaction. This can be developed in any individual. It occurs when one may be taking an antibiotic. The reaction requires a specific dose of the drug and a specific wavelength of ultraviolet. The reaction usually occurs within five days of the initial ingestion of the drug and appears only on the exposed areas of the body. A photoallergic reaction is an acquired altered capacity to respond to light energy and is dependent on an antigen-antibody relationship, the same type of mechanism responsible in producing other allergic reactions, for example to food and pollen. A complex interplay of body chemistry makes professional medical advice essential when there are doubts. Persons being treated for any form of cancer should also avoid sunbathing or other prolonged exposures to the sun. [668]

SWIMMING-POOL-TEST CHEMICAL. *See* Benzidine.

SYNESTROL. *See* Phenol.

TALCUM POWDER. Talc is finely ground magnesium silicate, a mineral. It is used in baby powders, dusting powders, face powders, eye shadows, liquid powders, protective creams, dry rouges, face masks, foundation cake makeups, skin fresheners, foot powders, and face creams. It gives a slippery sensation to powders and creams. It usually has small amounts of other powders such as boric acid or zinc oxide added as a mild antiseptic. Talcum powder is white to grayish white and is insoluble in water. It is also used as a coloring agent. Tremolite, a form of asbestos, can be found in nearly all talcum powder, since it is a naturally occurring contaminant in talc stone. A 1972 study by the Office of Product Technology of the FDA

d that of 40 cosmetic talcum-powder samples tested, 39 contained one
nt asbestos or less. Talc itself is similar in composition to asbestos and
efore inhalation is unwise.[669,670] *See also* Asbestos.

NNINS AND TANNIC ACID. *Gallotannic acid.* Tannic acid occurs
the bark and fruit of many plants, notably in the bark of the oak species,
sumac, cherry, wild bark, and in coffee and tea. It is used to clarify beer
and wine and as a refining agent for rendered fats. Tannins are used as a
flavoring in butter, caramel, fruit, brandy, maple and nut flavorings for
beverages, ice creams, ices, candy, baked goods, and liquors. They are used
medicinally as a mild astringent. When applied, they may turn the skin
brown. Tannic acid has a low toxicity when taken orally, but large doses
may cause gastric distress. During World War II, liver damage was observed in humans treated with tannic acids for burns. Subsequently, experiments with rats showed repeated subcutaneous injections of a water
solution of tannin led to liver toxicity, cirrhosis, and tumors.[671] But this has
not been associated with human cancer, with the exception of reports
of an association between hot-tea drinking and cancer of the esophagus in
Iran.[672]

TAR CAMPHOR. *See* Naphthalene.

2,4,5-T. The EPA declared this herbicide a potential health hazard to
humans on April 12, 1978. Findings of birth defects and cancerous tumors
among laboratory animals exposed to 2,4,5-T indicated that it might cause
the same problems among people. Then in March 1979, after a complaint
was filed by 10 Oregon women stating that they had discovered that among
them they could account for eight miscarriages all of which occurred after
nearby sprayings of 2,4,5-TCP, the EPA imposed a ban on this insecticide.
The Dow Chemical Company has protested the ban and plans to seek an
injunction against it.

The poison is commonly used on forests, rangeland, rice paddies, and
rights-of-way. Since 1970 its use around homes, lakes, or recreational areas
has been banned. It has been produced in this country since 1948 by Dow
Chemical of Midland, Michigan; the Thompson-Hayward Chemical Company of Kansas City, Kansas; and Transvaal, Inc., of Jacksonville, Arkansas. The agency said the area of concern involves the chemical contaminant
dioxin *(see)* that often shows up in 2,4,5-T.[673]

2,4,5-TCP. The EPA began a review of this widely used industrial pesticide
in 1978 because the compound contains the chemical contaminant dioxin
(see). The pesticide, which is produced mainly by Dow Chemical, has been
in use in the United States for more than 30 years. It is employed by textile
makers for preserving rayon and silk yarns and also hides and leathers; it
is used by adhesive makers to preserve emulsions; and by the auto industry
to kill slime, algae, and fungi in industrial processes. The chemical, which
is sold under the trade name Dowicide 2, is suspected of causing birth
defects and cancer. The EPA is concerned that workers or others who come

in contact with 2,4,5-TCP may be exposed to unsafe amounts through skin contact or by breathing the vapor. If these fears are confirmed, the agency may ban the pesticide or restrict its sale or use. Dow spokesmen claim that in all the years the chemical has been in use, there has been no indication of any hazard. Other producers of 2,4,5-TCP include North Eastern Pharmaceutical and Chemical Co., Occidental Petroleum Corp., Hooker Chemical Corp., and Transvaal, Inc.

TDE. **1,1-DICHLORO-2,2-BIS(p-CHLOROPHENYL) ethane.** *Dichlorodiphenyldichloroethane.* Colorless crystals derived from ethanol and chlorobenzene. Toxic when ingested, inhaled, or absorbed through the skin. Use in some states is restricted. It is similar to DDT and is used as dusts and wettable powders for the control of leaf rollers and other insects. It caused tumors when given orally to rats and mice in 10 to 39 milligram doses per kilogram of body weight.[674]

TELEVISION SETS. *See* Electromagnetic Radiation.

TELVAR. *Urea, 3-(p-chlorophenyl)-1,1-dimethyl-.* A weed killer for the control of preemergence weed control in cotton. It caused cancer when given orally to rats and mice.[675]

TEMARIL. *See* Chlorpromazine.

TEPA. *See* Triethylenephosphoramide.

TEQUINOL. *See* Hydroquinone.

TERPENE POLYCHLORINATES. These are mixed terpenes; they occur in most of the essential oils and oleoresins of plants to which chlorine has been added. They are used in insecticides and as mothproofers. Have been found to be carcinogenic in animals.[676] *See also* Strobane.

TESTOSTERONE. *Androlin, testiculosterone, testryl.* The male sex hormone produced by the testes. It has six times the androgenic (masculinizing) activity of its metabolic product, androsterone. Consists of white or cream-white crystals or powder, it is used in medicine, cosmetics, and biochemical research. It caused tumors when injected under the skin of mice in 30 milligram doses per kilogram of body weight.[677]

TETRACHLOROETHANE. A heavy, colorless corrosive liquid with a chloroformlike odor, it is derived from the distillation of a mixture of acetylene and chlorine. It is used as a solvent; as a cleansing and degreasing agent for metals; in paint removers, varnishes, lacquers, and photographic film. It is also used to extract oils and fats; as an alcohol denaturant (so you can't drink it); and as an insecticide, weed killer, and fumigant. Tetrachloroethane was the first chlorinated-hydrocarbon solvent to be manufactured on a large scale. In recent years it has been largely replaced by less-toxic solvents. Only one domestic manufacturer is currently producing it, and most of the compound is used at the same location as an intermediate *(see)* in the manufacture of trichloroethylene and tetrachloroethylene *(see* both*)*. Currently, minor uses of 1,1,2,2-tetrachloroethane include its use as a carrier or a solvent in manufacturing processes for other chemicals and as an analytical reagent to identify unknown chemicals. At one time 40 million pounds were produced and an estimated 5,000 workers were exposed to it each year. NCI tests showed it to be a liver carcinogen in mice when administered orally. The results were not conclusive in rats. The NCI, however, feels that tetrachloroethane has the potential of causing liver damage as well as gastrointestinal and neurological disturbances.[678]

TETRACHLOROETHYLENE. *Perchloroethylene, carbon dichloride.* In 1974 approximately 734 million pounds of this chemical were produced: 69 percent was used in the textile and dry-cleaning industries; 16 percent for metal cleaning and degreasing; 12 percent as chemical intermediates *(see);* and 3 percent for miscellaneous purposes. The last includes paint removers and other specific solvent forms, as well as a medicinal use as an antihookworm medicine. Human exposure is extensive at this writing. The greatest exposure is in the dry-cleaning establishments, especially when ventilation is inadequate. The chemical has also been found in water and food. Atmospheric concentrations as high as 1 to 10 micrograms per liter and concentrations in food have been found as high as 13 milligrams per kilogram in butter. It was found in New Orleans drinking water and in the blood of persons ingesting that water. Body fat has been found to contain as much as 29 milligrams per kilogram. Depression of the central nervous system is the primary effect of acute or chronic inhalation. When rats and mice were force-fed tetrachloroethylene for 78 weeks, it proved to be a liver carcinogen.[679]

TETRACHLOROMETHANE. *See* Carbon Tetrachloride.

TETRACHLORVINPHOS. An organophosphorous insecticide. Tetrachlorvinphos was given in feed to rats and mice for 80 weeks. The insecticide was associated with thyroid tumors in rats of both sexes, and with adrenal tumors in female rats. Tetrachlorvinphos caused liver cancer in male mice and liver tumors in female mice.[680]

TETRAETHYL LEAD. *Plumbane, lead, tetraethyl.* A colorless oily liquid with a pleasant odor that is soluble in all solvents. It is toxic when ingested, inhaled, or absorbed through the skin. Used in aviation and automotive gasoline. Consumption has declined because of United States air-pollution standards. There is an OSHA standard for it pertaining to both skin and air.

TETRAOXAHEXADECANE. *See* Triethylene Glycol Diglycidyl Ether.

TEXTILE DUSTS. The dustiest part of producing textiles is the cleaning of raw fibers. Raw wool, for example, may contain up to 55 percent nonfibrous material. The "dust" is removed from raw wool and raw cotton by beating and crushing it into fine particles that are shaken and blown or sucked away. Dust blows into workers' noses, mouths, and throats. Cancer of the tongue, mouth, and throat were found to be three times higher among textile workers in Britain than in the general population. Cancer appeared higher for those who worked with wool than with cotton. Raw wool often contains residues of a pesticide containing arsenic in which sheep are dipped.[681]

THALLIUM. Discovered in 1861, it occurs in crooksite (found in Sweden), in lorandite (found in Greece), and in hutchinsonite (found in Switzerland). It occurs in the earth's crust and forms alloys with other metals. It is used in semiconductor research, and its salts are used for rat poison. It caused tumors when given to rats in 0.8 milligram doses per kilogram of body weight.[682] Workers who manufacture industrial and scientific instruments are exposed to it and are considered by NIOSH to be at high risk for cancer.[683]

THEOPHYLLINE, 7-HYDROXY-. A white powder that occurs in small amounts in tea. Used in cosmetics. Caused tumors when injected under the skin of mice in 700 milligram doses per kilogram of body weight.[684]

THIAZOLE. A colorless or pale yellow liquid with a foul odor. There are thiazole dyes used in organic synthesis, in fungicides, and as rubber accelerators. They caused tumors when given orally to mice in doses as small as 7 milligrams per kilogram of body weight and cancer when given orally to rats in 36 milligram doses per kilogram of body weight.[685] Determined to be a positive animal carcinogen by a NIOSH review.[686]

THIOACETAMIDE. Colorless leaflets that are stable in solution and soluble in water, alcohol, ether, and benzene. Thioacetamide is combustible and moderately toxic when ingested or inhaled. It is used to replace gaseous hydrogen sulfide in qualitative analysis.

THIO-TEPA. A toxic agent of the alkylating type, it is related to nitrogen mustard. Its therapeutic action is believed to occur through the release of ethylenimine radicals that have a deleterious effect on actively dividing cells. It causes bone-marrow depression and has been found to cause lung tumors in mice.[687]

THIOUREA. Once used as a fungicide for dipping citrus fruits, it was banned because it caused liver and thyroid tumors. Thiourea and associated compounds, however, have been used for years to treat human thyroid disease. Whether or not it causes cancer in humans has not yet been determined.[688]

THORAZINE. *See* Chlorpromazine.

THORIUM DIOXIDE. *Thorium oxide, Thorotrast.* A heavy white powder derived from thorium nitrate. It is used in ceramics, as a nuclear fuel, in flame spraying, in crucibles, in medicine, in optical glass, as a catalyst for tungsten filaments in incandescent lamps, in cathodes in vacuum tubes, and in arc-melting electrodes. Caused cancer when injected under the skin of rats and mice and tumors when injected intramuscularly in mice in 800 milligram doses per kilogram of body weight.[689] *See also* Thorotrast.

THOROTRAST. A thorium-dioxide suspension used as a contrast medium for diagnostic X-rays between 1930 and 1950. It was found to be associated with a significant incidence of liver cancer in patients who received it.[690]

THROAT CANCER. There are 15,000 new cases of throat cancer and 7,500 people who die of this disease each year. Its symptoms are (1) a growth or persistent sore on the lip, tongue, or on the lining of the mouth or throat; (2) persistent pain or tenderness in the mouth; (3) difficulty swallowing. People who have had syphilis and people who have an irritation in the mouth due to sharp, broken, or ill-fitting dentures are more susceptible to the disease. Heavy alcohol intake is considered to be a contributing factor in the development of this form of cancer. Excessive use of cigarettes, cigars, or a pipe can lead to cancer of the mouth.

There is a condition called leukoplakia that causes white patches in the membranes of the mouth and throat; this condition is premalignant and requires treatment. Cancer of the lips is more common in farmers, sailors, or those with outdoor occupations. Throat cancer can be diagnosed by inspection and biopsy by a physician or dentist. Bad teeth, particularly those with sharp edges, and irritation from ill-fitting dentures should be corrected. All ulcerations of the mouth should be brought to the attention of a physician or dentist if they do not heal properly. It is essential that this disease be treated early before it spreads further into the mouth or still further into the glands of the neck.

THYROID CANCER. In 1976 mortality from this disease in the United States accounted for approximately 0.5 percent of all cancer deaths in women and 0.2 percent in men. The biologic behavior of thyroid cancer is extremely variable, and there is a need to identify important differences in epidemiology, natural history, prognosis, and rationale of therapy. Papillary carcinoma is the most common form of thyroid cancer, accounting for 64 percent of all principal, or first, malignant tumors. It occurs most often in people in their 30s and 40s and is three times more prevalent in women than in men. The disease is distinctly less malignant in children and young adults. The prognosis in patients with thyroid carcinoma is variable and correlates with type, extent of the disease, age at diagnosis, and sex. The survival rate is consistently better for women than for men.

Thyroid neoplasia develops predictably in experimental animals exposed to ionizing radiation or to any procedure that induces prolonged, excessive thyroid-stimulating hormone secretion. In experimental animals, chronic iodine deficiency may bring on thyroid cancer. More than one-third of the children with papillary and follicular cancer of the thyroid received radiation therapy to the head or the neck for some other condition. It has been known for several years that persons who received X-ray therapy to the head and neck—a common practice until the 1950s for such conditions as enlargement of the tonsils, acne, and sinusitis—are at increased risk for the development of thyroid cancer as late as 35 years after the time of treatment. Current follow-up data indicate that about 25 percent of those treated with such radiation will be found to have abnormalities of the thyroid, of which one-third will prove malignant. These malignancies are "slow growing" and curable by surgery. The Health, Education and Welfare Department has made the following recommendations:

- Any person who has been treated with radiation to the neck or head should be examined by a physician, who is expected to carefully inspect and feel the thyroid gland and its surrounding areas.
- If a suspicious growth can be seen or felt, a thyroid scan using radioactive tracers should be performed. There is controversy about routine scanning for all persons who have been treated with radiation; most reserve this test for persons with suspicious lumps.
- In those instances when an abnormal scan is found with no accompanying lump, surgery is not routinely advised. Most recommend treatment with a thyroid hormone, which will suppress the normal thyroid gland's activity, plus annual examination for the development of a growth.
- All experts agree that surgery should be done if both a lump and an abnormal scan are present. Such surgery should be performed only by a surgeon with competence in thyroid surgery.
- Persons with suspicious lumps who cannot undergo surgery, as well as those who have had surgery for removal of a growth, should be placed on continuous thyroid suppression therapy as a preventive measure.[691,692]

TITANOCENE, DICHLORIDE. An organo-metallic material, it consists of red crystals moderately soluble in toluene. Toxic when inhaled, and an irritant to the skin and mucous membranes, it is used in polymers, in ultraviolet absorbers, as a catalyst, as a reducing agent, as a free-radical scavenger, and in antiknock agents. It caused cancer when injected intramuscularly in rats in 1,000 milligram doses per kilogram of body weight.[693]

TOBACCO. In spite of decisions by at least 7 million Americans over the last decade to quit smoking, and in spite of persistent attacks by health organizations and the federal government, the $7 billion cigarette industry has managed not only to survive but, for the most part, to prosper. Members of the tobacco industry are one of the nation's most sophisticated and effective lobbying forces. According to health officials, someone in the United States dies every minute and a half as a result of smoking. But agents of the Tobacco Institute and tobacco-company executives deny that the health issue is conclusive. They spend considerable time and money attempting to discredit the antismoking forces by challenging their research, motives, accuracy, and objectivity. And they pump their own dollars into research—a good deal of it aimed at finding the other causes of cancer. Dr. Peter Bourne, former White House Medical Advisor, issued what was widely interpreted as a proindustry statement on cigarette smoking on the very day that Joseph A. Califano, Jr., secretary of Health, Education and Welfare, called for a $6 million government program on the dangers of smoking, restrictions against smoking in government buildings, and a possible increase in the federal excise tax on cigarettes.

Cigarette smoking is related to health hazards, being implicated in 80 percent of the cases of lung cancer and emphysema; a major factor in most cases of oral cancers and cancers of the larynx, pharynx, and bladder; and a major hazard for women who use oral contraceptives. Revenue from tobacco products in 1976 totaled about $12 million, and the habit costs smokers, their families, and society $18 billion in medical and hospital bills and lost wages—a net loss of $6 billion. The American Cancer Society urges teaching in schools of the dangers of cigarette smoking; a phasing out of the present tobacco price-support system; a large antismoking campaign; that smokers should be required to bear a greater part of the cost of their habit; a barring of advertising of cigarettes with more than 10 milligrams of tar and 0.7 milligrams of nicotine; that cigarettes be eliminated from the Food for Peace Program; that the tobacco industry be held accountable for the safety of its product; a ban on the sale of cigarettes to minors be strictly enforced; that state and local governments prohibit smoking in most public places and promote the separation of smokers and nonsmokers in such places as restaurants, trains, and buses; the banning of smoking in public schools by either students or teachers; the adoption of antismoking guidelines by all government and private hospitals and clinics and the promotion of healthful life-styles by physicians, health agencies, etc.; and other tactics they believe will slow down the sale and consumption of tobacco products. For now, both the rights of the smoker and of the nonsmoker must be taken into account. As members of a free society, we should recognize the rights of informed adults to smoke if they choose, because to suggest otherwise would be to imply prohibition, which is neither enforceable nor desirable in a democratic society.[694,695] *See* Smoking.

TOLBUTAMIDE. The first oral hypoglycemic used in the management of diabetes. It is one of a group of hypoglycemics that includes tolazamide, chlorpropamide, and acetohexamide. All stimulate insulin secretion by the pancreas and therefore are used only in patients with at least minimal pancreatic function, as in maturity-onset diabetes. Controlled studies have shown that the oral hypoglycemics may be no more effective than dietary modification in controlling the symptoms of maturity-onset diabetes, and on a long-term basis they may be associated with an increase in cardiovascular mortality. Since they are used over a long period of time, the NCI tested tolbutamide to see if it might be a carcinogen. It was given in feed to rats and mice for 78 weeks. It was found not to be carcinogenic for either rats or mice under the test conditions.[696]

o-TOLIDINE. *See* Benzidine.

TOLUAMIDE. *See* Procarbazine Hydrochloride.

TOLUENE. A widely used chemical, it is employed in the manufacture of benzoic acid, bezaldehyde, explosives, and dyes, and it is used as a solvent in saccharin, plastic toys, and model airplanes. It is used to extract various principles from plants. It may cause anemia but is considered less toxic than benzene *(see).* Toluene has been found in the drinking water in 20 American cities, according to the EPA. It can cause liver damage and is irritating to the skin and respiratory tract. While halogenated hydrocarbons like toluene are assumed to be responsible for health risks, long-term effects of low-level exposure to them in drinking water should be studied and assessed.[697,698,699]

TOLUENE,alpha-CHLORO-. *See* Benzyl Chloride.

TOLUENE-2,4-DIAMINE. *m-Toluenediamine.* Obtained from tar oil, it is a dye intermediate *(see),* and with direct oxidation it is used as a black dye for furs and hair. It is a skin irritant. It caused tumors when injected under the skin of mice in 280 milligram doses per kilogram of body weight.[700,701] *See* Hair Coloring.

p-TOLUENESULFONIC ACID, ETHYL ESTER AND METHYL ESTER. Colorless leaflet derived from treating toluene with chlorosulfonic acid. Used in dyes, organic synthesis, and as an acid catalyst. It is moderately toxic and a skin irritant. Caused tumors when injected subcutaneously in rats in 50 milligram doses per kilogram of body weight.[702]

alpha-TOLUENETHIOL. *Benzyl mercaptan, triobenzyl alcohol.* These cream to white moist crystals have a musty odor and can be toxic and irritating to the skin. Used in medicine as an intermediate *(see)* and as a bacteriostat. It caused tumors when painted on the skin of mice in 3 milligram doses per kilogram of body weight.[703]

o-TOLUIDINE, 5-CHLORO-. An aromatic amine *(see)* used as an intermediate *(see)* in the manufacture of dyes, it was given in feed to rats and mice for 78 weeks. It was found to cause cancers of the liver and blood vessels in male and female mice. The compound was not carcinogenic in rats under NCI test conditions. Compounds found to be carcinogenic in these animal tests are generally considered capable of causing cancer in humans. The tests do not provide information, however, that could be used to predict the frequency at which cancers might be produced in human populations under actual conditions of exposure.[704]

TOLUIDINE, m- and o-. Derived from nitrotoluene, it is used in dyes, printing textiles blue-black, and making various colors fast to acid in organic synthesis. It is toxic when inhaled or ingested, and it can be absorbed through the skin. It caused tumors when given orally to rats in 6,600 milligram doses per kilogram of body weight.[705,706]

o-TOLUIDINE, 4-(o-TOLYAZO)-. *C.I. solvent yellow 3, fat yellow B, oil yellow 21, tolabase fast garnet.* Caused cancer when given orally to rats, hamsters, and mice and when injected under the skin of mice.[707]

TOXAPHENE. Generic name for a chlorinated camphene, a substance that is a constituent of certain essential oils. An amber waxy solid with a mild odor of chlorine and camphor, it is used as a pesticide. Its standard commercial formulation is a dust containing 20 percent toxaphene. Emulsifiable concentrates contain up to eight pounds toxaphene per gallon; oil solutions are 90 percent toxaphene and wettable powders are 40 percent toxaphene. It is also mixed with other insecticide chemicals for a variety of uses. In 1976 toxaphene production in the United States amounted to more than 100 million pounds. The largest single use, about 85 percent, is on cotton crops. Other major uses are on cattle and swine, soybeans, corn, wheat, and peanuts. Substantial amounts are also used for lettuce, tomatoes, and other food crops.

Toxaphene has caused liver cancers in male and female mice given the compound in a feeding study. Test results also suggested that toxaphene caused thyroid cancers in rats. Toxaphene was tested because its chemical structure is similar to that of strobane *(see),* a known animal carcinogen, and because toxaphene is used extensively on food crops, where it may lead to long-term human exposure to residues in foods. No acceptable daily human intake has been established by the World Health Organization for toxaphene residues on food, because more knowledge is still being sought on the toxicity, including carcinogenicity, of the compound. The OSHA standards call for maximum tolerances of 7 parts per million in or on any of the fruits, vegetables, nuts, and meat products it has listed. A residue of 5 ppm is allowed on various grains, 3.5 ppm on soybeans in combined residues with DDT, and much smaller amounts in several other food products.

Toxaphene appears to be readily transported from its site of application, either by water or by air. Treated cotton fields are believed a common source of toxaphene contamination, polluting both the air and the surface water. In an ongoing survey of food and feed commodities by the FDA, toxaphene residues have been found steadily rising for the past five years. When a total of 4,228 food and feed samples were checked in 1976, toxaphene contamination was found in 261 of the samples tested—more than 6 percent—distributed over 16 different food and feed categories. In earlier years, leaf and stem vegetables were the most frequently contaminated by toxaphene, but since 1974 the highest rates of contamination have been found in fish. Investigation of fish in Louisiana in 1975 disclosed toxaphene residues in the fish tissues up to more than 10 ppm. The pesticide is persistent in the soil and water and accumulates at increased concentrations in aquatic life. One study revealed that catfish fry had concentrations in their tissues of as much as 91,000 times the toxaphene level of the surrounding water. The same study showed toxaphene to be the cause of retarded growth and decreased collagen in catfish bones, causing the "broken-back" syndrome.

A number of completed research projects indicating acute effects of toxaphene have led scientists at the EPA to conclude that exposure to toxaphene caused changes in bone composition and growth in fish, birds, and mammals. Because these effects occurred at dose levels similar to present-day human exposures, the agency has begun reviewing the risks and benefits of the pesticide. Between 1966 and 1976 there were 44 recorded episodes of abnormal exposure involving people, with 8 human fatalities. Reports of the 8 human fatalities related to toxaphene exposure were not linked exclusively with applications to crops or livestock: 5 involved application exposure, such as crop spraying or stock dipping, 2 of which were the result of crashes of aircraft engaged in the application of toxaphene and 3 of which were associated with mixtures of pesticides including toxaphene. Of the remaining 3 deaths, 2 were infants who ingested toxaphene, and in the third, circumstances were unknown.[708]

TOXIC SUBSTANCES CONTROL ACT (TSCA). The single major piece of environmental legislation. This act, clearly and for the first time, fully and directly acknowledges that cleaning up environmental residues after they have been produced is only a part of the job that lies ahead. The other, and in the long run the most difficult part, is to prevent or avert harmful residues in the first place. Under the Toxic Substances Control Act the EPA is required to insure the safe manufacture, use, and distribution of potentially dangerous chemicals. TSCA is the beginning of a long, difficult journey during which our society will learn how to prevent the introduction of harmful substances into our air, our water, our land, and our bodies.[709]

TRACE METALS. These are inorganic substances such as zinc, selenium, manganese, and probably even arsenic that occur in small amounts as components of living organisms. Some of these substances enhance tumor growth, while others apparently protect against cancer development. A dietary deficiency of the essential nutrient zinc decreases tumor growth in rats and mice. In some experiments transplanted tumors did not grow at all in zinc-deficient animals, whereas animals with normal diets developed tumors. Clinical studies indicate that cancer patients with low levels of zinc in their blood fail to respond to anticancer drugs, which usually act when cells are dividing. It has been suggested that zinc therapy might be used in patients to increase tumor-cell division temporarily, thereby possibly increasing the responsiveness of the tumors to anticancer drugs.

Contrasting with zinc's stimulation of cancer growth, the trace element selenium apparently prevents tumor development in experimental animals and in people. A study was conducted that added different concentrations of selenium to the drinking water of a strain of mice that develop mammary tumors spontaneously. With only 0.1 part per million selenium in their drinking water, 94 percent of the mice developed tumors. This is about the spontaneous rate. Among mice with 1 ppm selenium in their drinking water, only 3 percent developed tumors. The protective effect of selenium against tumor development disappeared when the mice also received supplemental zinc. Selenium intake and cancer mortality are inversely related. In areas where people have relatively high levels of selenium in their blood, or eat diets rich in selenium, overall cancer death rates are lower than in those areas where populations ingest little of this element. The optimum amount of selenium in an adult diet is 0.3 milligrams per day, and Americans on the average get half this amount. Cereal grains and seafood contain relatively large amounts of this element. Cadmium is toxic to the body and concentrates mainly in the liver and kidneys, and to a lesser extent in other organs. Further statistical studies of cancer suggest additional relationships between dietary trace elements and cancer mortality. Whereas selenium, and possibly manganese, are associated with low cancer-mortality rates, zinc, chromium, and cadmium are generally associated with higher cancer mortality. The antagonistic effects of zinc and selenium seen in cancer development in mice also seem to apply to people.[710,711]

TRIALLYL PHOSPHATE. *Phosphoric acid, tri-2-propenyl ester, allyl phosphate, triallyl phosphate.* Water-white liquid used as an intermediate *(see).* Causes tumors when injected under the skin of mice in 200 milligram doses per kilogram of body weight.[712]

TRIAZENE, 3,3-DIMETHYL-1-PHENYL-, AND 2-CHLORO-4,6-BIS-(ETHYLAMINO)-. Herbicide that is a suspected carcinogen. The EPA has determined it a candidate for additional carcinogenesis studies.[713]

s-TRIAZINE,2,4,6-TRIS(1-AZIRIDINYL)-. See Ethylenimine.

s-TRIAZOLE, 3-AMINO-. See Aminotriazole.

TRIBUTYRIN. *Glyceryl tributyrate.* Prepared from glycerol with butyric acid, it is a colorless liquid with a characteristic odor and bitter taste. It occurs naturally in butter. It is soluble in alcohol and is used as a flavoring agent in beverages, ice cream, candy, baked goods, margarine, and puddings. Causes tumors when given orally to rats in doses of 150 milligrams per kilogram of body weight.[714]

TRICHLOROETHYLENE (TCE). *Trichloroethene.* Tests conducted by the NCI showed that this chlorinated hydrocarbon caused cancer of the liver in mice. Rats failed to show significant response, a fact which may be attributed to the cancer-resistance of the strain used. Despite the species difference in cancer response, the NCI concluded that the TCE test clearly showed the compound caused liver cancer in mice. The findings are considered definitive for animal studies and serve as a warning of possible human carcinogenicity in humans. However, the extent of possible human risk cannot be predicted reliably on the basis of these studies alone. A related compound, vinyl chloride *(see)* does cause cancer in humans.

Trichloroethylene is used in the United States mainly as a degreasing solvent for machine parts. It is also used in industrial dry-cleaning and extraction processes, in the manufacture of other chemical products, in retail cleaning products, and in the extraction of caffeine from coffee. Consumers may be exposed to the chemical in pesticides, waxes, gums, resins, tars, paints, varnish, spot removers, rug-cleaning products, air fresheners, and metal cleaners. The chemical is also used as an anesthetic in some dental and surgical procedures, and as an analgesic in the treatment of trigeminal neuralgia. An estimated 5,000 medical and dental workers are exposed to it as an anesthetic gas each year. In addition, 280,000 industrial workers are also exposed to it. Trichloroethylene can penetrate the skin and cause irregularities in heartbeat and breathing. It can cross the placenta in pregnant women. Other chlorinated solvents, such as methyl chloroform, perchloroethylene and ethylene chloride have been proposed or employed as replacements for trichloroethylene but such replacements are viewed with caution because they also have potential toxicological hazards.[715]

2,4,6-TRICHLOROPHENOL. A germicide and a wood and glue preservative. Also a textile antimildew agent. Fed to rats and mice for 105 to 107 weeks. It caused lymphomas and luekemias in male rats and liver cancer in male and female mice.

TRIETHYLENE GLYCOL DIGLYCIDYL ETHER. *Tetraoxahexadecane.* An alkylating antineoplastic agent that causes bone-marrow depression and nausea. Has been determined to be an animal carcinogen by a NIOSH review.[716]

TRIETHYLENEPHOSPHORAMIDE. *Phosphine oxide, tris (1-aziridinyl), aphoxide, APO, ENT, acid triethyleneimide.* Colorless crystals derived from ethylenimine that are highly toxic and are irritating to the skin. Used in nitrogen mustards, insect sterilants, and formerly in flameproofing cotton. Caused cancer when given orally to rats in 110 milligram doses per kilogram of body weight.[717]

TRIETHYLENETHIOPHOSPHORAMIDE. *Phosphine sulfide, Tris (1-aziridinyl), TEPA, tespamin, TSPA.* Crystals from pentane or ether used as an antineoplastic agent. Causes cancer when given intravenously to rats in 52 milligram doses per kilogram of body weight and when injected in mice in 11 milligram doses per kilogram of body weight.[718]

TRIFLURALIN. A teriary aromatic amine, it is a derivative of dinitrotoluene and is one of several widely used agricultural pesticides selected for testing by the NCI. Introduced in 1960 as a selective preemergence herbicide, it is presently used for weed control on a variety of field crops, such as fruits, vegetables, and ornamentals. In 1971, the most recent statistics available, approximately 16.6 million acres of agricultural land were treated with 11.4 million pounds of the herbicide. Weed control of grasses in soybean and cotton fields accounted for 92 percent of the total consumption. It was the single herbicide most frequently used on cotton in 1971 and was listed among those products identified by distributors as having increased most rapidly in use between 1971 and 1975. An estimated 25 million pounds per year are currently used.

Although it is considered nontoxic in mammals, trifluralin has been found to cause potential chromosomal damage in workers' cells. Agricultural workers have the greatest exposure through pesticide application and in manufacturing plants. It has three to four times more effect when incorporated in soil where it may persist three to six months. Workers using it, and 13 other pesticides, were found to have four times the number of chromosomal gaps and 25 times the number of breaks in cells than nonexposed workers. When trifluralin was fed to rats and mice for 78 weeks, it was found to be a liver carcinogen in female mice. It has also been associated with an increased number of benign tumors in the lung and windpipe tissues of female mice.[719]

TRIMETHYLTHIOUREA. This chemical has a variety of industrial uses and is a relative of thiourea (see). A rat-liver carcinogen, it was given in feed to rats and mice for 77 weeks. It caused thyroid cancers in female rats under NCI test conditions, but the tests did not provide evidence for carcinogenicity in male rats or in mice of either sex.[720]

TRIS. A fabric flame retardant. It was given in feed to rats and mice for 103 weeks. Tris was carcinogenic in rats and mice, causing liver, lung, and stomach tumors in female mice; kidney, lung, and stomach tumors in male mice; and kidney tumors in rats of both sexes. Tris appeared in the urine of children wearing treated garments. The tris product dibromoproponal appeared in all of the children who wore treated and washed pajamas for 5 to 7 days. Urinary concentrations of the compound, in the 10 parts per billion range, are low but indicate that more is present elsewhere in the body. Levels of the poison in children's urine declined with time, although the substance was present 12 days after exposure to the sleepwear had ended. Sleepwear with Tris was being sold in late 1977, despite a ban against its sale.[721,722]

TRISODIUM ETHYLENEDIAMINETETRACETATE TRIHYDRATE (EDTA). Chelating agent used extensively as a food additive to remove trace metals that catalyze the oxidation of oils, vitamins, and unsaturated fats and cause rancidity flavor changes and discoloration. The acceptable daily intake, according to a World Health Organization Expert Committee on Food Additives, is 25 to 800 parts per million, or 2.5 milligrams per kilogram of body weight. Also used in liquid soaps, cosmetics, pharmaceuticals, metalworking, pulp and paper processing, rubber and polymer chemistry, textile processing and dyeing, and in the treatment of metal poisoning (although it can be toxic and is poorly absorbed by the body when taken orally). Under conditions of an NCI study, using concentrations of 3,500 ppm and 7,500 ppm in feed, it was not demonstrated to be a carcinogen. However, intervals for all tumor sites indicate a positive value; this indicates that the possibility of tumorogenicity is not theoretically precluded.[723]

TRISTEARIN. *Steric acid; 2,3-epoxypropyl ester and 12 hydroxy- and 12 hydrozy-; methyl ester; glyceryl tristearate; and glycidyl stearate.* Constituent of most fats. Used in textile sizes. Formerly used in making candles, it is still used in metal polishing, in waterproofing papers, and in soaps. Caused tumors when injected under the skin of mice in doses of from 26 to 2,000 milligrams per kilogram of body weight.[724]

TRYPAFLAVINE. *Acriflavine.* Deep reddish brown crystalline powder used to treat animal wounds. Formerly used as an udder infusion for bovine mastitis. Caused cancer when injected under the skin of rats in 160 milligram doses per kilogram of body weight.[725]

TRYPTOPHAN Certain metabolites of tryptophan have been implicated in cancers of the urinary bladder in humans. There is no direct evidence that tryptophan metabolites produce bladder cancer in man, but there is evidence from animal studies that suggests that they may act as co-carcinogens in the presence of cancer-causing agents. In one study, elevated levels of tryptophan metabolites were detected in about half the bladder-cancer patients.[726]

TUBERCULOSIS DRUG. *See* Isoniazid.

TURNIPS. *See* Antithyroid Compounds.

ULTRAVIOLET RADIATION. The cancer-producing effects of ultraviolet radiation appear to be limited to the skin, probably because of its low penetration. In thin-skinned animals, such as albino mice, sarcomas are initiated, as well as other cancers.[727] *See also* Sun and Skin Cancer.

URACIL, 5-FLURO-. *See* 5-Fluorouracil.

URACIL, 6-METHYL-2-THIO-. *See* Methylthiouracil.

URACIL MUSTARD. *5-(Bis(2-chloroethyl)amino) uracil, aminouracil mustard, Demethyldopan.* An alkylating anticancer agent (*see* Anticancer Drugs) used in biochemical research. It is derived from urea and is eight times as active as thio-tepa *(see)*. It is a potent inducer of lung tumors in mice and caused cancer when implanted in extremely small doses.[728,729]

URACIL,6-PROPYL-2-THIO-. *See* Propylthiouracil.

URANIUM. Occurs in earth crust. It is chiefly found in Colorado; Utah; Canada; Zaire; Czechoslovakia; and Cornwall, England. Used in atomic and hydrogen bombs and nuclear powder, it is a highly toxic radiation hazard. Radioactive uranium produces ionizing radiation. Uranium compounds are toxic to animals and may be able to penetrate normal human skin. The kidneys and liver are the principle sites of absorption and often become diseased. Uranium hexachloride fumes irritate the lungs and can cause severe chemical pneumonia or emphysema. Exposed workers have also developed anemia and intestinal troubles. Uranium workers are exposed to radioactive dusts from the mining and machining of uranium. Radioactive uranium decays to form radon gas, which is also radioactive. As a result of inhaling these gases and dusts, uranium workers have a high incidence of lung cancer. In fact, the Public Health Service has recently estimated that between 600 and 1,100 of the 6,000 uranium miners will die of lung cancer during the next 20 years.

UREA, ETHYL NITROSO (ENU). Determined by a NIOSH review to be a definite animal carcinogen, it is a NIOSH candidate for hazard review for carcinogenesis.[730] *See also* Urea, Methyl Nitroso-.

UREA, METHYL NITROSO-(MNU) (NMU). *N-Methyl-N-nitrosourea, nitrosomethylurea.* One of the most powerful cancer-causing agents known, it is used in cancer research. It causes cancer in rats, mice, rabbits, guinea pigs, hamsters, and dogs.[731] Urea is the chief end product of nitrogen metabolism in mammals and is excreted in human urine. In combination with nitrogen, oxygen, and alcohol, it forms a powerful carcinogen.

URETHAN. *See* Urethane.

URETHANE. *Ethyl carbamate.* Urethane induces liver tumors and tumors of the lung in experimental animals. It was the first carcinogen demonstrated to pass through the placenta and affect the fetus. For several years urethane was used as a chemotherapeutic agent in leukemia and multiple myeloma, but there are no definite reports of a cancer hazard to humans.[732]

VABROCID. *See* Nitrofurazone.

VALERIC ACID, 4,5-EPOXY-2-(2,3-EPOXYPROPYL)- METHYL ESTER. It is used in the manufacture of perfumes and as a synthetic flavoring, and some of its salts are used in medicine. It occurs naturally in apples, cocoa, coffee, oil of lavender, peaches, and strawberries. Colorless with an unpleasant odor, it is usually distilled from valerian root. Inhalation caused tumors in mice in 3,700 milligram doses per kilogram of body weight.[733]

VAPONA. *See* Dichlorvos.

VEREL. *See* Acrylonitrile.

VESPRIN. *See* Chlorpromazine.

VINYL CHLORIDE. The most frequently used vinyl monomer, it is usually handled as a liquid and employed in the making of plastics. Vinyl chloride has caused cancer in laboratory animals and in humans. In laboratory tests, animals who inhaled vinyl chloride vapors were found to have adenomas and adenocarcinomas of the lung; lymphomas; neuroblastomas of the brain; and angiosarcomas of the liver. Subsequent epidemiological investigations of workers exposed to vinyl chloride demonstrated an excessive number of deaths due to cancer of the brain, liver, lung, and lymphatic systems. Vinyl chloride was also found to induce tumors in pregnant rats and their offspring. Subsequent studies of children born in communities contiguous to vinyl-chloride polymerization facilities were shown to have an increased risk of birth defects, particularly of the central nervous system, upper digestive tract, and genital organs. A significant number of deaths from central nervous system tumors were found among adult men. Workers in vinyl-chloride plants were found to have angiosarcomas, an extremely rare and fatal liver cancer. Exposure to small quantities of vinyl chloride was determined to cause fibrotic lesions of the liver after only one year. The livers of workers did not return to normal for up to two and a half years after the workers were removed from exposure to the chemical. Those at risk of liver damage from vinyl chloride are not just the estimated 6,500 workers in the United States who produce it but thousands of others who work in plants where the polymer is heated before being used to make containers and other products.

Exposure to aerosols containing 50 to 10,000 parts per million of vinyl chloride regularly induces tumors in rats, mice, and hamsters, not only in the liver but in other tissues as well. Trichloroethylene *(see)* is a higher order structural compound similar to vinyl chloride and has been used for many years as an anesthetic. It is also widely used as a degreasing agent for metals and as an extractant in the foodstuff industry. Chloroprene *(see)*, another related compound, is used extensively in the chemical industry, being the starting material for synthetic rubber polychloroprene. Residues of vinyl chloride have been found in such products as vegetable oil, mouthwashes, meats, and medicines. Certainly, the red flag should be up on this common and potent carcinogen.[734,735,736,737,738]

At this writing, two federal occupational health agencies were investigating two Houston-area chemical plants following reports of 15 deaths from rare brain cancer among workers at both facilities. The major investigation centers on the Union Carbide plant, where 11 cases of brain cancer have been discovered, and all but one of the affected workers are dead. At the Monsanto plant, five employees have died of brain cancers.

On death certificates from 1962–1978, 9 of the 11 cancers among Union Carbide employees and 2 of the 5 Monsanto cases were reported to be glioblastoma multiforme, a type of brain cancer that has been linked in previous human studies to vinyl chloride.

Both vinyl chloride and acrylonitrile (the latter is a chemical that has been shown to cause brain tumors in animals) have been used at both plants at various times. According to OSHA and NIOSH, both chemicals are suspect.

The 11 brain cancers among Union Carbide's Texas City workers came to light after an employee filed a complaint with the local OSHA office, November 22, 1978, alleging a high incidence of such tumors among employees in the chemical shipping area of the plant. The Monsanto plant came under investigation because of the findings at Union Carbide. The investigators said that in addition to vinyl chloride, other chemicals which may be carcinogens in the plant include ethylene oxide and acrylonitrile.[739]

VINYLIDENE CHLORIDE. Similar to vinyl chloride *(see)*, which has caused a rare form of liver cancer among workers, vinylidene chloride is used to make Saran Wrap and other transparent plastic wrappings and coatings. It is a colorless liquid, insoluble in water. Flammable and explosive, it is copolymerized from vinyl chloride or acrylonitrile to form various kinds of Saran adhesives. It is a component of synthetic fibers, upholstery, curtain and drapery fabrics. It is largely resistent to most chemicals and solvents, and to weather, moths, and mildew. At present it is not known to have caused ill effects among persons exposed to it. It should be easier to control and less hazardous than vinyl chloride because it is a liquid rather than a gas in its natural state. It is also produced in much smaller quantities and is used for far fewer plastic products. Little, in fact, is known of the chemical's hazards, but it is believed that the dangers are confined to the production process. It is considered inert by the time it appears in consumers' products.[740]

VIOLETS. *Those with ammonium bases include acid violet, acid fast violet, C.I. food violet 2, D & C violet.* These acid dyes remain fast during washing and exposure to light. They are widely used in dyes for plastics, varnishes, and some pigments. They cause neoplasms when injected under the skin of rats.[741]

VIRUSES. Viruses have been proven to be the cause of cancer in fowl, mice, frogs, and rabbits. Filtrates from viral-infected cancer tissue have been injected into healthy animals, and they have induced cancer in these animals. As to the viral cause of cancer in man, there is only a suspicion, but a strong one, that is backed by persuasive evidence and by the knowledge that in many other fundamental respects the development of cancer in the higher animals and in man is generally very similar.

It is hypothesized that an unconventional C-type RNA virus that does not infect cells from the outside is responsible for cancer. The organism is harbored in the cell from the time of embryotic development. The virus is repressed in normal cells, but when the tumor-inducing genetic material of the virus, the oncogene, is activated, it transforms the normal cells into cancer cells. This can come naturally, through aging; in association with genetic defects or genetic predispositions; or through outside influences such as chemicals or radiation. It is hypothesized that both spontaneous cancers and those induced by chemical or physical agents are caused when the type-C virus genome, or hereditary information, becomes activated. This viral information, called the oncogene, serves as the source of the genetic information that transforms normal cells into tumor cells. That part of the viral genetic material responsible for the virus particle becoming activated is called the viragene.

These RNA viruses, or type-C particles, cause cancer in several animals. The particle has been found in cancers in 10 animal species and in the embryos and newborns of 5. When an animal or an individual gets cancer, according to the theory, it is because the virus becomes overt or expressed. The virus is transmitted through inheritance, rather than by communication with a diseased individual. The outcome of infection by a particular virus depends on species, strain, age, and differences in susceptibility of the host, as well as on hormonal status, route of infection, and specific immunologic factors. Some of the type-C viruses also have the ability to transform cells grown in cultures. This transformation is thought to be similar to the way normal cells become malignant or cancerous in the body. Both transformed and cancerous cells are often capable of multiplying under conditions in which normal ones are not. They are usually locked into a more primitive state of development than their normal counterparts. In some of the viruses, investigations have identified a specific gene that is necessary for transformation to occur, and they have also identified the proteins involved. Several of the type-C viruses apparently gain the ability to transform, or at least to increase, their malignant potential as a result of acquiring new genetic information from the cells they infect. Virus-free mouse cells grown in the laboratory for several months have been found to produce tumor viruses as a product of spontaneous transformation by some of the cells into tumor cells. Many such experiments have led to the conclusion that the virus must be present in masked form in the original embryo cells, and probably all other cells of the mouse's body, just waiting to be "turned on." This same ability of viruses to transform cells has been found in tests on chicken, hamster, rat, cat, and pig cells.

What about human cells? The Epstein-Barr Virus (EBV) transforms human cells. When a person is infected with EBV, a few white blood cells are altered—the cells undergo unlimited cell division. EBV has been associated with mononucleosis, a usually mild infection of the glands in young people. It has also been associated with human nose and throat cancer and Burkitt's lymphoma, a rapidly fatal cancer found in children of tropical Africa. The multiple tumors of Burkitt's lymphoma appear so rapidly that scientists believe an infectious agent rather than metastasis is involved. Age distribution also lends weight to the theory of a viral infection. The disease is unknown in children under 2 when they are receiving antibodies through their mother's milk: incidences of it rise to a peak between the ages of 3 and 8; and it is again virtually unknown past the age of 12. EBV is a type of herpes virus and so is another virus associated with human cancer. Many researchers think the long-suspected link between sexual intercourse and cervical cancer may be the herpes simplex virus, type 2, a common virus that causes a venereal disease. One out of four women who had the virus infection go on to develop cancer or a precancerous condition of the cervix. Women with type-2 herpes are six times more likely to get cervical cancer than women who had never had herpes infection. It has been suggested that once a person is infected the virus might persist for years in a dormant state. Then, at some point, it might subvert the cells of the cervix and, either alone or with some chemical assistant, initiate the development of cancer. There is some evidence that the virus might be abetted by female sex hormones, because though herpes infection is common in men, penile cancer is a rarity. Men may be the transmitters of herpes, because the virus has been found in the genital and urinary tracts of men, and the virus is most probably transmitted through sexual intercourse.

Particles suspected of being pieces of viruses have also been found in the breast tissue and milk of some breast-cancer patients. This does not prove, however, that these particles are cancer-causing viruses.

Viruses have also been associated with human sarcomas—cancers that arise in the bone, fat, and connective tissues. Antibodies have given telltale evidence of the presence of a virus in 80 percent of the blood specimens from six patients with a type of bone cancer and two patients with cartilage cancer. Interestingly, antibodies were also found in the blood samples of 80 percent of the healthy friends and families of the patients. However, antibodies were detected in only 25 percent of the normal blood donors.

In mice, harmless viruses, "proviruses," that have become part of the genetic blueprint have been suspected of exchanging genetic material and acquiring the knowledge to make blood cells turn leukemic. Morever, proviruses that are potential gene swappers may number in the hundreds. Therefore, instead of one or a few viruses being responsible for leukemia, the theory goes, there many be many viruses responsible. Whether this will prove the case in human leukemia, no one is certain. There is still no evidence that humans harbor proviruses that can turn into cancer viruses.

An animal-cancer virus has been used to immunize cancer patient. Twenty patients with advanced cancers were given a vaccine made up of a virus that causes leukemia in mice. As a result, two-thirds of the patients developed cellular immunity specifically against the virus. Half of the patients also developed antibodies specifically against the cancer virus. Although all the patients had advanced cancer, some of them experienced long-lasting remissions of their disease. However, investigators believe that the remissions were due to chemotherapy and treatment with an antibody-inducing tuberculosis vaccine, BCG, rather than to the cancer-virus immunization. They continue to hope that virus immunization will eventually be used, along with other therapy, to boost patients' resistance to cancer.[742,743,744,745,746, 747,748,749,750,751,752,753,754,755,756,757,758,759]

Some animal cancers caused by viruses:

Date	Investigators	Animals	Cancers
1908	Ellerman and Bang	Chickens	Leukemia
1911	Rous	Chickens	Sarcoma
1933	Shope	Rabbits	Skin cancer
1934	Lucke	Frogs	Kidney cancer
1936	Bittner	Mice	Breast cancer
1951	Gross	Mice	Leukemia
1957	Stewart et al.	Mice to mice, rats, rabbits	Multiple cancers
1961	Eddy et al.	Monkeys to hamsters	Sarcoma
1962	Trentin et al.	Man to hamsters	Sarcoma
1964	Harvey	Mice	Sarcoma
1964	Jarrett et al.	Cats	Leukemia
1965	Hull et al.	Monkeys to hamsters	Sarcoma-lymphoma
1965	Sarma et al.	Chickens to hamsters	Fibrosarcoma
1966	Darbyshire	Bovines to hamsters	Sarcoma
1967	Opler	Guinea pigs	Leukemia
1967	Sarma et al.	Dogs to hamsters	Fibrosarcoma
1968	Melendez et al.	Monkeys	Lymphoma
1968	Graffi et al.	Hamsters	Lymphoma
1969	Snyder and Theilen	Cats	Fibrosarcoma
1972	Wolfe et al.	Monkeys	Fibrosarcoma

Source: Michael B. Shimkin, M.D., *Science and Cancer,* Public Health Service Publication, no. 1162, Washington, D.C., 1969.

VITAMINS A AND C. Dr. Michael Sporn and his colleagues from the NCI in Bethesda reported in *Science,* February 4, 1977, that a chemical modification of vitamin A—13-cis-retinoic acid—inhibits the incidence and extent of bladder cancer in rats previously exposed to N-methyl-N-nitrosourea, one of the most potent carcinogens known. Although it is still not proven, it is suspected that some forms of cancer found in human beings may be at least partially due to nitroso compounds introduced into our system from many different natural and man-made sources. Dr. Sporn says that the NCI studies were prompted by earlier findings that indicated that a dietary deficiency of vitamin A greatly increased the susceptibility of chemically-induced bladder cancers. Animal studies have also shown that man-made modifications of the vitamin inhibit cancer of the skin, lungs, and breast.

The NCI researchers found that when rats were fed a diet containing the vitamin derivative, it reduced not only the number and extent of bladder tumors, but also the nonmalignant cellular changes that usually precede the onset of bladder cancer in animals. At this writing, Dr. Sporn and his colleagues say they don't know how the vitamin derivative protects the rats against the chemically induced cancers, but they hope that a recently developed organ-culture system, in which both normal and carcinogen-treated bladder tissue can be maintained for long periods of time, may help them come up with some of the key answers.

In another report in *Nature,* June 16, 1977, Dr. Sporn and another group of collaborators wrote that natural vitamin A—retinyl acetate—in large doses inhibits the development of breast tumors in rats that had been treated with N-methyl-N-nitrosourea. Tumors appeared in 50 percent of the rats that were given a high dose of N-methyl-N-nitrosourea and fed with a vitamin A supplemented diet, compared to a mammary cancer incidence of 83 percent in animals that did not receive the vitamin. At lower doses of the carcinogen, none of the vitamin-fed rats developed breast tumors, compared to 20 percent of the rats in the other group.

Other reports have suggested that vitamin C—ascorbic acid—protects laboratory animals against carcinogen-induced skin and bladder tumors. Dr. Joseph B. Guttenplan wrote in *Nature,* July 28, 1977, that the normal mutagenic effects, that is, effects causing genetic change, of two N-nitroso compounds are inhibited by vitamin C. The Ames Test (*see* Introduction, page 7) uses mutagenicity in bacteria to predict carcinogenicity. Vitamin C is now being added to bacon to prevent or retard the formation of nitrosoamines in the product.

VITAMIN B.   Riboflavin deficiency has been shown to retard the growth of certain spontaneous and transplanted tumors. The mechanism underlying the antitumor effect of riboflavin deficiency is not known, but one possible explanation is the starvation of the rapidly multiplying tumor of the flavin coenzymes that are vital for metabolism. In contrast, riboflavin deficiency enhanced the carcinogenicity of azo dyes in the liver, perhaps because flavin cofactors are involved in the degradation of these carcinogens. Riboflavin-rich diets have been reported to inhibit hepatic-tumor formation in rats. A deficiency of lipotropic agents—folic acid, vitamin B_{12}, choline, and the amino acid methionine—enhances the chemical induction of tumors in the liver, colon, and esophagus. This deficiency has been used as an experimental model for human alcoholic cirrhosis, a disease associated with increased cancer of the liver and esophagus. In another study, vitamin B_{12} enhanced markedly the carcinogenic effect of p-dimethyl-aminoazobenzene in rats receiving a methionine-deficient diet.[760]

WATCHES. *See* Radioluminescent Paint.

WATER. Drinking water that comes into your home may be the greatest source of cancer-causing agents to which you are exposed. There are thousands of organic chemicals potentially present in our water supplies due to industrial discharges and spills, the use of agricultural chemicals, and the runoff of rainwater from cities. Groundwater—subsurface water which supplies springs, lakes, and rivers—can be polluted by surface waters, deep-well disposal, seepage from mines, landfills, septic tanks, feedlots, and pesticides. Groundwater supplies 20 percent of the freshwater used in the United States and constitutes the entire water supply of more than 95 percent of the rural population and 20 percent of the 100 largest cities in the country; the semiarid Southwest is almost completely dependent upon groundwater. It is estimated that 10 million barrels of brine are injected into underground reservoirs by the gas and oil industry. While relatively little is known about the chemicals that pollute our water, it is known that many of them do cause cancer in test animals.

The Safe Drinking Water Act of 1974 required that the administrator of the EPA arrange with the National Academy of Sciences for a study to determine the safety of American drinking water. The academy's 1975 study revealed thousands of organic chemicals in the drinking water of 80 cities.

The academy committee found volatile organic compounds made up about 10 percent by weight of the total organic matter in the water. They examined 74 nonpesticides from among the more than 300 volatile organic compounds identified. They also examined 55 pesticides, some of which had not yet been detected in water but may be expected to show up because of their use in large quantities.

The committee judged 22 of those compounds to be known or suspected carcinogens for humans or animals. "There is no hard evidence that low-level oral exposure to any of these chemicals produce cancer, but present data and methods of calculating risks to large populations are uncertain," said the committee. "Even more uncertainty exists when one considers the possibility that some of these chemicals may also be mutagenic and teratogenic."

The NAS committee noted that chlorination, a primary control of water-borne infection, may result in the formation of suspected carcinogens for humans and that substitute disinfectants have been proposed.

The committee also presented data that indicated that although there may be no immediate hazard to public health from ingesting asbestos in drinking water, more must be known about asbestos and other mineral fibers in water, and mineral-fiber contamination should be controlled to the extent possible by means of appropriate water treatment. Lead *(see)* toxicity, the committee said, is a particular risk for inner-city children. Consequently, the interim drinking-water regulations for lead—established under the Safe Drinking Water Act in 1974—may provide an adequate margin of safety for adults but not for urban children.

Similarly, they noted, present data support reexamination of the margins of safety provided by interim drinking-water limits for nitrate, arsenic, and selenium (*see* all).

The committee also strongly urged research on the problems of contamination by viruses, because knowledge of the scale of potential viral contamination is scanty and because there is no rigorous basis for establishing a harmless level of viral contamination in water. While water systems test for bacteria, they do not test for viral contamination. Although cancer-causing viruses have not been identified in humans, it is known that viruses can cause cancer in animals.

The pollution of the waterways where we get our drinking water evidently has become a looming peril. The Hudson River, which currently supplies drinking water to 150,000 persons, is laced with cancer-causing chemicals, including polychlorinated biphenyls (PCBs). The Hudson is not even a heavily industrialized river, and similar tests in other waterways would probably turn up more serious pollutants. Studies in New Orleans and Cincinnati showed similar chemical pollution with statistical correlation to increased bladder and gastrointestinal cancers.

In one study of Mississippi River water, it was found that it contained significant amounts of cancer-causing compounds that may represent a potential threat to public health. Fifty-one percent of the unconcentrated river-water samples contained such potential carcinogens. In earlier studies of the lower Mississippi, the EPA found a broad spectrum of heavy metals and inorganic and organic compounds in concentrates of the river water, as well as in finished water obtained from water-treatment plants. At least three of the organic compounds were identified in finished waters as either carcinogenic or potentially carcinogenic. The lower Mississippi serves as the source of 40 water utilities that provide potable water for approximately 1.5 million people.

A few months after the National Academy of Sciences Committee report on water, the EPA Administrator, Douglas Costle, announced regulations to limit dangerous chemicals in drinking water. He said: "The proposed program marks the start of the first large scale effort in history to deal with organic chemical contaminants in drinking water. It will initiate changes in our approach to regulating the quality of the water we drink and will give the American public an 'insurance policy' against the dangers associated with chemicals in our water. . . ."

"The widespread contamination of our environment by synthetic chemicals is a relatively recent development. We're taking this step-by-step approach because there are still many gaps in our knowledge about organic contaminants and the fact that our proposals would result in American water-treatment practices. We know that some of these chemicals are dangerous. The lifetime exposure of our population to these chemicals poses a serious threat to public health. We are especially concerned about the increase in cancer risk."

The proposed EPA standard is for chloroform (see) and related organic chemicals of the trihalomethane (THM) group that are formed during the disinfection process at the treatment plant. They also call for some water systems to install a special treatment technique—filtration with granular activated carbon—to control other organics that are present in untreated water due to upstream pollution of drinking-water sources. Such pollution comes from industrial and municipal waste discharges and spills and from agricultural and urban runoff. The proposed standard for chloroform and other THMs is 0.10 parts per billion. The THMs are formed at the drinking-water treatment plant when chlorine is added to kill disease-causing bacteria. They are an unwanted by-product of chlorine's reaction with naturally occurring organic substances in the untreated water. Most public water systems use chlorine to disinfect water, and THMs are present in virtually every supply EPA has tested. EPA is concerned about chloroform because it has caused cancer in test animals and may pose the same risk to humans. Toluene (see), another THM, is also suspect. The THM standard would apply initially only to community water systems serving over 75,000 people and within five years will use granular activated carbon to deal with other chemicals.

In the meantime, agency officials warned citizens against relying on home charcoal-filtering systems. Activated charcoal requires careful and constant maintenance and replacement. Otherwise it can be ineffective and even become a breeding ground for the kind of bacterial diseases that chlorinated water was originally designed to eliminate. In the past, officials focused on removing carriers of communicable diseases from the water. Now it is evident they must also consider those chemicals that may cause cancer and other noncommunicable diseases.[761,762,763,764]

WATER SOFTENERS. See Zeolite.

WOOD. Workers in the wood-products industry have an unusually high rate of certain types of cancer. Although the types of malignancy varied among occupations, nearly all the groups surveyed—carpenters, loggers, professional foresters, pulp and papermill workers—had high rates of cancer of the stomach and of the lymph and blood-forming tissues. It is thought that stomach cancer could result from swallowing wood particles. The blood and lymphatic cancers—especially among pulp and paper-mill and plywood-mill workers—might be caused by the chemical-breakdown products of wood. Loggers have a high rate of prostate cancer. Professional foresters, who have a variety of exposures in mills and offices as well as forests, often develop cancer of the rectum, pancreas, and lungs; pulp and paper-mill workers develop cancer of the small intestines; sawmill workers and those involved in other wood-machining operations develop cancer of the pancreas and testes.

People who work in sawmills, or where wood is simply machined, do not have as high a cancer risk as those in the paper and pulp and plywood industries. The British have found cancer of the nasal passages and sinuses among furniture workers. No such cancer turned up in a Washington State study of 3 million death records, but British workers handle mostly hardwoods while Washington workers deal with softwood. Another study has indicated cedar can cause cancer in laboratory mice.

Swedish scientists have discovered an extraordinarily high rate of sinus cancer among woodworkers in that country and numerous stomach cancers among woodworkers who live in urban areas. Approximately 45 percent of nasal-sinus cancer in the Swedish cancer registry occurred in woodworkers.

Whatever the actual carcinogen, whether wood dust itself, which is a breakdown product of wood, or some chemical used in processing or treating wood, there is still a high cancer risk for workers throughout the wood-products industry.[765]

XANTHINE. *Dioxopurine, xanthin.* First isolated from gallstones, it occurs in animal organs, and in yeast, potatoes, coffee, beans, tea, and in human blood and urine. The drugs, theophylline and theobromine, the alkaloids of tea and cocoa respectively, are both dimethylxanthines. Caffeine in coffee is trimethylxanthine. It is used in organic synthesis and in medicines. It causes tumors when injected under the skin of rats in 3,600 milligram doses per kilogram of body weight and when implanted in mice in 80 milligram doses per kilogram of body weight.[766]

X-RAY. The diagnostic uses of X-rays is one of the greatest boons to health that has been developed in the past 50 years. But, too much exposure to X-rays can be hazardous to your health. Medical and dental patients are far too frequently exposed to potentially harmful levels of radiation. In 1968 the American Dental Association reported that it knew of no one mention in the scientific literature of a death or any serious injury resulting to a patient from a dental radiographic examination. At the time there was no conclusive proof that radiation exposures at low levels have caused injury to humans. Radiological experts acknowledge the link between ionizing radiation and potential damage to the body and its reproductive mechanisms. On the basis of research, this potential danger becomes apparent only at high levels of exposure to radiation. Experts do concur that, in itself, any measurable radiation is more likely to be harmful than helpful.

Having recognized the risk, doctors and dentists are striving to reduce this potential hazard. Federal officials have found that about one-third of all X-ray examinations are totally unnecessary. The cumulative effect of too much exposure to X-rays can cause cancer and birth defects. The developing embryo is particularly sensitive to the carcinogenic effect of radiation. A one-third reduction in X-ray tests for pregnant women would avoid approximately 90 cases of childhood cancer annually. Thirty percent of all new X-ray equipment is defective and emits too much radiation. And older equipment may also be leaking too much radiation. At fault too are doctors who use faulty techniques: setting X-ray levels too high; repeating one X-ray test in 10, thus subjecting the patient to twice the amount of radiation he would get in a normal exam. Many doctors with their own X-ray machines recommend tests for their patients because it means more money or because they want to protect themselves against future malpractice suits in case they fail to spot an injury.

Organs which have been associated with the effects of radiation include the lens of the eye (because of the possible relationship between radiation and cataract formation), bone marrow (because of the possible link between radiation and leukemia), and the thyroid (because of the possible relationship between radiation and thyroid cancer). Over 400 hospitals are now seeking patients given X-rays decades ago. A recent study has found that some face the risk of developing cancer of the thyroid from earlier X-ray treatment. Researchers discovered abnormal thyroids in more than 25 percent of the initial former patients located. A radioactive material called Thorotrast, which was once used to outline the abdominal organs for diagnostic X-rays, decades later resulted in unexpected cancers of the bone, liver, and kidney. Young patients who received radiation therapy for such conditions as acne, ringworm, inflamed tonsils, or enlargement of the thymus gland have increased rates of leukemia and cancers of the head and neck regions, including the brain and thyroid. Similarly, doctors were unaware of the potential hazards of a then common practice of fluoroscopy, an X-ray procedure in which the area to be studied is viewed directly instead of on film. The old fluoroscopy machines gave off many hundreds of times more radiation than modern X-ray machines do.

Experts point out that radiation has cumulative effects over the years, so that any exposure adds to a person's risk of cancer. Children are 5 to 10 times more sensitive to radiation-induced cancer than adults, and the fetus is 10 to 150 times more sensitive. The incidence of benign and malignant breast tumors in 606 women treated with X-rays for acute postpartum mastitis (inflammation of the breast) was investigated. Thirteen confirmed cases of breast cancer were observed instead of the 5.86 cases that were expected in a comparable group of women. In 5 of the 13 women with cancer, only one breast was treated; in each case, the cancer arose in the irradiated breast. The incidence of benign tumors appeared to have increased in the untreated as well as in the treated breasts. It was concluded that at least some breast cancers in this series of women could have been induced by the prior X-ray exposures. While diagnostic X-rays generally deliver extremely low levels of radiation, there is some evidence that the children of women who get diagnostic X-rays during pregnancy face a somewhat greater than average chance of developing leukemia or other cancers. Therefore, X-rays during pregnancies should be limited to those circumstances where the benefit of the knowledge to be gained clearly outweighs any possible risk to the unborn child.

A new diagnostic tool is sharply reducing the X-ray exposure patients receive during dental examinations. Called a Novar fiber optic transilluminator, the instrument uses an ultrahigh-intensity light that shines through, over, or around a tooth to provide information even an X-ray cannot. The transilluminator delivers light with great efficiency along thousands of tiny internally reflective glass fibers, which remain cool despite the lights intensity. It is particularly important to curtail X-ray exposure for children. Dentists can routinely use the transilluminator when examining children and use X-rays selectively to corroborate data. The transilluminator also can be used in conjunction with the panoramic X-ray technique, which cuts X-ray exposure significantly but sometimes fails to spot problems between teeth. By using both panoramic X-rays and a transilluminator, dentists can make a thorough examination. In addition, dentists who might otherwise hesitate to take X-rays because of their danger are able to make examinations with the transilluminator instead. In addition, if each dentist gave one less X-ray each day, there would be 300 million X-rays less each year. The FDA estimates 30 percent of all X-rays are unnecessary.

In the meantime, while government experts are working to increase protection against radiation exposure, you can help keep your personal exposure down. Since medical procedures constitute an estimated 90 percent of exposure, avoiding unnecessary X-rays could make a major contribution towards reducing your body burden.

There may or may not be a threshold below which cancer risk is near zero. However, current theory is that each dose of radiation adds to the body burden. Some people will be more affected than others and reach the cancer-causing threshold more quickly. While the scientists try to develop methods of protecting us from harmful effects, here's what you can do in the meantime:

- *Question the need for an X-ray.* In this day of lawsuit-happy patients, doctors will often order an X-ray as a defense against a malpractice suit. These are "just in case" X-rays and are unnecessary. Dental X-rays should not be taken routinely. X-rays should be taken only to diagnose a suspected problem.

- *Keep a record of your X-rays.* Tell your physician of your past X-rays. He/she may be able to use them instead of taking new ones. The FDA has printed cards for this purpose.
- *Ask for protection.* Ask for lead gonad shields to protect your reproductive organs whenever X-rays are taken.
- *If you're pregnant.* If there is any possibility that you may be pregnant, inform your physician or dentist before X-rays are taken.
- *Ask if the technician is certified and when the X-ray machine was last inspected.* If you don't like the answers, have your X-rays taken elsewhere.
- *Don't insist on X-rays.* If your doctor doesn't suggest an X-ray, don't you.

XYLENE. *Dimethylbenzene, xylol.* Derived from coal tar or coal-tar gas, it is considered less toxic than benzene, but it is suspect. It can cause a decrease in the number of red and white blood cells, irritate the skin, and it is narcotic in high doses. It can cause women to develop menstruation problems and repeated exposure to it can lead to heart problems. It is used in aviation gasolines; in protective coatings; and as a solvent in lacquers, enamels, and rubber cement. It has been found to be present in drinking water in about 20 cities. A recent investigation showed that there is a 44 percent higher incidence of gastrointestinal and urinary-tract cancer in populations drinking chlorinated water than in matched cohort groups drinking nonchlorinated water. Since xylene is an aromatic hydrocarbon as chlorene is, it certainly warrants further investigation, although there is no definite cancer-xylene link. There was an association between xylene USG, an ethyl ammonium compost, which caused cancer in rats when given orally, subcutaneously, and by injection.[767,768]

2,4-XYLENOL. 2-4-Dimethylphenol. A white crystalline solid that is derived from coal tar and is toxic by ingestion and skin absorption. It is used as a disinfectant and as a solvent in pharmaceuticals, as a solvent in insecticides and rubber manufacture, and as a wetting agent for dyestuffs. It caused cancer when painted on the skin of mice at 5,600 milligrams per kilogram of body weight.[769] It has been selected by EPA for priority attention as a water pollutant.[770]

XYLITOL. Made from birchwood, it is used in chewing gum as an artificial sweetener. It has been reported to sharply reduce cavities in teeth, but it costs more than sugar; it also has calories. FDA preliminary reports from England cited it as a cancer-causing agent. The data from the Huntingdon Research Center there, under the sponsorship of Hoffmann-La Roche, showed that several mice in the group fed a diet of 10 to 20 percent xylitol developed tumors in their adrenal glands.[771] Gum manufacturers' representatives disputed the significance of the Huntingdon study, noting that the ill effects in mice occurred at consumption levels equal to a human chewing nearly 200,000 sticks of gum a year.

YELLOWS. *Those deriving from aniline, N,N,-dimethyl-p-phenylazo include: cerasine yellow GG; C.I. solvent yellow, fat yellow A, methyl yellow, oil yellow, fast oil yellow, orient oil yellow, brilliant oil yellow, resinol yellow AD.* They cause cancer when given orally and when painted on the skin of rats. They also cause tumors when given orally and intramuscularly in rats and orally in hamsters. There is an OSHA standard for these dyes as carcinogens.

YELLOWS. *A.F. yellow 2, cerisol yellow, C.I. solvent yellow 5, oil yellow A, yellow AB.* A phenylazo-2-Naphthalamine dye made from aniline *(see)*

YTTERBIUM. A dark gray metal used in nuclear technology and with iron and other alloys. It is also used as a deoxidizer for vanadium and other nonferrous metals. Used in microwave ferrites and as a coating on high-temperature alloys. Causes tumors when implanted in mice in doses of 25 milligrams per kilogram of body weight.[772]

ZEOLITE. A natural hydrated silicate of aluminum. Both natural and artificial zeolites are used extensively for water softening. Artifical zeolites are made in a variety of forms, ranging from gelatinous to porous and sandlike, and are used as gas adsorbents, drying agents, catalysts, and water softeners.

Turkish researchers reported a cluster of 50 cases in two villages of the rare lung cancer mesothelioma, usually associated with asbestos. There was no asbestos in the two small villages, but the Turkish researchers suspected zeolite. An American mineralogist found another village with a soil just as rich in zeolite where there were no mesotheliomas. The researchers now believe that a certain zeolite, which appears as inorganic fibers in the soil around the cluster of mesotheliomas, may be the cause. Dr. Irving Selikoff, director of environmental medicine at New York's Mount Sinai School of Medicine, and the man who conducted the mesothelioma-asbestos research, said, "The significance of the Turkish findings is that fine fibers with a chemistry and structure different from asbestos can apparently also cause mesothelioma."[773]

ZINC CHLORIDE. *Butter of zinc.* It is white and odorless and composed of very deliquescent granules. The substance is used as a deodorant, disinfecting and embalming material, and also alone or with phenol and other antiseptics for preserving railway ties. It is also used in etching metals; in fireproofing lumber; with ammonium chloride as a flux for soldering; in manufacturing parchment paper and artificial silks; and activating cold-water glues. Its diversified uses include being used as an antiseptic for the skin and as a cement for metals, along with its use as a solvent for cellulose and a dehydrating agent in chemical synthesis. It causes tumors when injected in hamsters and chickens in doses of only 15 to 17 milligrams per kilogram of body weight. There is an OSHA standard for it pertaining to air.[774]

ZINC, (ETHYLENEBIS (DITHIOCARBAMATO))-. *See* Zineb.

ZINC SULFATE. *Sulfuric acid, zinc salt, zinc vitriol.* A yellowish white lustrous metal known since early times. Its a mineral source for many products. It is used as a pigment in opaque glass; as a base for color lakes; in rubber, plastics, dyeing; in phosphor, which is used in X-rays; in TV screens; and in luminous watch faces. Causes tumors when injected under the skin of rabbits in 6,170 milligrams per kilogram of body weight. [775]

ZINC VITRIOL. *See* Zinc Sulfate.

ZINEB (ETHYLENEBIS(DITHIOCARBAMATO))ZINC. *Lonacol, parzate, dithane Z-78.* Powder or crystals derived from chloroform plus alcohol. The powder spreads easily. It is used as an agricultural fungicide. Zineb is less toxic than ziram *(see)*. It causes cancer when given orally or implanted in rats in doses from 84 to 54 milligrams per kilogram of body weight.[776]

ZIRAM, BIS (DIMETHYLDITHIOCARBAMATO)-ZINC. *Methasan.* This is white and odorless, and when pure is used as a fungicide and as a rubber accelerator. It is moderately toxic and a strong irritant to eyes and mucous membranes. It caused cancer when given orally in 13 milligram doses per kilogram of body weight and when implanted in rats in 60 milligram doses per kilogram of body weight.[777]

ZIRCONIUM LACTATE. This is a white slightly moist pulp that decomposes without melting. It is used as a body deodorant and as a source of zirconia. It has been found moderately toxic to animals, but there are no known reports of industrial toxicity. It caused tumors in mice when injected in doses of 240 milligrams per kilogram of body weight.[778]

NOTES

With the exception of the following twelve references, all references in the Notes are listed in full.

- *A Consumer's Dictionary of Cosmetic Ingredients* by Ruth Winter, Crown Publishers, Inc., 1976. (Listed in Notes as *A Consumer's Dictionary of Cosmetic Ingredients.*)
- *A Consumer's Dictionary of Food Additives* by Ruth Winter, Crown Publishers, Inc., 1978. (Listed in Notes as *A Consumer's Dictionary of Food Additives.*)
- *The Condensed Chemical Dictionary* by Gessner G. Hawley, 9th ed. rev., Van Nostrand Reinhold Company, New York, 1977. (Listed in Notes as *Chemical Dictionary.*)
- *Federal Register,* published daily by the executive branch of government and contains all the proposed and final rules of federal departments and agencies. (Listed in Notes as *Federal Register.*)
- *Inserm Symposia Series: World Health Organization International Agency for Research on Cancer,* Institut National de la Santé et de la Recherche Médicale, Environmental Pollution and Carcinogenic Risks, Inserm Symposia Series, vol. 52, IARC Scientific Publications, no. 13, 1976. (Listed in Notes as Inserm Symposia Series.)
- *The Merck Index,* 8th ed., Rahway, N.J., Merck, Sharp and Dohme Research Laboratories, 1968. (Listed in Notes as *Merck.*)
- *Physicians' Desk Reference,* Medical Economics, Oradell, N.J., 1970. (Listed in Notes as *Physicians' Desk Reference.*)
- Gary Stoner, Michael B. Shimkin, Alexis Kniazeff, John Weisburger, Elizabeth Weisburger, and Gio B. Gori, "Test for Carcinogenicity of Food Additives and Chemotherapeutic Agents by the Pulmonary Tumor Response in a Strain of

227

Mice," *Cancer Research,* vol. 33, December 1973. (Listed in Notes as Gary Stoner et al.)
• *Suspected Carcinogens: A Subfile of the National Institute for Occupational Safety and Health,* Rockville, Md., 1975 and 1978. (Listed in Notes as *Suspected Carcinogens.*)
• *Toxicants Occurring Naturally in Foods,* 2d ed., National Academy of Sciences, Washington, D.C., 1973. (Listed in Notes as *Toxicants in Foods.*)
• *Toxic Substances List,* 1974 ed., U.S. Department of Health, Education and Welfare, Public Health Service Center for Disease Control, National Institute for Occupational Safety and Health, Rockville, Md. (Listed in Notes as *Toxic Substances List.*)
• *Work Is Dangerous to Your Health* by Jeanne Stellman, Ph.D., and Susan Baum, M.D., Pantheon Books, New York, 1973. (Listed in Notes as *Work Is Dangerous to Your Health.*)

The following abbreviations of government agencies are used in the Notes: EPA (Environmental Protection Agency), HEW (Health, Education and Welfare), WHO (World Health Organization), NCI (National Cancer Institute), ACS (American Cancer Society), NIH (National Institutes of Health), OSHA (Occupational Safety and Health Administration), NIOSH (National Institute for Occupational Safety and Health).

1. *Merck,* p. 4.   **2.** *Toxic Substances List.*   **3.** *Work Is Dangerous to Your Health,* p. 213.   **4.** *Toxic Substances List.*   **5.** *Toxic Substances List.*   **6.** Michael B. Shimkin, M.D., *Contrary to Nature,* HEW, Washington, D.C., 1977, p. 338.   **7.** *Toxic Substances List.*   **8.** *Toxic Substances List* and *Chemical Dictionary,* pp. 12–13.   **9.** *Toxic Substances List.*   **10.** "U.S. Moves Against Carcinogenic Fiber Substance," *New York Times,* January 17, 1978, p. 15.   **11.** *Toxicants in Foods,* p. 52.   **12.** *Toxic Substances List.*   **13.** *Suspected Carcinogens.*   **14.** *Toxic Substances List* and *Toxicants in Foods,* pp. 522–23.   **15.** *Suspected Carcinogens.*   **16.** *Toxic Substances List.*   **17.** Cesare Maltoni, "Occupational Chemical Carcinogenesis; New Facts, Priorities and Perspectives," Inserm Symposia Series, pp. 127–50.   **18.** *Journal of Agricultural and Food Chemistry,* November/December 1974.   **19.** "Carcinogens," *Medical World News,* March 10, 1972, p. 6.   **20.** *Toxicants in Foods,* pp. 517–18.   **21.** "Research Report on Agent Orange," University of Illinois Medical Center Campus, February 14, 1979.   **22.** "EPA Citing Miscarriages, Restricts 2 Herbicides," *New York Times,* March 2, 1979.   **23.** L. M. Shabad and G. A. Smirnov, "Aviation and Environmental Benzopyrene Pollution," Inserm Symposia Series, pp. 53–60.   **24.** *Science,* vol. 169, August 21, 1970.   **25.** *Health Effects of Air Pollutants,* EPA bulletin, June 1976.   **26.** "Epidemiology Statistics and Cancer Control," *Journal of American Medical Women's Association,* October 1976.   **27.** *Environmental Science and Technology,* vol. 12, May 1976.   **28.** *A Consumer's Dictionary of Food Additives,* p. 22.   **29.** *Toxic Substances List.*   **30.** International Research Agency Bulletin, no. 69372, Lyon, Cedex 2, France, September, 1977.   **31.** "Report on Carcinogenesis Bioassays of Aldrin and Dieldrin," HEW, Technical Report Series, no. 21, Washington, D.C., 1978.   **32.** *Health Hazards of the Human Environment,* WHO, Washington, D.C., 1972, p. 225.   **33.** *Federal Register,* October 27, 1978.   **34.** *Toxic Substances List.*   **35.** "Diet, Nutrition, and Cancer," *The American Journal of Clinical Nutrition,* September 1976.   **36.** *Federal Register,* November 3, 1978.

37. *Washington Post,* July 8, 1978.   38. Philippe Shubik, "Potential Carcinogenicity of Food Additives and Contaminants," *Cancer Research,* vol. 35, November 1975, pp. 3475–3480.   39. *Minnesota Science,* vol. 32, Fall 1976, p. 14.   40. EPA news release, Washington, D.C., January 15, 1979.   41. *Toxic Substances List.*   42. *Chemical Dictionary,* p. 59.   43. *Toxic Substances List.*   44. *Toxic Substances List.*   45. Thomas Corbett, M.D., "Cancer, Miscarriages and Birth Defects Associated with Operating Room Exposure," *Cancer and Chemicals,* Nelson-Hall, Inc., Chicago, 1976.   46. "Anesthesiologists Tend to Be Long Lived," *Journal of the American Medical Association,* November 28, 1977, p. 2340.   47. *Toxic Substances List.*   48. *Toxic Substances List.*   49. *A Consumer's Dictionary of Cosmetic Ingredients,* p. 33.   50. *Merck,* p. 86.   51. *Toxic Substances List.*   52. *Toxic Substances List.*   53. Alvin Segal, Ph.D., Charlene Katz, Ph.D., and Benjamin L. Van Duuren, Ph.D., *Journal of Medicinal Chemistry,* November 3, 1971.   54. "Report on Carcinogenesis Bioassay of Anthranilic Acid," HEW, Technical Report Series, no. 36, Washington, D.C., 1978.   55. *Merck,* p. 88.   56. *Toxic Substances List.*   57. *Toxic Substances List.*   58. "Report on Carcinogenesis Bioassay of Isophosphamide," HEW, Technical Report Series, no. 32, Washington, D.C., January 20, 1978.   59. *Toxicants in Foods,* p. 535.   60. *Merck,* p. 98.   61. *Toxic Substances List.*   62. "Bioassay of Aroclor 1254 for Possible Carcinogenicity," *Federal Register,* April 21, 1978.   63. *Health Hazards of the Human Environment,* WHO, Geneva, Switzerland, 1972, p. 223.   64. *Toxic Substances List.*   65. Richard K. Vitek of Bio-Metal Analysis Inc.; William C. Houser, M.D., of Milwaukee County Hospital; Stanton Deeley and James Bors of Wauwatosa, Wisconsin. Paper presented at the One hundred seventy-second National Meeting of the American Chemical Society, San Francisco, September 3, 1976.   66. "Arsenic: Poison Turned Carcinogen," *Science News,* September 7, 1974, p. 155.   67. *Cancer and the Worker,* New York Academy of Sciences, 1977, pp. 243–45.   68. *Toxic Substances List.*   69. *Toxic Substances List.*   70. E. Cuyler Hammond, Sc.D., and J. Selikoff, M. D., "Relation of Cigarette Smoking to Risk of Death of Asbestos-Associated Disease Among Insulation Workers in the United States," American Cancer Society report, 1978.   71. "Asbestos, An Occupational Environmental Hazard," *Journal of the American Medical Association,* August 17, 1970, p. 1249.   72. *Work Is Dangerous to Your Health,* pp. 178–79.   73. "Asbestos Exposure and Cancer Risk: Long Ago but Not Far Away," *Journal of the American Medical Association,* May 26, 1978, p. 2215.   74. "Asbestos: Environmental Time Bomb?" *Current Health,* September 1978, pp. 29–30.   75. Dr. Irving Selikoff, Waksman Institute of Microbiology. Symposium on carcinogens, Piscataway, N.J., November 8, 1978.   76. *Work Is Dangerous to Your Health,* pp. 202–3.   77. Anthony Polednak, Ph.D., "College Athletics, Body Size and Cancer Mortality," *Cancer,* vol. 38, 1976, pp. 382–87. 78. Michael B. Shimkin, M.D., *Science and Cancer,* OSHA, Washington, D.C., 1973.   79. N. Lee Wolfe, Ph.D., and Richard Zepp, Ph.D., of the EPA. Paper presented at the One hundred seventieth Annual Meeting of the American Chemical Society, August 26, 1975.   80. Gary Stoner et al.   81. "Are Auto Brakes a Danger to Health?" *University of California Clipsheet,* March 21, 1978.   82. Gary Stoner et al.   83. *Toxic Substances List.*   84. *Suspected Carcinogens.*   85. *Toxic Substances List.*   86. *Toxic Substances List.*   87. University of Notre Dame news report, February 6, 1978.   88. "Beef Believed Key Factor in Bowel Cancer," *Medical Tribune,* November 7, 1973, p. 4.   89. "Beef and Bowel Cancer," *Newsweek,* February 18, 1974, p. 80.   90. *Toxic Substances List.*   91. *Toxic Substances List.*   92. EPA news release, May 31, 1977.   93. *Wall Street Journal,* March 14, 1978.   94. *Science News,* October 8, 1977.   95. *Toxic Sub-*

stances List. **96.** "Carcinogens," Job Health Hazard Series, OSHA, Washington, D.C., pp. 11–12. **97.** *Toxic Substances List.* **98.** *U.S. Occupational Standard Carcinogens,* OSHA. **99.** "Carcinogens," Job Health Hazard Series, OSHA, Washington, D.C., p. 12. **100.** P. D. Moore, Ph.D., and M. Koreeda, Ph.D. Paper presented to the American Chemical Society, Chicago, September 1, 1977. **101.** *Toxic Substances List.* **102.** Inserm Symposia Series. **103.** *Work Is Dangerous to Your Health.* **104.** *Toxic Substances List.* **105.** *Chemical Dictionary,* p. 740. **106.** *Toxic Substances List.* **107.** *Toxic Substances List.* **108.** *Toxic Substances List* and *Chemical Dictionary,* p. 100. **109.** *Chemical Dictionary,* p. 138. **110.** *Toxic Substances List.* **111.** *Chemical Dictionary,* p. 101. **112.** *Toxic Substances List.* **113.** *Suspected Carcinogens.* **114.** *Suspected Carcinogens.* **115.** "Beryllium: Carcinogenicity Studies," *Science,* vol. 201, July 1978, pp. 298–99. **116.** *Toxic Substances List.* **117.** *U.S. Occupational Standard Carcinogens,* OSHA, 1975, pp. 13–14. **118.** "Chewers and Critics Gird for a Showdown in the Betel Battle." *Wall Street Journal,* February 8, 1978. **119.** *Toxic Substances List.* **120.** *Merck,* p. 150. **121.** "Carcinogens," Job Health Hazards Series, OSHA, Washington, D.C., 1975, p. 10. **122.** *Cancer and the Worker,* New York Academy of Sciences, New York, 1977, p. 24. **123.** *Toxic Substances List.* **124.** *Medical Information for Laymen,* Strang Clinic, New York, 1976. **125.** *Toxic Substances List.* **126.** *Consumer's Dictionary of Cosmetic Ingredients,* p. 48. **127.** *Toxic Substances List.* **128.** *Toxicants in Foods,* pp. 533–34. **129.** *Science News,* February 18, 1978, p. 104. **130.** Benjamin Rush, M.D., "To Health," New Jersey College of Medicine report, July 12, 1978. **131.** Frances Goodnight, "Breast Cancer Risk High in Sisters of Familial Disease Patient," *Medical Tribune,* April 17, 1974, p. 1. **132.** "Closer to the Cause of Breast Cancer?" *Medical World News,* December 3, 1971, pp. 15–18. **133.** *A Report to the Profession from the Breast Cancer Task Force,* HEW bulletin, Bethesda, Md., September 30, 1974. **134.** Brian E. Henderson, M.D., et al., "Elevated Serum Levels of Estrogen and Prolactin in Daughters of Patients with Breast Cancer," *New England Journal of Medicine,* October 16, 1975, pp. 100–105. **135.** "Factors That Influence Mammary Carcinogenesis," *New England Journal of Medicine,* May 1, 1975, p. 974. **136.** "Virus Found in Monkey Breast Cancer," *Journal of the American Medical Association,* May 4, 1970 , pp. 718–19. **137.** NCI, Office of Cancer Communication, Bethesda, Md., May 30, 1978. **138.** H. Stott et al., *British Medical Journal,* December 10, 1977, pp. 1513–1516. **139.** *Work Is Dangerous to Your Health,* p. 228. **140.** *Toxic Substances List.* **141.** *Suspected Carcinogens.* **142.** *Toxic Substances List.* **143.** *Toxic Substances List.* **144.** *Toxic Substances List.* **145.** *Suspected Carcinogens.* **146.** *Toxic Substances List.* **147.** EPA review report, November 4, 1977. **148.** Rob Warden and Ward Sinclair, "EPA in Dispute over Cadmium in Sludge," *Washington Post,* July 16, 1978. **149.** *Work Is Dangerous to Your Health,* p. 248. **150.** *Toxic Substances List.* **151.** *Suspected Carcinogens.* **152.** *Toxic Substances List.* **153.** *Toxic Substances List.* **154.** *Suspected Carcinogens.* **155.** *Toxic Substances List.* **156.** *Suspected Carcinogens.* **157.** *Toxicants in Foods,* p. 530. **158.** *Toxic Substances List.* **159.** *Toxic Substances List.* **160.** *Toxic Substances List.* **161.** *Merck,* p. 209. **162.** *Toxic Substances List.* **163.** *Suspected Carcinogens.* **164.** *A Consumer's Dictionary of Cosmetic Ingredients,* p. 58. **165.** *Toxicants in Foods,* p. 536. **166.** Padman Sarma, Robert J. Huebner et al., "Feline Leukemia and Sarcoma Viruses; Susceptibility of Human Cells to Infection," *Science,* May 1970, pp. 1098–1099. **167.** Glyn Caldwell, M.D., Chronic Diseases Division, Bureau of Epidemiology report, March 29, 1978. **168.** *Toxic Substances List.*

169. "Sex at an Early Age a Prime Factor in Cervical Cancer," University of Illinois at the Medical Center Campus, November 20, 1972. **170.** "Incidence of Cervical Cancer Related to Genital Secretions," The Institute of Community Studies, Inc., December 10, 1961. **171.** Arthur Upton, Ph.D., *Issues and Answers*—ABC Radio, December 25, 1977. **172.** The American Chemical Society News Service, June 29, 1976. **173.** *Medical World News,* May 8, 1970. **174.** *Toxic Substances List.* **175.** *Physicians' Desk Reference,* pp. 1240–1241. **176.** EPA news release, March 6, 1978. **177.** EPA news release, March 30, 1978. **178.** *Health Hazards of the Human Environment,* WHO, Geneva, Switzerland, 1972, p. 223. **179.** James Barron, EPA. Report before the American Chemical Society's Middle Atlantic Regional Meeting, Baltimore, April 5–7, 1978. **180.** Gary Eiceman et al., University of Colorado. Report before the American Chemical Society's Fourth Biennial Rocky Mountain Regional Meeting, June 6, 1978. **181.** *Merck,* p. 239. **182.** *Toxic Substances List.* **183.** *Suspected Carcinogens.* **184.** NIH, Cancer Communications Office announcement, October 17, 1978. **185.** EPA news release, February 13, 1979. **186.** HEW news release, June 10, 1976 and NIOSH *Recommended Standards,* August 14, 1975. **187.** *Merck,* p. 246. **188.** *Cancer and the Worker,* New York Academy of Sciences, New York, p. 28. **189.** *Physicians' Desk Reference,* p. 1582. **190.** Sigmund Deutscher, M.D., *Journal of the National Cancer Institute,* 1971, pp. 217–24. **191.** Fred Ederer et al., "Cancer Among Men on Cholesterol Lowering Diets," *The Lancet,* July 24, 1971. **192.** "Can You Predict When the Cure for Cancer Will Come Along," Jackson Laboratory report, Winter 1978. **193.** *Suspected Carcinogens.* **194.** *Toxic Substances List.* **195.** *Suspected Carcinogens.* **196.** Inserm Symposia Series, p. 249. **197.** *Toxic Substances List.* **198.** *Suspected Carcinogens.* **199.** American Lung Association report, May 15, 1978. **200.** W. Weiss, "Mortality of a Cohort Exposed to Chrysotile Asbestos," *Journal of Occupational Medicine,* November 1977, pp. 737–40. **201.** "Bioassay of C.I. Vat Yellow for Possible Carcinogenicity," NCI, Office of Cancer Communications, Bethesda, Md., December 1, 1978. **202.** Gary Stoner et al. **203.** "Narrowing the Search," ACS, 1961, p. 7. **204.** *Consumer's Dictionary of Food Additives,* p. 77. **205.** *Toxic Substances List.* **206.** *Work Is Dangerous to Your Health,* pp. 202–4. **207.** P. J. Lawther and R. E. Waller, "Coal Fires, Industrial Emissions and Motor Vehicles as Sources of Environmental Carcinogens," Inserm Symposia Series, pp. 27–40. **208.** *Toxicants in Foods,* p. 538. **209.** *Toxic Substances List.* **210.** *Toxicants in Foods,* p. 537. **211.** *Work Is Dangerous to Your Health,* p. 25. **212.** *City of Hope Quarterly,* vol. 7, Spring 1978. **213.** *Toxic Substances List.* **214.** William Cole, "The Cancer Nobody Talks About," *Family Circle,* July 10, 1978. **215.** *General Accounting Office Survey of Cosmetics,* presented to the House Subcommittee on Interstate and Foreign Commerce Oversight, February 3, 1978. **216.** *Newark Star-Ledger,* April 2, 1978. **217.** *Toxic Substances List.* **218.** *Toxic Substances List.* **219.** Michael B. Shimkin, M.D., *Contrary to Nature,* HEW, Washington, D.C., p. 345. **220.** *Toxic Substances List.* **221.** *Federal Register,* October 27, 1978. **222.** *Toxicants in Foods,* p. 531. **223.** *Physicians' Desk Reference,* p. 1097. **224.** "Report on Carcinogenesis Bioassay of Dapsone," HEW, Technical Report Series, no. 20, Washington, D.C., 1977. **225.** "Drug Tested on Troops in Vietnam Is Found to Cause Cancer in Rats," *New York Times,* December 6, 1977. **226.** *Toxic Substances List.* **227.** *Suspected Carcinogens.* **228.** *Federal Register,* February 28, 1978. **229.** EPA news release, October 28, 1977. **230.** *New York Times,* July 13, 1972. **231.** *Journal of the American Medical Association,* August 23, 1971. **232.** *Toxic Substances List.* **233.** Gary Stoner et al. **234.** *American Medical News,*

March 20, 1978. **235.** *Physicians' Desk Reference,* p. 1697. **236.** Cesare Maltoni, "Occupational Chemical Carcinogenesis; New Facts, Priorities and Perspectives," Inserm Symposia Series, pp. 127–50. **237.** FDA *Bulletin,* March–April 1978. **238.** *Toxic Substances List.* **239.** "Report on Carcinogenesis Bioassay of 2,4-Diaminoanisole Sulfate," HEW, Technical Background Information Series, Bethesda, Md., April 18, 1978. **240.** "Report on Carcinogenesis Bioassay of Diarylanilide Yellow," HEW, Technical Report Series, no. 30, Washington, D.C., 1978. **241.** *Toxic Substances List.* **242.** *Physicians' Desk Reference,* p. 1563. **243.** Gary Stoner et al. **244.** "Carcinogens," Job Health Hazards Series, OSHA, Washington, D.C., 1975, pp. 8–9. **245.** "Animal Tests of 2,7-Dichlorodibenzo-p-Dioxin for Cancer-Causing Activity," *Federal Register,* February 13, 1979. **246.** "Report on Carcinogenesis Bioassay of Dichlorvos," HEW, Technical Report Series, no. 10, Washington, D.C., 1977. **247.** *Toxic Substances List.* **248.** *Toxic Substances List.* **249.** NCI, Office of Cancer Communications, Bethesda, Md., May 30, 1978. **250.** "Report on Carcinogenesis Bioassay of Dieldrin," HEW, Technical Report Series, no. 22, Washington, D.C., 1978. **251.** *New York Times,* November 13, 1977. **252.** *Toxic Substances List.* **253.** *Toxic Substances List.* **254.** "Bioassay of N,N'-Diethylthiourea for Possible Carcinogenicity," NIH, Washington, D.C., November 17, 1978. **255.** *Journal of the American Medical Association,* May 5, 1978, p. 1849. **256.** "Report on Carcinogenesis Bioassay of Dimethoate," HEW, Technical Report Series, no. 4, Washington, D.C., January 1977. **257.** "Tests of 3,3'-Dimethoxybenzidine-4,4'-Diisocyanate for Cancer-Causing Activity by the National Cancer Institute," *Federal Register,* January 9, 1979. **258.** "Carcinogens," Job Health Hazards Series, OSHA, Washington, D.C., 1975, p. 15. **259.** Michael B. Shimkin, M.D., *Contrary to Nature,* HEW, Washington, D.C., 1977, p. 399. **260.** *Chemical Dictionary,* p. 310. **261.** *Toxic Substances List.* **262.** *Federal Register,* May 1978. **263.** *Merck,* p. 384. **264.** *Toxic Substances List.* **265.** Dr. Barry Commoner, "Toxicologic Time Bomb," *Hospital Practice,* June 1978, p. 56. **266.** University of Illinois Medical Center Campus research report, February 14, 1979. **267.** *Merck,* p. 387. **268.** *Toxic Substances List.* **269.** *Work Is Dangerous to Your Health,* pp. 192, 265. **270.** *Toxic Substances List.* **271.** NIOSH and NCI *Current Intelligence Bulletin 24,* HEW, Rockville and Bethesda, Md., April 17, 1978. **272.** *Physicians' Desk Reference,* p. 591. **273.** Ralph Yodaiken, M.D., "Ethylene Dibromide and Disulfiram —A Lethal Combination," *Journal of the American Medical Association,* June 30, 1978, p. 2783. **274.** *Federal Register,* January 26, 1979. **275.** *Toxic Substances List.* **276.** *Toxic Substances List.* **277.** Philippe Shubik, "Potential Carcinogenicity of Food Additives and Contaminants," *Cancer Research,* vol. 35, November 1975, pp. 3475–3480. **278.** *Work Is Dangerous to Your Health,* pp. 167–81. **279.** *The Post,* Frederick, Md., May 31, 1978. **280.** Lowell Ponte, *The Killer Electric,* June 1978. **281.** "Report on Carcinogenesis Bioassay of Emetine," HEW, Technical Report Series, no. 43, Washington, D.C., 1978. **282.** "Emotion and Cancer," *Medical World News,* December 12, 1978, p. 108. **283.** *Frontiers of Clinical Psychiatry,* published by Hoffmann-La Roche Inc., June 1, 1969. **284.** *Science,* vol. 200, June 23, 1978. **285.** Saul Gusberg, M.D., "Postmenopausal Estrogens and Endometrial Cancer," *CA: A Cancer Journal for Clinicians,* January/February 1977, pp. 47–49. **286.** "Estrogen Is Linked to Uterine Cancer," *New York Times,* December 4, 1975. **287.** Laman A. Gray, Sr., M.D., et al., "Estrogens and Endometrial Carcinoma," *Obstetrics and Gynecology,* vol. 49, pp. 385–89, 1977. **288.** HEW news release, June 9, 1978. **289.** *A Consumer's Dictionary of Food Additives,* p. 96. **290.** *Wall Street Journal,* December 6, 1978.

291. *Science News,* December 9, 1978. 292. Eugene Cliffton, M.D., "The Diagnosis and Treatment of Esophageal Cancer," *CA: A Cancer Journal For Clinicians,* 1976, pp. 107–9. 293. Harold Schmeck, Jr., "Chinese Study Involving Chickens Links Cancer to Food of Humans," *New York Times,* November 9, 1977. 294. "Chasing Chinese Chicken Cancer," *Science News,* November 19, 1977, pp. 342–43. 295. Janez Kmet and Ezattollah Mahboubi, "Esophageal Cancer in the Caspian Littoral of Iran," *Science,* February 25, 1972, pp. 175–78. 296. Gary Stoner et al. 297. Elwood V. Jensen, Ph.D., editorial, *New England Journal of Medicine,* vol. 291, July 27, 1978. 298. Johanna Perlmutter, M.D., *The Medical Forum,* May 1978. 299. Special Communication National Cancer Program, May 22, 1978. 300. "Estrogens and Cancer Change the Way You Treat Postmenopausal Patients," *Modern Medicine,* March 1, 1977. 301. *Physicians' Desk Reference,* supplement A, pp. A56–58. 302. *Toxic Substances List.* 303. *Toxicants in Foods,* p. 525. 304. *Toxic Substances List.* 305. *Toxic Substances List.* 306. *Federal Register,* August 9, 1977. 307. "Report on Carcinogenesis Bioassay of 1,2-Dibromoethane (EDB), HEW, Technical Background Information Series, Bethesda, Md., November 14, 1978. 308. "Report on Carcinogenesis Bioassay of 1,2-Dichloroethane," HEW, Technical Background Information Series, Bethesda, Md., September 26, 1978. 309. *Consumer's Dictionary of Cosmetic Ingredients,* p. 104. 310. *Toxic Substances List.* 311. *Federal Register,* June 23, 1978. 312. *U.S. Occupational Standard Carcinogens,* OSHA, 1975. 313. "Medical News," *Journal of the American Medical Association,* July 4, 1977, pp. 19–20. 314. Robert W. Miller, M.D., "Bedside Etiology of Childhood Cancer," *CA: A Cancer Journal for Clinicians,* vol. 27, September/October 1977, pp. 273–80. 315. *Merck,* p. 717. 316. *Medical World News,* October 17, 1977. 317. *Modern Medicine,* June 15, 1977. 318. *The Lancet,* March 6, 1971. 319. The American Chemical Society News Service, August 31, 1977. 320. *Journal of the American Medical Association,* vol. 239, January 30, 1978. 321. *A Consumer's Dictionary of Food Additives,* p. 109. 322. *Toxic Substances List.* 323. *A Consumer's Dictionary of Food Additives,* pp. 108–9. 324. EPA news release, July 10, 1978. 325. *Consumer's Dictionary of Food Additives,* p. 137. 326. *Toxic Substances List.* 327. *Toxic Substances List.* 328. University of Illinois news release, June 8, 1978. 329. *Work Is Dangerous to Your Health,* p. 175. 330. Paul Shinoff, "Insulate Your Lungs—Use Fiber Glass," *New York Times,* September 30, 1977. 331. NCI news release, January 3, 1972. 332. Deedee Pendleton, "Fish Tumors, Carcinogenic Indicators?" *Science News,* vol. 107, March 8, 1975, pp. 157–58. 333. University of Health Sciences, University of Chicago Medical School report, June 5, 1978. 334. *Physicians' Desk Reference,* p. 1547. 335. *Toxic Substances List.* 336. *Toxic Substances List.* 337. *Toxic Substances List.* 338. American Dental Association News, October 3, 1977. 339. *Physicians' Desk Reference,* p. 1387. 340. *Toxic Substances List.* 341. *Toxic Substances List.* 342. *Toxic Substances List.* 343. *Toxic Substances List.* 344. *Toxic Substances List.* 345. *Occupational Cancer,* WHO, no. 23, December 1972. 346. *Toxicants in Foods,* p. 515. 347. Warren Bontoyan and Jack Looker, EPA. American Chemical Society presentation, August 31, 1973. 348. *Toxic Substances List.* 349. *Toxic Substances List.* 350. *Toxic Substances List.* 351. *Toxicants in Foods,* p. 521. 352. *Physicians' Desk Reference,* p. 1081. 353. *Toxic Substances List.* 354. *Suspected Carcinogens.* 355. *Toxic Substances List.* 356. S. Venitt and C. E. Searle, "Mutagenicity and Possible Carcinogenicity of Hair Colourants and Constituents," Inserm Symposia Series, p. 263. 357. Jane E. Brody, *New York Times,* November 9, 1978, p. A14. 358. *A Consumer's Dictionary of Cosmetic Ingredi-*

ents, pp. 123–24.   **359.** *Cancer News,* ACS, vol. 32, Spring 1978.   **360.** University of Notre Dame news report, February 6, 1978.   **361.** *Medical World News,* June 12, 1978.   **362.** John Weisburger, M.D., "Cooking Methods and Cancer." Paper presented at the American Health Foundation Conference on Nutritional Factors and Cancer, Oregon, June 29, 1978.   **363.** *Toxic Substances List.*   **364.** Susan Fogg, "Hepatitis Virus May Surface as Cancer Link," *Newark Star-Ledger,* March 11, 1978.   **365.** "Report on Carcinogenesis Bioassay of Heptachlor," HEW, Technical Report Series, no. 9, Washington, D.C., September 23, 1978. **366.** Jane E. Brody, *You Can Fight Cancer and Win,* McGraw Hill, New York, 1977, pp. 259–61.   **367.** "Scientists Recommend Dropping Dye-Light Treatment of Herpes Infections," National Institute Research Advances report, October 25, 1975.   **368.** National Academy of Sciences news report, August 1978, p. 4.   **369.** Henry Trochimowicz, Sc.D., Du Pont de Nemours. "Steps Taken to Protect Workers Against Hexymethylphosphoramide." Paper presented at the American Occupational Health Conference, Anaheim, Calif., May 1, 1979.   **370.** *Toxic Substances List.*   **371.** *Consumer's Dictionary of Cosmetic Ingredients,* p. 131.   **372.** The American Chemical Society News Service, November 1, 1977. **373.** *Science News,* vol. 112, November 5, 1977.   **374.** *Toxic Substances List.* **375.** *News from NIH,* March 1, 1972.   **376.** Mortimer Lipsett, M.D., "Estrogen Use and Cancer Risk," *Journal of the American Medical Association,* March 14, 1977.   **377.** Elwood V. Jensen, Ph.D., "Some Newer Aspects of Breast Cancer," *New England Journal of Medicine,* vol. 291, October 8, 1974.   **378.** *Medical World News,* May 1977, pp. 222–23.   **379.** Michael B. Shimkin, M.D., *Science and Cancer,* OSHA, Washington, D.C., 1973.   **380.** "Household Products and Industrial Chemicals," *Chemicals and Health.* Report of the panel on Chemicals and Health, President's Science Advisory Committee, September 1973, p. 77.   **381.** *Medical World News,* July 10, 1978, p. 41.   **382.** *Toxic Substances List.*   **383.** *Toxic Substances List.*   **384.** *Toxic Substances List.*   **385.** *Toxic Substances List.*   **386.** *Consumer's Dictionary of Cosmetic Ingredients,* p. 135.   **387.** *Toxic Substances List.*   **388.** Gary Stoner et al.   **389.** HEW news release, October 25, 1974.   **390.** Harvard University news release, April 15, 1971.   **391.** *Physicians' Desk Reference,* p. 718.   **392.** *Toxic Substances List.*   **393.** *Toxic Substances List.*   **394.** *Chemical Dictionary,* p. 742.   **395.** "Report on Carcinogenesis Bioassay on IPD," HEW, Technical Report Series, no. 18, Washington, D.C., 1978. **396.** *Physicians' Desk Reference,* p. 1176.   **397.** *Suspected Carcinogens.*   **398.** *Toxic Substances List.*   **399.** *Suspected Carcinogens.*   **400.** *Physicians' Desk Reference,* p. 770.   **401.** *Toxic Substances List.*   **402.** *Merck,* p. 586.   **403.** *Toxic Substances List.*   **404.** "Report on Carcinogenesis Bioassay of Isophosphamide," HEW, Technical Report Series, no. 32, Washington, D.C., 1977.   **405.** *Occupational Cancer,* WHO, no. 23, December 1972.   **406.** Philippe Shubik, "Potential Carcinogenicity of Food Additives and Contaminants," *Cancer Research,* vol. 35, November 1975, pp. 3475–3480.   **407.** *Toxic Substances List.*   **408.** The American Chemical Society News Service, September 16, 1971.   **409.** "Report on Carcinogenesis Bioassay of Technical Grade Chlordecone (Kepone)," HEW, Technical Background Information Series, Bethesda, Md., January 1976.   **410.** National Academy of Science news report, August 1978, p. 4.   **411.** *Toxic Substances List.* **412.** *Physicians' Desk Reference,* p. 1339.   **413.** Barbara Scherr Trenk, American Lung Association bulletin, May 1977, p. 4.   **414.** *Toxic Substances List.*   **415.** "Report on Carcinogenesis Bioassay of Lasiocarpine," HEW, Technical Report Series, no. 39, Washington, D.C., 1978.   **416.** *Chemical Dictionary,* p. 502.   **417.** *Toxic Substances List.*   **418.** *Toxicants in Foods,* p. 538.   **419.** *Toxic Sub-*

stances List. **420.** *Toxic Substances List.* **421.** *Toxic Substances List.* **422.** *Toxic Substances List.* **423.** *Merck,* p. 621. **424.** *Toxic Substances List.* **425.** *SEER Program: Cancer Incidence and Mortality in the U.S.,* 1973–76, HEW, Bethesda, Md., October 20, 1978. **426.** *Cancer Rates and Risks,* 2d ed., HEW, Washington, D.C., 1974. **427.** *Toxicants in Foods,* pp. 515–16. **428.** *Toxic Substances List.* **429.** *Federal Register,* March 24, 1978. **430.** *Toxic Substances List.* **431.** EPA news release, November 4, 1977. **432.** R. J. Shamberger, B. A. Shamberger, and C. E. Willis, "Malonaldehyde Content of Food," *Journal of Nutrition,* vol. 107, 1977, pp. 1401–1419. **433.** *Toxic Substances List.* **434.** *American Medical News,* March 20, 1978. **435.** *Medical World News,* May 1, 1978. **436.** *Toxic Substances List.* **437.** *Physicians' Desk Reference,* p. 1102. **438.** *Suspected Carcinogens.* **439.** David Stein, M.D., et al., "Melanomas of the Skin," *Journal of the New Jersey Medical Society,* May 1978, pp. 391–92. **440.** *Merck Manual,* 11th ed., Merck, Sharp and Dohme Research Laboratories, Rahway, N.J., pp. 1481–1482. **441.** *Suspected Carcinogens.* **442.** *Toxic Substances List.* **443.** *Toxic Substances List.* **444.** *Toxicants in Foods,* p. 538. **445.** *Toxic Substances List.* **446.** *Suspected Carcinogens.* **447.** "FDA Intends to Ban Cancer-Linked Item," *Wall Street Journal,* June 13, 1978. **448.** *Physicians' Desk Reference,* p. 1014. **449.** *Toxic Substances List.* **450.** *Toxic Substances List.* **451.** *Physicians' Desk Reference,* p. 954. **452.** "Report on Carcinogenesis Bioassay of Methoxychlor," HEW, Technical Background Information Series, Bethesda, Md., March 21, 1978. **453.** "Carcinogens," Job Health Hazards Series, OSHA, Washington, D.C., 1975. pp. 7–8. **454.** "Carcinogens," Job Health Hazards Series, OSHA, Washington, D.C., 1975, p. 7. **455.** *Wall Street Journal,* July 19, 1978. **456.** *Toxic Substances List.* **457.** "Report on Carcinogenesis Bioassay of 2-Methyl-1-Nitroanthraquinone," HEW, Technical Report Series, no. 29, Washington, D.C., 1978. **458.** *Merck,* p. 693. **459.** *Toxic Substances List.* **460.** *Science News,* vol. 96, October 25, 1969. **461.** *Science News,* April 12, 1978. **462.** *New York Times,* April 14, 1978. **463.** *New York Times,* March 6, 1978. **464.** World Book Science Service, March 8, 1970. **465.** *Work Is Dangerous to Your Health,* p. 63. **466.** *Occupational Cancer,* WHO, no. 23, December 1973. **467.** C. Thony et al., "Hydrocarbures Polycycliques Aromatiques Cancérogènes dans les Produits Pétroliers Prévention Possibles du Cancer des Huiles Minérales," Inserm Symposia Series, pp. 165–70. **468.** *Toxic Substances List.* **469.** National Academy of Sciences news report, August 1978, p. 4. **470.** *Toxicants in Foods,* p. 523. **471.** *Merck,* p. 703. **472.** *Toxic Substances List.* **473.** "Cancer From Mushrooms?" *Science News,* vol. 114, July 15, 1978. **474.** I. T. T. Higgins, "Epidemiological Evidence on the Carcinogenic Risk of Air Pollution," Inserm Symposia Series, p. 42. **475.** "Carcinogens," Job Health Hazard Series, OSHA, Washington, D.C., 1975, p. 6. **476.** *Merck,* p. 717. **477.** *Toxic Substances List.* **478.** *Merck,* p. 717. **479.** *Merck,* p. 717. **480.** *Toxic Substances List.* **481.** *Toxic Substances List.* **482.** *Suspected Carcinogens.* **483.** *Suspected Carcinogens.* **484.** *Suspected Carcinogens.* **485.** *Toxic Substances List.* **486.** *Toxic Substances List.* **487.** *Suspected Carcinogens.* **488.** *Suspected Carcinogens.* **489.** *Toxic Substances List.* **490.** *Work Is Dangerous to Your Health,* p. 214. **491.** *Suspected Carcinogens.* **492.** *Toxic Substances List.* **493.** *Suspected Carcinogens.* **494.** *Toxic Substances List.* **495.** *Suspected Carcinogens.* **496.** *Toxic Substances List.* **497.** *Toxic Substances List.* **498.** *Merck,* p. 717. **499.** *Toxic Substances List.* **500.** *Toxic Substances List.* **501.** *Environmental Pollution and Carcinogenic Risk,* WHO, France, 1976. **502.** *Toxicants in Foods,* p. 538. **503.** *Toxic Substances List.* **504.** *Toxic Substances List.* **505.** *Toxic*

Substances List. **506.** A Consumer's Dictionary of Food Additives, p. 168. **507.** Federal Register, October 31, 1978. **508.** Federal Register, October 24, 1978. **509.** "Carcinogens," Job Health Hazards Series, OSHA, Washington, D.C., 1975, p. 5. **510.** "Report on Carcinogenesis Bioassay of Nitrofen," HEW, Technical Report Series, no. 26, Washington, D.C., 1978. **511.** Physicians' Desk Reference, p. 840. **512.** FDA Consumer, December 1978–January 1979, p. 7. **513.** Michael B. Shimkin, M.D., Contrary to Nature, HEW, Washington, D.C., 1977, p. 401. **514.** Toxic Substances List. **515.** Toxic Substances List. **516.** "Report of the National Cancer Institute's Test on 2-nitro-p-phenylenediamine," Federal Register, January 9, 1979. **517.** NCI, Office of Cancer Communications, Bethesda, Md., May 19, 1978. **518.** U. Morh and J. Hilfrich, "Effects of a Single Dose of N-Diethynitrosamine on the Rat Kidney," Journal of the National Cancer Institute, 1972, pp. 1729–1731. **519.** Deborah Shapley, "Nitrosamines; Scientists on the Trail of Prime Suspect in Urban Cancer," Science, January 23, 1976, pp. 266–67. **520.** "Carcinogens," Job Health Hazards Series, OSHA, Washington, D.C., 1975, p. 16. **521.** Toxic Substances List. **522.** Toxic Substances List. **523.** Michael B. Shimkin, M.D., Science and Cancer, OSHA, Washington, D.C., 1973. **524.** "Study Reportedly Links Leukemia to Bomb Test," New York Times, February 14, 1979. **525.** "4,300 Sheep Near Nevada Nuclear Tests Died in '53," New York Times, February 15, 1979. **526.** Toxic Substances List. **527.** Thomas Maugh II, "Carcinogens in the Workplace: Where to Start Cleaning Up," Science, September 23, 1977, pp. 1268–1269. **528.** Toxic Substances List. **529.** Consumer's Dictionary of Food Additives, p. 173. **530.** Toxic Substances List. **531.** Science News, vol. 113, no. 20, May 20, 1978. **532.** Washington Star, June 21, 1978. **533.** Physicians' Desk Reference, p. 1646. **534.** Toxic Substances List. **535.** Toxic Substances List. **536.** "Bioassay of Parathion for Possible Carcinogenicity," NCI, Office of Cancer Communications, Bethesda, Md., November 28, 1978. **537.** Joseph D. Rosen, M.D., and Stephen Pareles, M.D., "An Improved Method to Measure Patulin," Journal of Agricultural and Food Chemistry, November 26, 1974. **538.** Dr. Yvonne Greichus et al. Paper presented at the One-hundred seventy-second National Meeting of the American Chemical Society, San Francisco, September 3, 1976. **539.** EPA news release, June 7, 1978; April 27, 1978. **540.** Dr. Ralph Doughtery and Krystyna Piotrowskia, Florida State University. Paper presented before the American Chemical Society, August 28, 1975. **541.** Toxic Substances List. **542.** Toxic Substances List. **543.** Toxic Substances List. **544.** Merck, p. 670. **545.** Toxic Substances List. **546.** Toxic Substances List. **547.** Science, June 23, 1978, p. 1363. **548.** Science News, vol. 108, September 20, 1975. **549.** "Report on Animal Tests of p,p'-Ethyl-DDD for Cancer-Causing Activity," Federal Register, February 13, 1979. **550.** EPA news release, February 15, 1978. **551.** Work Is Dangerous to Your Health, pp. 221–23. **552.** National Research Council news report, November 16, 1977. **553.** Minnesota Science, vol. 32, Fall 1976. **554.** Southeast Farm Press, November 23, 1977. **555.** Toxic Substances List. **556.** Memorial Sloan-Kettering News, February 11, 1978. **557.** Miles R. Chedekel, Ph.D., R. M. Deibel, Ph.D., and M. Kalus, Ph.D., Ohio State Medical College, "Destruction of the Human Pigment by Ultra-Violet Light." Paper presented at the American Chemical Society meeting, August 29, 1977. **558.** "Urinary Tumors Linked to Abuse of Phenacetin," Medical Tribune, February 16, 1974. **559.** "Phenacetin Studies, Pedro Cuatre Casas, Wellcome Research Laboratories," Science, January 5, 1979. **560.** Toxic Substances List. **561.** Toxic Substances List. **562.** Gary Stoner et al. **563.** "Report on Carcinogenesis of Bioassay of Phenformin," HEW, Technical Report Series, no. 7, Washington, D.C., January 1977.   **564.** *Consumer's Dictionary of Cosmetic Ingredients,* p. 181.   **565.** *Toxic Substances List.*   **566.** *Consumer's Dictionary of Cosmetic Ingredients,* p. 182.   **567.** *Toxic Substances List.*   **568.** *Suspected Carcinogens.* **569.** *Toxic Substances List.*   **570.** "Report on Carcinogenesis Bioassay of Photodieldrin," HEW, Technical Report Series, no. 17, Washington, D.C., 1977. **571.** *Federal Register,* February 7, 1978.   **572.** National Cancer Program special communication, May 22, 1978.   **573.** Dr. Johanna Perlmutter, *The Medical Forum,* May 1978.   **574.** *Physicians' Desk Reference,* supplement A, 1978, pp. A56–58.   **575.** "High Hematoma Risk for Women on Pill Four Years or More," *Medical World News,* July 24, 1978.   **576.** "Bioassay for Possible Carcinogenicity of Piperonyl Sulfoxide," NCI, Office of Cancer Communications, Bethesda, Md., December 1, 1978.   **577.** *Federal Register,* October 31, 1978.   **578.** *Harvard University Morning,* no. 53, January 17, 1964.   **579.** Dr. Roland E. Lehr et al. Paper presented before the American Chemical Society Meeting, March 21, 1978. **580.** *Toxic Substances List.*   **581.** *Toxic Substances List.*   **582.** *Consumer's Dictionary of Food Additives,* p. 192.   **583.** *Toxic Substances List.*   **584.** *Health Hazards of the Human Environment,* WHO, Geneva, Switzerland, 1972, pp. 222–23. **585.** *Toxic Substances List.*   **586.** *Toxic Substances List.*   **587.** Robert J. Rubin, *Chemical and Engineering News,* February 17, 1971.   **588.** *Toxic Substances List.* **589.** *Consumer's Dictionary of Food Additives,* p. 192.   **590.** Simon Soumeral, M.D., "Pseudo-Tumors of the Arm Following Injections of Polyvinyl Pyrrolidinone," *Journal of the Medical Society of New Jersey,* May 1978, pp. 407–08.   **591.** Jane E. Brody, *You Can Fight Cancer and Win,* McGraw-Hill, New York, 1977, p. 76.   **592.** Robert W. Miller, M.D., "Bedside Etiology of Childhood Cancer," *CA: A Cancer Journal for Clinicians,* vol. 27, no. 5, September/October 1977, pp. 273–80.   **593.** H. King, "Cancer Risk and Life-Style." Paper presented at the meeting of the American Association for the Advancement of Science, Boston, Mass., February 1976.   **594.** "Report on Carcinogenesis Bioassay of Proflavine," HEW, Technical Report Series, no. 5, Washington, D.C., 1977.   **595.** *Physicians' Desk Reference,* pp. 1720–1721.   **596.** Dr. Ernest Wynder, "Nutrition and Cancer," *Federation Proceedings,* vol. 35, 1977, p. 1309.   **597.** EPA *Review of Herbicide Used with Lettuce and Alfalfa,* January 15, 1979.   **598.** Gary Stoner et al.   **599.** *Toxic Substances List.*   **600.** *Toxic Substances List.*   **601.** *Science,* vol. 200, June 9, 1978.   **602.** "Prostate Cancer," *CA: A Cancer Journal for Clinicians,* vol. 28, no. 2, March/April 1978.   **603.** "Diet, Nutrition, and Cancer," *The American Journal of Clinical Nutrition,* September 1976.   **604.** *Federal Register,* May 12, 1978.   **605.** *Toxic Substances List.*   **606.** *Suspected Carcinogens.*   **607.** *Physicians' Desk Reference,* pp. 715–16.   **608.** Gary Stoner et al.   **609.** *Toxicants in Food,* pp. 527–28.   **610.** *Toxic Substances List.*   **611.** *Toxic Substances List.* **612.** *Merck,* p. 901.   **613.** *Toxic Substances List.*   **614.** *Toxic Substances List.* **615.** *Toxic Substances List.*   **616.** *Federal Register,* January 26, 1979.   **617.** *South Bay Daily Breeze,* March 24, 1970.   **618.** "Fallout: Its Effects on Air, Water and Foods," *Science News,* August 21, 1962.   **619.** *Medical World News,* September 11, 1970.   **620.** *Journal of the American Medical Association,* vol. 239, May 5, 1978.   **621.** Vilma Hunt, Pennsylvania State University, "Radiation Exposure and Protection." Paper presented before the Occupational Health Association, 1978.   **622.** *Medical Tribune,* vol. 3, 1962.   **623.** The American Chemical Society News Service, September 17, 1977.   **624.** HEW, Public Health Service, National Center for Radiological Health, April 24, 1968.   **625.** *Science News,* vol. 113, March 4, 1978.   **626.** *Journal of the American Medical Association,* vol. 228, June 10, 1974.   **627.** "The Carcinogenic Effect of Antenatal Radiography and Some

Implications," Inserm Symposia Series. **628.** Stephen Zemelman, *Nuclear Information, Radiation and Childhood Cancer,* Greater St. Louis Committee for Nuclear Information, 1973. **629.** *New York Times,* January 25, 1978. **630.** *Work Is Dangerous to Your Health,* pp. 18, 36, 132, 133, 134, 145–53, 227. **631.** *Occupational Cancer Feature,* HEW, December 1972. **632.** *Cancer and the Worker,* New York Academy of Sciences, New York, 1977, pp. 39–40. **633.** "Radiation Dose Estimates from Timepieces Containing Tritium or Promethium-147 in Radioluminous Paints," NUREG/CRO216m, January 24, 1979. **634.** Hyman Fisher et al., "Validity of Radiation Protection Standards," *Journal of the Medical Society of New Jersey,* November 1961, pp. 536–37. **635.** *Wall street Journal,* September 23, 1974. **636.** *Physicians' Desk Reference,* pp. 576, 774, 1151. **637.** *Suspected Carcinogens.* **638.** *Toxic Substances List.* **639.** *Toxic Substances List.* **640.** *Medical World News,* September 6, 1974. **641.** H. King, "Cancer Risks and Life-Style." Paper presented at the meeting of the American Association for the Advancement of Science, Boston, Mass., February 1976. **642.** Robert Batzinger et al., "Saccharin añd Other Sweeteners, Mutagenic Properties," *Science,* December 2, 1977, pp. 942–46. **643.** Hazel B. Matthews, Minerva Fields, and Lawrence Fishbein, "Saccharin Distribution and Excretion of a Limited Dose in Rat," *Journal of Agricultural Food Chemistry,* vol. 21, 1973. **644.** *Toxicants in Foods,* p. 535. **645.** *Toxic Substances List.* **646.** H. King, "Cancer Risk and Life-Style." Paper presented at meeting of the American Association for the Advancement of Science, Boston, Mass., February 1976. **647.** *Toxic Substances List.* **648.** "Silica May Cause Cancer, Study Shows," UCLA news release, May 24, 1974. **649.** *Toxic Substances List.* **650.** *Merck,* p. 436. **651.** *Suspected Carcinogens.* **652.** "Cancer of the Skin," *Medical Information for Laymen,* Preventive Medicine Institute, Strang Clinic, New York, 1976. **653.** "New Mexico Out to Detect, Prevent Skin Cancers," *Journal of the American Medical Association,* May 4, 1978, p. 184. **654.** "The Development of an Engineering Control Research and Development Plan for Carcinogenic Materials," *Science,* September 23, 1978, p. 1268. **655.** *Toxic Substances List.* **656.** *Cancer and the Worker,* The New York Academy of Sciences, New York, 1977. **657.** *Toxicants in Foods.* **658.** *Toxic Substances List.* **659.** *Merck,* p. 986. **660.** *Toxic Substances List.* **661.** *Work Is Dangerous to Your Health,* pp. 132–36. **662.** *Toxic Substances List.* **663.** Gary Eiceman et al., University of Colorado. Report before the American Chemical Society's Fourth Biennial Rocky Mountain Regional Meeting, June 6, 1978. **664.** *Toxic Substances List.* **665.** *Toxicants in Foods,* p. 536. **666.** *Physicians' Desk Reference,* pp. 1192–1193. **667.** *Toxic Substances List.* **668.** FDA *Consumer,* May 1974. **669.** *Emergency Medicine,* August 1977. **670.** *Modern Medicine,* September 30, 1977. **671.** *Toxicants in Foods,* pp. 535–36. **672.** Philippe Shubik, "Potential Carcinogenicity of Food Additives and Contaminants," *Cancer Research,* vol. 35, November 1975, pp. 3475–3480. **673.** EPA news release, April 12, 1978. **674.** *Toxic Substances List.* **675.** *Toxic Substances List.* **676.** *Suspected Carcinogens.* **677.** *Toxic Substances List.* **678.** "Report on Carcinogenesis Bioassay of Tetrachloroethane," HEW, Technical Report Series, no. 27, Washington, D.C., 1978. **679.** "Report on Carcinogenesis Bioassay of Tetrachloroethylene," HEW, Technical Report Series, no. 13, Washington, D.C., 1977. **680.** "Report on Carcinogenesis Bioassay of Tetrachloromethane," HEW, Technical Background Information Series, Bethesda, Md., 1978. **681.** *Cancer and the Worker,* New York Academy of Sciences, New York, 1977, p. 41. **682.** *Merck,* p. 1031. **683.** *Science,* September 23, 1977, p. 1269. **684.** *Toxic Substances List.* **685.** *Toxic Substances List.* **686.** *Suspected Carcinogens.* **687.** Gary Stoner et al. **688.** Philippe Shubik, "Potential Carcinogenicity of Food Additives and Contaminants," *Cancer Research,* vol. 35, November 1975, pp. 3475–3480. **689.** *Toxic Substances List.* **690.** *Merck,* p. 1048. **691.** *The Harvard Medical School Health Letter,* vol. III, no. 7, May 1978. **692.** *CA: A Cancer Journal for Clinicians,* vol. 28, no. 2, March/April 1978. **693.** *Toxic Substances List.* **694.** American Cancer Society News Service, January 31, 1978. **695.** *New York Times,* February 19, 1978. **696.** *Federal Register,* December 9, 1977. **697.** Gary Eiceman et al., University of Colorado. Report before the American Chemical Society's Fourth Biennial Meeting, Rocky Mountain Regional Meeting, June 6, 1978. **698.** *Merck,* p. 1058. **699.** *Work Is Dangerous to Your Health,* pp. 39, 190. **700.** *Toxic Substances List.* **701.** *Merck,* p. 1058. **702.** *Chemical Dictionary,* p. 869. **703.** *Chemical Dictionary,* p. 869. **704.** *Federal Register,* January 26, 1979. **705.** *Toxic Substances List.* **706.** *Chemical Dictionary,* p. 870. **707.** *Toxic Substances List.* **708.** "Report on Carcinogenesis Bioassay of Toxaphene," HEW, Technical Background Information Series, Bethesda, Md., March 16, 1979. **709.** *On the Threshold of a New Environmental Era,* EPA bulletin, April 1978. **710.** Federation of American Societies for Experimental Biology, Fifty-fifth Annual Meeting, April 13, 1976. **711.** *Science News,* vol. 111, January 15, 1977. **712.** *Toxic Substances List.* **713.** *Suspected Carcinogens.* **714.** *Toxic Substances List.* **715.** "Report on Carcinogenesis Bioassay of Trichloroethylene," HEW, Technical Report Series, no. 2, June 14, 1976. **716.** *Suspected Carcinogens.* **717.** *Toxic Substances List.* **718.** *Toxic Substances List.* **719.** "Report on Carcinogenesis Bioassay of Trifluralin," HEW, Technical Report Series, no. 34, Washington, D.C., 1978. **720.** "Bioassay of Trimethylthiourea for Possible Carcinogenicity," NCI Office of Cancer Communications, Bethesda, Md., November 21, 1978. **721.** The American Chemical Society News Service, May 27, 1977. **722.** *Federal Register,* May 5, 1978. **723.** "Report on Carcinogenesis Bioassay of EDTA," HEW, Technical Report Series, no. 11, Washington, D.C., 1977. **724.** *Toxic Substances List.* **725.** *Toxic Substances List.* **726.** *Toxicants in Foods,* p. 142. **727.** Michael B. Shimkin, M.D., *Science and Cancer,* OSHA, Washington, D.C., 1973. **728.** Gary Stoner et al. **729.** *Toxic Substances List.* **730.** *Suspected Carcinogens.* **731.** *Toxic Substances List.* **732.** Michael B. Shimkin, M.D., *Contrary to Nature,* HEW, Washington, D.C., p. 399. **733.** *Toxic Substances List.* **734.** John Wagner et al., "Genetic Effects Associated with Industrial Chemicals," NIOSH, 1978. **735.** M. Bolt et al., "Metabolism of ^{14}C-Vinyl Chloride in Vitro and in Vivo," Inserm Symposia Series. **736.** NIOSH Recommended Standard for Occupational Exposure to Vinyl Chloride. **737.** *Science News,* vol. 106, September 7, 1974. **738.** *Journal of the American Medical Association,* vol. 228, June 10, 1974. **739.** *American Medical News,* March 16, 1979. **740.** *New York Times,* October 5, 1974. **741.** *Toxic Substances List.* **742.** *Medical World News,* June 8, 1962. **743.** G. Klein, "Herpes Viruses & Oncogenesis," *Proceedings National Academy of Sciences,* vol. 69, April 1972, pp. 1056–1064. **744.** *Wall Street Journal,* February 12, 1973. **745.** Sloan-Kettering Institute report, April 11, 1970. **746.** *News from* NIH, October 1, 1969. **747.** Information File, *Science News,* April 1976. **748.** *New York Times,* April 4, 1973. **749.** *Baltimore Sun,* April 5, 1973. **750.** *Science,* vol. 199, January 13, 1978. **751.** *Medical Tribune,* December 17, 1962. **752.** *Science News,* vol. 112, October 6, 1977. **753.** *Cancer Questions,* HEW, Bethesda, Md., 1975. **754.** *New York Times,* April 23, 1973. **755.** Roger Johnson, *Viral Transformation of Cancer Cells.* **756.** *Livermore, California, Herald News,* April 3, 1973. **757.** D. Allen and P. Cole, "Viruses & Human Cancer," *New England Journal of Medicine,* pp. 70–82, January 13, 1972.

758. *Medical World News,* December 19, 1969. **759.** *Science News,* vol. 11, no. 19, May 13, 1978. **760.** "Diet, Nutrition, and Cancer," *The American Journal of Clinical Nutrition,* September 1976. **761.** "Is the Water Safe to Drink?" *National Academy of Sciences News Report,* vol. 27, August 1977. **762.** EPA Proposes Controls on Suspected Carcinogens in Drinking Water," *Environmental News,* EPA, January 25, 1978. **763.** William Pelon et al., "Reversion of Histidine-Dependent Mutant Strains of Salmonella Typhimurium by Mississippi River Water Samples," *Environmental Science and Technology,* vol. 11, June 1977, pp. 619–23. **764.** "NCI Supports Reduction of Chemicals in Drinking Water," *Environmental News,* EPA, June 12, 1978. **765.** *Cancer and the Worker,* New York Academy of Sciences, New York, 1977, pp. 40–41. **766.** *Toxic Substances List.* **767.** *Toxic Substances List.* **768.** Gary Eiceman et al., University of Colorado. Report before the American Chemical Society's Fourth Biennial Rocky Mountain Regional Meeting, June 6, 1978. **769.** *Toxic Substances List.* **770.** *Suspected Carcinogens.* **771.** "Xylitol; Another Sweetener Turns Sour," *Science,* February 1978, p. 670. **772.** *Toxic Substances List.* **773.** "New Mineral Linked to Mesothelioma Cluster in Turkey," *Medical World News,* July 24, 1978, p. 12. **774.** *Toxic Substances List.* **775.** *Toxic Substances List.* **776.** *Merck,* p. 1131. **777.** *Toxic Substances List.* **778.** *Toxic Substances List.*

INDEX

NOTE: See *and* see also *references in small capitals (e.g.* VITAMIN*) are to main entries in the book. Those in lower case (e.g. Rubber cement) to other entries in this index.*